Introduction to Athletic Training

Second Edition

Athletic Training Education Series

Susan Kay Hillman, ATC, PT

Arizona School of Health Sciences
A Division of the A.T. Still University

David H. Perrin, PhD, ATC

Series Editor
University of North Carolina at Greensboro

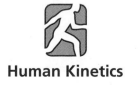

Human Kinetics

Library of Congress Cataloging-in-Publication Data

Hillman, Susan Kay, 1952-
  Introduction to athletic training / Susan Kay Hillman.-- 2nd ed.
     p. ; cm. -- (Athletic training education series)
  Includes bibliographical references and index.
  ISBN 0-7360-5292-5 (hardcover)
  1. Athletic trainers. 2. Physical education and training. 3. Sports medicine.
  [DNLM: 1. Sports Medicine. 2. Athletic Injuries--prevention & control. 3. Physical
Education and Training. QT 261 H654i 2005] I. Title. II. Series.
  RC1210.H49 2005
  617.1'027--dc22

                         2004012974

ISBN: 0-7360-5292-5

Permission notices for material reprinted in this book from other sources can be found on page(s) xi-xii.

The Web addresses cited in this text were current as of September 24, 2004, unless otherwise noted.

Acquisitions Editor: Loarn D. Robertson, PhD; **Series Development Editor:** Elaine H. Mustain; **Developmental Editor:** Maggie Schwarzentraub; **Assistant Editors:** Amanda M. Eastin and Lee Alexander; **Copyeditor:** Joyce Sexton; **Proofreader:** Anne Rogers; **Indexer:** Sharon Duffy; **Permission Manager:** Dalene Reeder; **Graphic Designer:** Fred Starbird; **Graphic Artist:** Yvonne Griffith; **Photo Manager:** Kareema McLendon; **Cover Designer:** Keith Blomberg; **Photographer (cover):** Tom Roberts; **Photographer (interior):** All photos by Tom Roberts unless otherwise noted; figures 5.1, 7.19, and 9.5 by Kelly J. Huff; **Art Manager:** Kelly Hendren; **Illustrator:** Argosy and Kareema McLendon; **Printer:** Edwards Brothers.

Printed in the United States of America   10 9 8 7 6 5 4 3 2 1

Human Kinetics
Web site: www.HumanKinetics.com

United States: Human Kinetics, P.O. Box 5076, Champaign, IL 61825-5076
800-747-4457
e-mail: humank@hkusa.com

Canada: Human Kinetics, 475 Devonshire Road Unit 100, Windsor, ON N8Y 2L5
800-465-7301 (in Canada only)
e-mail: orders@hkcanada.com

Europe: Human Kinetics, 107 Bradford Road; Stanningley, Leeds LS28 6AT, United Kingdom
+44 (0) 113 255 5665
e-mail: hk@hkeurope.com

Australia: Human Kinetics, 57A Price Avenue; Lower Mitcham, South Australia 5062
08 8277 1555
e-mail: liaw@hkaustralia.com

New Zealand: Human Kinetics, Division of Sports Distributors NZ Ltd., P.O. Box 300 226 Albany
North Shore City, Auckland
0064 9 448 1207
e-mail: blairc@hknewz.com

To my mother. You are the wind beneath my wings. You have stood by me through all my efforts and challenges and I am blessed to have you as my most loyal friend. You make every one of my tasks easier to accomplish through your never-ending support. God bless you and keep you safe and healthy.

Contents

Introduction to the Athletic Training Education Series

The five textbooks of the Athletic Training Education Series—*Introduction to Athletic Training, Examination of Musculoskeletal Injuries* (formerly *Assessment of Athletic Injuries*), *Therapeutic Exercise for Musculoskeletal Injuries* (formerly *Therapeutic Exercise for Athletic Injuries*), *Therapeutic Modalities for Musculoskeletal Injuries* (formerly *Therapeutic Modalities for Athletic Injuries*), and *Management Strategies in Athletic Training*—were written for athletic training students and as a reference for practicing certified athletic trainers. Other allied health care professionals, such as physical therapists, physician's assistants, and occupational therapists, will also find these texts to be an invaluable resource in the prevention, examination, treatment, and rehabilitation of injuries to physically active people.

The rapidly evolving profession of athletic training necessitates a continual updating of the educational resources available to educators, students, and practitioners. The authors of the five new editions in the series have made key improvements and have added important information. *Introduction to Athletic Training* includes a revised and simplified chapter on pharmacology. A new part I in *Examination of Musculoskeletal Injuries* makes this text one of the most comprehensive presentations of the foundational techniques for each assessment tool used in injury examination. Updated information on proprioceptive neuromuscular facilitation and sacroiliac joint evaluation and treatment is included in *Therapeutic Exercise for Musculoskeletal Injuries*, and a section on Pilates has been added. In *Therapeutic Modalities for Musculoskeletal Injuries*, a new chapter on evidence-based practice has been added, and the FDA's approval of laser treatment for selected injuries has led to a new chapter on this topic. Finally, the impact of the Health Insurance Portability and Accountability Act and the appropriate medical coverage model of the National Athletic Trainers' Association (NATA) are now addressed in *Management Strategies in Athletic Training*.

The Athletic Training Education Series offers a coordinated approach to the process of preparing students for the NATA Board of Certification examination. If you are a student of athletic training, you must master the material in each of the content areas delineated in the NATA publication *Competencies in Athletic Training*. The Athletic Training Education Series addresses these competencies comprehensively and sequentially while avoiding unnecessary duplication.

The series covers the educational content areas developed by the Education Council of the National Athletic Trainers' Association for accredited curriculum development. These content areas and the texts that address each content area are as follows:

- Risk management and injury prevention (*Introduction* and *Management Strategies*)
- Pathology of injury and illnesses (*Introduction, Examination, Therapeutic Exercise*, and *Therapeutic Modalities*)
- Assessment and evaluation (*Examination* and *Therapeutic Exercise*)
- Acute care of injury and illness (*Introduction, Examination*, and *Management Strategies*)
- Pharmacology (*Introduction* and *Therapeutic Modalities*)
- Therapeutic exercise (*Therapeutic Exercise*)
- General medical conditions and disabilities (*Introduction* and *Examination*)
- Nutritional aspects of injury and illness (*Introduction*)
- Psychosocial intervention and referral (*Introduction, Therapeutic Modalities*, and *Therapeutic Exercise*)
- Health care administration (*Management Strategies*)
- Professional development and responsibilities (*Introduction* and *Management Strategies*)

The authors for this series—Craig Denegar, Susan Hillman, Peggy Houglum, Richard Ray, Ethan Saliba, Susan Saliba, Sandra Shultz, and I—are eight certified athletic trainers with well over a century of collective experience as clinicians, educators, and leaders in the athletic training profession. The clinical experience of the authors spans virtually every setting in which athletic trainers practice, including the high school, sports medicine clinic, college, professional sport, hospital, and industrial settings. The professional positions of the authors include undergraduate and graduate curriculum director, head athletic trainer, professor, clinic director, and researcher. The authors have chaired or served on the NATA's most important committees, including the Professional Education Committee, the Education Task Force, Education Council, Research Committee of the Research and Education Foundation, Journal Committee, Appropriate Medical Coverage for Intercollegiate Athletics Task Force, and Continuing Education Committee.

This series is the most progressive collection of texts and related instructional materials currently available to athletic training students and educators. Several elements are present in all the books in the series:

- Chapter objectives and summaries are tied to one another so that students will know and achieve their learning goals.
- Chapter-opening scenarios illustrate the importance and relevance of the chapter content.
- Cross-referencing among texts offers a complete education on the subject.
- Thorough reference lists allow for further reading and research.

To enhance instruction, each text includes an instructor guide and test bank. *Therapeutic Exercise for Musculoskeletal Injuries*, *Therapeutic Modalities for Musculoskeletal Injuries*, and *Examination of Musculoskeletal Injuries* each includes a presentation package. Presentation packages (formerly known as graphics packages) are usually in Microsoft PowerPoint format and delivered via CD-ROM. They contain selected illustrations, photos, and tables from the text. Instructors can use these to enhance lectures and demonstration sessions. Other features vary from book to book, depending on the subject matter; but all include various aids for assimilation and review of information, extensive illustrations, and material to help students apply the facts in the text to real-world situations.

Beyond the introductory text by Hillman, the order in which the books should be used is determined by the philosophy of each curriculum director. In any case, each book can stand alone so that a curriculum director does not need to revamp an entire curriculum in order to use one or more parts of the series.

When I entered the profession of athletic training over 25 years ago, one text—*Prevention and Care of Athletic Injuries* by Klafs and Arnheim—covered nearly all the subject matter required for passing the NATA Board of Certification examination and practice as an entry-level athletic trainer. Since that time we have witnessed an amazing expansion of the information and skills one must master in order to practice athletic training, along with an equally impressive growth of practice settings in which athletic trainers work. You will find these updated editions of the Athletic Training Education Series textbooks to be invaluable resources as you prepare for a career as a certified athletic trainer, and you will find them to be useful references in your professional practice.

David H. Perrin, PhD, ATC
Series Editor

Preface

This second edition of *Introduction to Athletic Training* reflects the continuing belief that the day-to-day tasks of injury evaluation and treatment are the tasks that keep most athletic trainers busy. Consequently, many athletic training courses mirror the amount of time most athletic trainers spend in those functions. Often, introductory athletic training courses provide an overview of the physical skills of bracing and taping and of other tasks like assessing and evaluating injuries, but give little attention to the aspects that set athletic training apart from other professions: the prevention of injury and the emergency management of acute injury and illness.

Prevention and management of injury are critical in the health care of the physically active individual. Simple prevention methods, such as designing protective equipment or altering game rules, protect participants from injury. Carefully designed emergency management procedures may prevent even serious injuries from having a catastrophic outcome. Much of the basis of these prevention and management measures comes from research in sport injury rates and injury types. From the viewpoint of the athletic trainer, these sport-related data help them do their job by allowing organizers to identify the kinds of health care needed at various practices and competitions. Such knowledge then creates a safer environment for play. Other data point to risk factors found in sport participation. Risk factors alert coaches, administrators, and athletic trainers to potential injury situations; assist strength and conditioning professionals in the development of prevention programs aimed at reducing risks; and alert people who are more susceptible to a particular injury or condition when a sport is a high-risk endeavor for them.

Newly featured in this second edition of *Introduction to Athletic Training* is a revised chapter on pharmacology. This new chapter simplifies this difficult material and eliminates the depth of technical pharmacokinetics and drug information, instead focusing on practical application of the information in relation to banned substances lists and drug-testing policies. Other new information appears throughout the text, with updated and expanded information in every chapter. In addition to the discussion questions provided in each chapter, new critical thinking questions have been added to each. Discussion topics become more abundant in this second edition.

The second edition of *Introduction to Athletic Training* is packaged with a Primal Pictures software product titled *Essentials of Interactive Functional Anatomy*. This CD-ROM will help you thoroughly review components of structural anatomy with a complete high-resolution 3-D model of the human musculature. The model can be rotated and allows for 11 layers of anatomy to be visually removed—from arteries down to major ligaments. The CD also includes 32 animations showing clinical muscle function and joint motion.

Introduction to Athletic Training not only provides you with the theoretical basis of the work of an athletic trainer as part of a sports medicine team; it also supplies valuable information related to the prevention and management of sport injuries and illnesses. This book is written primarily for the college student pursuing a degree in athletic training, but could be used as a professional resource by certified athletic trainers as well as sport physical therapists, clinical exercise physiologists, sport orthopedists, sport chiropractors, sport massage therapists, and personal trainers.

Introduction to Athletic Training begins with an examination of athletic training as a profession, its characteristics, history, and employment opportunities. This material segues to the role and relationship most athletic trainers have with other sports medicine professionals and allied heath workers and the ways in which a sports medicine team operates (chapter 1).

Next comes a thorough discussion of epidemiology of athletic injuries through description of sport injury surveillance systems, injury trends, high-risk sports, and intrinsic risk factors (chapter 2). This is followed by information regarding the essential elements of the preparticipation physical examination—health status information, physical fitness or performance testing, and facility setup for a group preparticipation physical examination (chapter 3). Fundamental fitness-testing procedures and parameters are presented, as are the basics of developing a strength training and conditioning program designed to prevent injury (chapter 4).

The next chapter is totally revised from the first edition of this text and now introduces the reader to medicinal and street drugs that one may see used in athletics. Regulations governing drug use are discussed and various drug-testing policies are presented (chapter 5).

Other significant topics include the prevention and care of heat- and cold-related illnesses in addition to other environmental factors influencing sport participation (chapter 6).

Attention then turns to an area related to the outcomes of epidemiological research: protective devices, sport regulations, and subsequent laws. This discussion includes a look at the standards for equipment design and reconditioning and maintenance of athletic headgear; agencies for development of sport safety rules; legal concerns and determination of liability; and information on protecting oneself from legal misfortune (chapter 7).

The topic of legal liability in health care brings to mind consideration of the emergency care and medical management of athletic injury. This includes background information on first aid, emergency care, and cardiopulmonary resuscitation; the emergency care plan; legal and ethical issues in treatment; community-based emergency medical services and facilities; and prevention of the transmission of bloodborne pathogens (chapter 8).

The book concludes with a discussion of nutritional concerns for the physically active. Nutritional needs and fluid replacement concepts are covered in order to aid in planning the athlete's diet as well as the pre-event meal. Carbohydrates, fats, and proteins are analyzed with respect to the extent to which they are needed in the athlete's diet as well as various sources for obtaining the necessary calories. Attention is given to weight gain and loss through nutrition, and concerns including specific nutritional needs associated with selected medical problems are discussed. Sources for obtaining sound nutritional advice are provided to aid the athlete throughout his or her career (chapter 9).

With careful thought and attention, athletic trainers may be able to keep athletes doing what they like to do—that is, playing! Understanding the many aspects of preventing sport-related medical problems would actually require several volumes of text, not just one book. However, *Introduction to Athletic Training* provides the theoretical information and foundation you'll need to advance and hone your skills as a student learner, succeed in your courses and training, and eventually find your calling as a certified athletic trainer.

Credits

Figure 2.2, a and b Reprinted with permission from the NCAA. http://www1.ncaa.org/membership/ed_outreach/health-safety/iss/Injury_Reports_2004/Football_Summary_2004.pdf.

Figure 2.10 Reprinted, by permission, from NCAA. http://www1.ncaa.org/membership/ed_outreach/health-safety/iss/Injury_Reports_2004/Football_Summary_2004.pdf.

Form on p. 39 (Weekly Exposure Form) Reprinted with permission from the NCAA.

Form on p. 40 (Individual Injury Form) Reprinted with permission from the NCAA.

Text on p. 66 (1996 In-Line Skating Injuries–All Age Groups) Adapted, by permission, from International Inline Skating Association, 1999.

Table 2.2 Data from 2002-2003 NCAA Injury Surveillance System from 123 reporting schools.

Form on pp. 94–96 (Health Status Questionnaire) Reprinted, by permission, from E.T. Howley and B.D. Franks, 1986, *Health fitness instructor's handbook*, 3rd ed. (Champaign, IL: Human Kinetics), 34.

Form on p. 97 Physical Activity Readiness Questionnaire (PAR-Q) © 2002. Reprinted with permission from the Canadian Society for Exercise Physiology. Http://www.csep.ca/forms.asp

Form on p. 104 (Fitness Evaluation Form) Reprinted, by permission, from Club Corporation of American, 1995, *Standards of design and construction of an athletic facility*, (Dallas, TX: Club Corporation of America).

Form on pp. 108–110 (Preparticipation Physical Evaluation) Reprinted from the *Preparticipation Physical Evaluation* (monograph) Second Edition. Leawood, Kansas: American Academy of Family Physicians, American Academy of Pediatrics, American Medical Society for Sports Medicine, American Osteopathic Academy of Sports Medicine, The Physician and Sportsmedicine © 2004 The McGraw-Hill Companies.

Text on p. 89 (Classification of Sports by Contact) Reproduced with permission from *Pediatrics*, Vol. 107, Page(s) 1205-1209, Copyright 2001.

Text on pp. 91–92 (NCAA Guidelines 1B: Medical Evaluations, Immunizations, and Records) Reprinted with permission from the NCAA.

Figure 4.13 Adapted, by permission, from S.J. Fleck and W.J. Kraemer, 1997, *Designing resistance training programs*, 2nd ed. (Champaign, IL: Human Kinetics), 89.

Figure 4.21 Reprinted, by permission, from S.J. Fleck and W.J. Kraemer, 2004, *Designing resistance training programs*, 3rd ed. (Champaign, IL: Human Kinetics), 31.

Figure 4.25 Reprinted, by permission, from S.J. Fleck and W.J. Kraemer, 2004, *Designing resistance training programs*, 3rd ed. (Champaign, IL: Human Kinetics), 140.

Text on p. 128 (Aerobic Tests) Reprinted, by permission, from K.H. Cooper, 1968, *Journal of the American Medical Association* 203: 201-204.

Text on p. 129 (Three-Minute Step Test) Reprinted, by permission, from W.D. McArdle et al., 1972, "Reliability and interrelationships between maximal oxygen uptake, physical work capacity and step test scores in college women," *Exercise and Sport Science Reviews* 4: 182-186.

Figure 5.3 Copyright © 1993 From *Molecular biology of the cell* by B. Alberts, et al. Reproduced by permission of Garland Science/Taylor & Francis Books, Inc.

Figure 5.5 Reprinted from *Journal of the American Academy of Dermatology*, Vol. 9(5), A.K. Bronner and A.F. Hood, Cutaneous complications of chemotherapeutic agents, Page(s) 645-663, Copyright (1983), with permission from The American Academy of Dermatology.

Figure 5.7 Adapted, by permission, A.A. White III, 1989, The 1980 symposium and beyond. In *Perspectives in low back pain*, edited by J.W. Frymoyer and S.W. Gordon (Park Ridge, IL: American Academy of Orthopaedic Surgeons).

Figure 6.1 Adapted, by permission, from J.H. Wilmore and D.L. Costill, 1994, *Physiology of sport and exercise* (Champaign, IL: Human Kinetics), 246.

Figure 6.2 Reprinted, by permission, from W. Fink, et al., 1975, "Muscle metabolism during exercise in the heat and cold," *European Journal of Applied Physiology* 34: 183-190.

Figure 6.5 Adapted, by permission, from J.H Wilmore and D.L.Costill, 2004, *Physiology of sport and exercise*, 3rd ed. (Champaign, IL: Human Kinetics), 308.

Figure 6.13 Reprinted, by permission, from NCAA, 1999, *NCAA Guideline 2C: Prevention of heat illness* (Indianapolis, IN: NCAA).

Figure 6.15 Reprinted, by permission; from National Collegiate Athletic Association, 1999, *NCAA guideline 2M: Cold stress* (Indianapolis, IN: NCAA).

Text on p. 216 (National Collegiate Athletic Association Recommendations for Preventing Cold Injuries) Reprinted with permission from the NCAA.

Text on p. 217 (Decision Tree for Personal Lightning Safety) Reprinted, by permission, from National Lightning Safety Institute, 1999, Available: http://www.issa.org/tips.safety.com/nlsi_pls/1st.html. Accessed October 1999.

Form on p. 266 (National Youth Sports Safety Foundation, Inc. Emergency Plan) Reprinted, with permission of the National Youth Sports Safety Foundation, Inc. All rights reserved.

Form on p. 274 (Emergency Medical Authorization) Reprinted, by permission, from D. Herbert, 1994, *Legal aspects of sports medicine*, 2nd ed. (Canton, OH: PRC Publishing).

Form on pp. 291–292 (Report of Exposure to Human Blood or Other Potentially Infectious Materials) Reprinted, by permission, from T. Zeigler, 1997, *Management of bloodborne infections in sport*, (Champaign, IL: Human Kinetics), 41.

Table 9.4 Adapted from McArdle, Katch and Katch 1999.

Appendix A Reprinted, by permission, from National Athletic Trainers' Association 2004.

CHAPTER 1

Athletic Training: The Profession and Its History

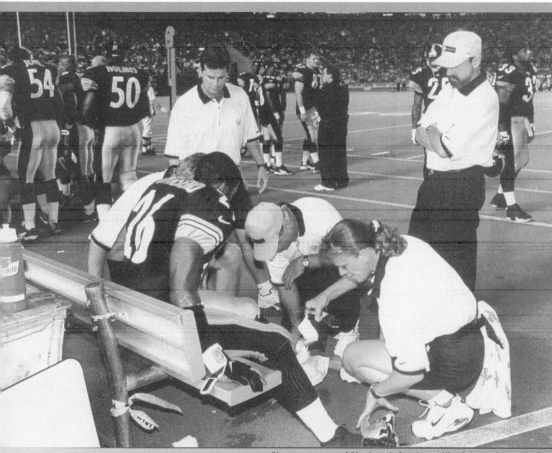

Photo courtesy of Pittsburgh Steelers, Mike Fabus, photographer.

Objectives

After reading this chapter, the student should be able to do the following:

1. List the characteristics of athletic training that identify it as a profession.

2. Discuss five major historical events that shaped the current structure of the National Athletic Trainers' Association.

3. Identify the members of a sports medicine team.

4. Identify job opportunities for certified athletic trainers and explain his or her own ideal job setting.

5. Identify the courses at his or her own school that a person interested in athletic training should take.

6. Explain how the most recent changes in the education of athletic trainers might affect college and university programs in the United States.

Chris considered himself very fortunate to have landed his "dream" job just three short years after completing his master's degree. College athletic trainer, then on into professional sports! He had never thought the dream would come true.

After three seasons in the pros, Chris found himself looking for some different challenges. Working with the professional athlete was fun, but demanding; free time was limited and, worst of all, the injuries always seemed to be the same, over and over again. He was worried he was becoming stale.

"Hey, Chris! How's life in the big leagues?" queried an enthusiastic voice on the telephone.

"It's great," Chris replied, hesitantly. "Is this Pete?" he asked.

"Yeah, I graduated last year and now I'm working with the Special Olympics! We have a huge meet in Philly next month and I want you to come help!"

"Special Olympics? How'd you go from athletic training to that?" Chris asked.

"I got into it while in graduate school. I volunteered to work some events and just fell in love with it. But I'm still an athletic trainer. I help the kids with their injuries, and believe me, they get hurt!"

"Dang, that sounds like it could be a real challenge!" Chris said, deep in thought.

"You can't believe the feeling you get watching some of these kids run a race. They all feel like winners . . . first through last place. It's so rewarding to help them achieve things even they never dreamed they could!"

"Say no more—just tell me where to be and when to be there. Count me in!" Chris replied.

It was perfect. The Special Olympics had its national championships in Philadelphia, and Chris was in his off-season with the professional team. He spent the better part of four days working with Pete and the medical staff for the Special Olympics, and he had never felt so appreciated in his life.

After that experience, Chris decided to get involved in local events and even found a course at a nearby community college that helped him understand more about working with disabilities: adaptive physical education. With a renewed focus on health care for the physically active, Chris's enthusiasm for learning more and helping others not only improved his outlook, it also infected others around him. Now, life for Chris was really in the "big leagues."

As we begin the task of understanding the quite diverse career field of athletic training, we might first ask a few questions. Is athletic training a profession? Does health care of the physically active meet the criteria for classification as a profession? Would the fact that people in this field work with disabled athletes, professional athletes, college athletes, or recreational athletes qualify the field to be considered a profession? To discuss this topic—one that engenders considerable debate—we must start with a definition of "profession."

WHAT ARE THE CHARACTERISTICS OF A PROFESSION?

Sociologists have repeatedly attempted to identify the components of a "profession." No single description is completely satisfactory, yet service occupations have attempted to justify their status in society by the fact that they are considered a profession. Other groups of individuals (occupations) have tried to remodel their organizational structures to more closely resemble that of a profession in the hope that this would raise their social status. Because there are no firm rules or regulations regarding what occupations can be considered professions, and because of the status associated with professions, much debate surrounds the issue.

In 1964, noted sociologist Geoffry Millerson analyzed the ideas of 21 writers on this topic and found six characteristics that were most often mentioned as key components of a profession (Mitchell 1973).

- A profession involves a skill based on theoretical knowledge.
- A profession involves a skill that requires training and education.

- The professional must demonstrate competence by passing a test.
- The professional's integrity is maintained by adherence to a code of conduct.
- The professional's service is provided for the public good.
- The profession is organized.

Some people may feel that occupations not possessing all six characteristics should not be considered true professions; others would argue that fields such as medicine, law, and divinity that are regarded as professions do not meet all six criteria.

As we examine aspects of the field of athletic training and consider the labeling of the occupation as a profession, there is much to take into account. Certainly the field of athletic training has developed a broader base than the original group of athletic trainers envisioned. In the following sections we'll examine these six criteria (see figure 1.1).

Theoretical Knowledge

A profession involves a skill based on theoretical knowledge. Looking at medicine as an example, we see that the medical disciplines apply skills based on empirical information. The first time a physician encountered a patient with lupus or Hodgkin's disease, he or she may not have had the skills to treat this exact condition. However, the physician would have been

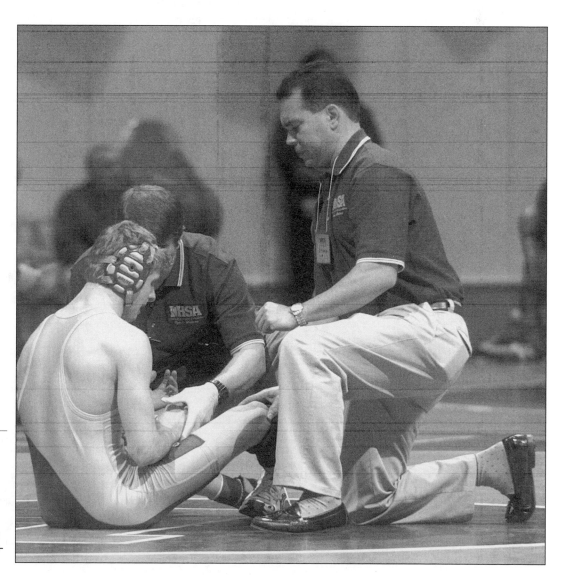

Figure 1.1 To be considered a profession, an occupation requires skill-based knowledge, specialized training, standard licensing or accreditation, a code of conduct, and organization.

able to determine a treatment method based on prior studies of immunosuppressive disease. Therefore, the idea of a true profession should not be so limited as to suggest that all the required information and knowledge must be available in one tight package. The professional's knowledge is "theoretical" in that it is based on sound reasoning and thinking drawn from scientific knowledge and fact. As another example, consider the practice of law. After lawyers gather facts and observations from testimony, they use deductive reasoning to present their theory on the "who, what, and why" of the case. This case in all its particulars has never happened before, but the lawyer continues to seek plausible answers. Although an exact match may never be encountered, most professionals are able to extrapolate information related to theory-based knowledge from other sources and apply that wisdom to a particular case.

Training and Education

Keeping the practice of law in mind, let's consider the probing, somewhat argumentative nature of the work of a lawyer. One of the characteristics of a profession that we have noted is that it involves specialized skills that must be taught. For a physician, taking a patient's blood pressure or listening to heart sounds is a learned skill. Those who might suggest that law is not truly a profession may believe that the practice of law does not require "unique skills." Lawyers, however, would argue that oration and debate are truly skills requiring training and education. Perhaps the debate would construe the attainment of legal knowledge as the acquisition of skill. Thus, this characteristic may not be universal for all established professions. A "skill" may be defined differently by different groups. The training and education of a profession should be quite evident in the areas of skills and knowledge (see figure 1.2).

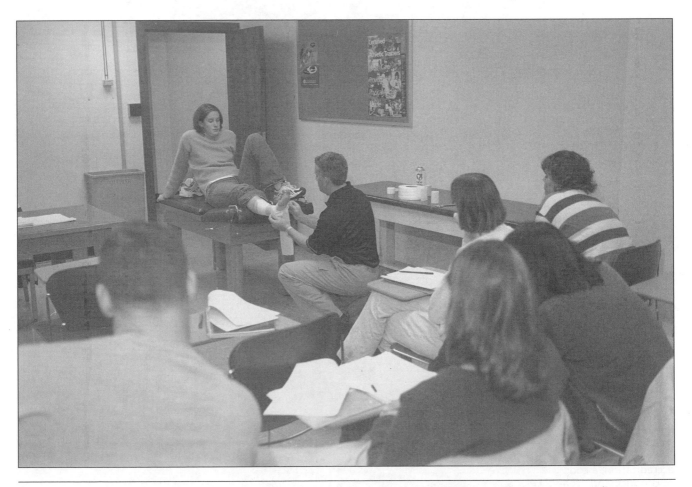

Figure 1.2 Training and education transmit the specialized skills and knowledge that an athletic trainer must have.

Certification and Examinations

The professional must demonstrate competence by passing a test (see figure 1.3). Many fields require a test for licensing or certification; educators must obtain certification to teach; an RN is a registered nurse; and even the plumber must pass a test to become licensed. But not all occupations that require a license or certification can also satisfy all five of the other criteria. The requirement of passing a test is just one of the six elements that we look for in occupations representing themselves as professions.

Integrity and a Code of Ethics

Integrity is maintained by adherence to a code of conduct. Thus, the **ethics** of a profession outline the way in which the members of the association or field should conduct themselves. It may include areas of interpersonal skills, honesty, and service. The physician must obey the Hippocratic Oath; scientists work within a set of informal rules of fair and equal collaboration with other researchers and prompt and public dissemination of their results. Most professions and organizations have a committee to investigate and review breach-of-conduct reports concerning their members and take punitive measures for any behaviors deemed in violation of the code; for example, an unprincipled attorney is brought before the bar association for formal review. The integrity of the professional is measured by the ability of the ethics committees to review and act on a fellow member's unethical behavior.

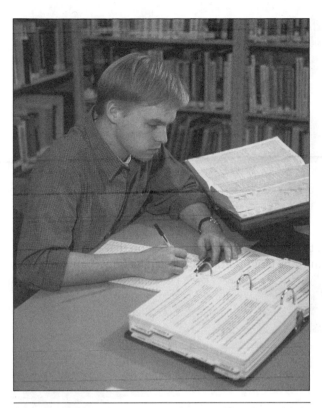

Figure 1.3 In addition to meeting specific educational and experience requirements, a student athletic trainer must pass a national certification exam to become an athletic trainer.

Public Good

The professional's service is for the public good. This means that the service is available, not just to certain individuals, but to everyone (see figure 1.4). An organization should not be considered a profession unless it provides a service for all. This is not to say that because an individual remains healthy, or for other reasons never visits a physician, the medical profession does not serve the public good. If the service of a profession is available and accessible to the public, it is considered to be "for the public good." It is doubtful that anyone could successfully argue that medicine, law, and divinity are reserved for only a sector of society. All are available and usually accessible to everyone, thus providing a service for the public good.

Organizations and Associations

For an occupation to be considered a profession, it must be organized. Organization implies more than a systematically arranged list of persons in the field; instead, most professions have highly organized associations. Medicine may present the best example of organization. The membership of the American Medical Association (AMA) is very large; most of the members are also involved in smaller committees, societies, academies, and colleges, all of which bring together individuals with common medical specialty interests. Medicine has also been long recognized as a field that has excellent representation in the political arena and that has a strong organization dedicated to exerting political influence.

However, the term organization implies much more than politics and presidents. Organization of a profession indicates that there are committees, task forces, and other special groups of members that function within the larger structure, all working toward a common goal. Just within the realm of sports medicine there are a number of specialty groups in addition to the governing agency, the **AMA:** the American Academy of Orthopaedic Surgeons, the

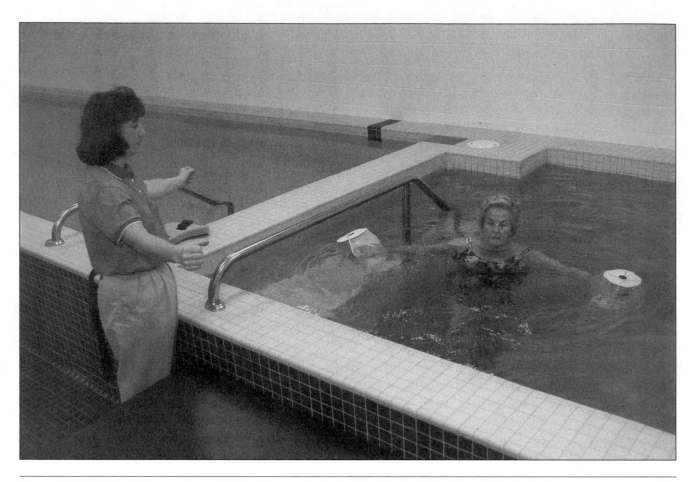

Figure 1.4   Athletic trainers enhance the health care of physically active individuals and elderly and young persons, as well as of professional and recreational athletes.

American College of Sports Medicine, and the American Orthopaedic Society for Sports Medicine. The larger the membership, the more effective the organizational structure must become. A profession would not, then, exist merely by virtue of having a number of people interested or involved in the same activity or service; the group must show a purpose beyond that of a club or a collection of people with a job in common. For example, the United Food Workers (UFW) is a union comprising people with a common job, but would the UFW be classified as a profession by virtue of its organization?

WHAT MAKES ATHLETIC TRAINING A PROFESSION?

In evaluating athletic training in terms of the list of characteristics presented, one could consider the field a true profession. Athletic training does not satisfy all of the characteristics, but it does satisfy a majority of them. Next we'll look at the six characteristics of a profession in relation to athletic training.

Skill-Based Theoretical Knowledge

Similar to medicine, athletic training involves the skill of evaluating a patient problem. The evaluation is based on theoretical knowledge—knowledge drawn from sound scientific information. Just as a physician does, the athletic trainer encounters situations that call for the use of deductive reasoning to solve a problem. Beyond the skills involved in injury care, **rehabilitation**, and counseling, the skills of an athletic trainer transcend many disciplines, each providing the framework for analysis of the athlete's particular problem or situation. For example, a young female distance runner is experiencing chronic stress syndrome in the lower extremities. One may merely treat the injury or irritation, or one may proceed further in attempting to find a cause of the problem (in the athlete's dietary habits, or perhaps the presence of amenorrhea) as well as providing rehabilitation to correct any muscular imbalances, structural problems, or other discoverable factors.

The National Athletic Trainers' Asssociation **(NATA)** enjoys a strong research emphasis within its membership. Students seeking scientific evidence of the value of particular treatments or the outcome of certain protocols can often find that information through the research efforts of NATA members and associates. Through continued research, athletic training will continue to exemplify skills based on theoretical knowledge.

Training and Education

Athletic training requires at least four years of college education plus hands-on practice in evaluation, prevention, and management of athletic injuries. Without completing the required course work in a specified period of time and accumulating hours of experience under the guidance of a certified athletic trainer, the individual seeking to become certified would not meet the standards set by the NATA.

Colleges and universities offering athletic training programs for students must undergo accreditation by the Commission on Accreditation of Allied Health Higher Education Programs, or CAAHEP. Accreditation may be sought by the institution upon recommendation of the JRC-AT of the NATA. The JRC-AT (Joint Review Committee-Athletic Training) is the NATA committee endorsed by the CAAHEP that evaluates and recommends NATA educational programs for CAAHEP accreditation. The CAAHEP is a nonprofit allied health education organization whose purpose is to accredit entry-level allied health education programs. The profession of athletic training is one of the many allied health professions accredited by this agency.

Certification

To become certified as an athletic trainer, the student not only must satisfy the educational and experience requirements, but also must pass a national certification exam. The certification exam includes a written test of didactic information; a practical demonstration of athletic training skills; and a written simulation that tests problem solving, decision making, and critical thinking in the management of selected patient problems. The satisfactory completion of all three exams is required for entrance into the field of athletic training and earning the designation of **ATC** (Certified Athletic Trainer). Once certified, athletic trainers must continue their education through any combination of continuing education programs and activities. The certified athletic trainer must verify accumulation of a predetermined number

Athletic Training Curriculum Subject Matter Requirements

- Prevention of athletic injuries/illnesses
- Evaluation of athletic injuries/illnesses
- First aid and emergency care
- Therapeutic modalities
- Therapeutic exercise
- Administration of athletic training programs
- Human anatomy*

- Human physiology
- Exercise physiology
- Kinesiology/biomechanics
- Nutrition
- Psychology
- Personal/community health
- Instructional methods

*You should note that anatomy is a consistent element of the athletic trainer's education. Take some time to explore *Essentials of Interactive Functional Anatomy*, the CD provided with this book.

of CEUs during each three-year "term" of membership. In addition to CEUs, the athletic trainer must show proof of having a current cardiopulmonary **resuscitation** (CPR) certificate. Members must adhere to the NATA Board of Certification (**NATABOC**) Standard of Professional Practice as well as remain current in the payment of annual professional dues (see www.bocatc.org/athtrainer/STDS).

Code of Ethics

As with other professions, the NATA—the governing body for athletic trainers—has a well-established code of ethics (see appendix A). The Code of Ethics was one of the first steps the NATA took as it became organized early in the 1950s. This code was written by athletic trainers and is enforced by fellow members of the organization. A system of evaluating infractions of the code is well established and ready for immediate activation. Infractions of the Code of Ethics may result in loss of certification privileges.

Public Good

The next question one might ask is whether the service performed by athletic trainers is for the public good. This issue is debatable, not only for athletic training, but, as previously mentioned, for other established professions also. As athletic training service enlarges its focus into workplace and industrial settings, continues to expand its role in physical therapy service, and maintains its strong base in school and professional athletic programs, the public is more fully served. Athletic trainers are licensed health care providers in some states, and most other states are working toward a similar goal. "To enhance the health care of the physically active through funding and support of research and education" is central to the mission of the NATA Research and Education Foundation (the Foundation).

Organization

Although the committee dealing with the Code of Ethics is one of the oldest committees within the NATA, it is far from the only sign of organization. The number of committees, subcommittees, and organizations within the NATA is staggering. No area within athletic training is without representation in the NATA. Each state is represented within one of the 10 NATA districts. Figure 1.5 illustrates the division of these 10 districts. A district chair represents each district. The district also has a leadership structure like that of the total organization (see figure 1.6). Athletic trainers may serve on committees locally in the

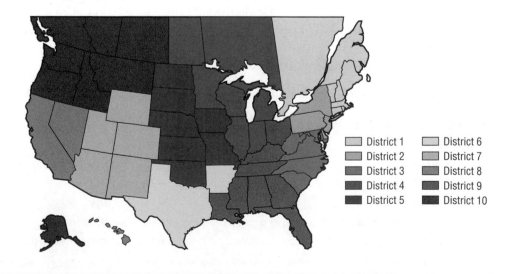

Figure 1.5 National Athletic Trainers' Association districts.

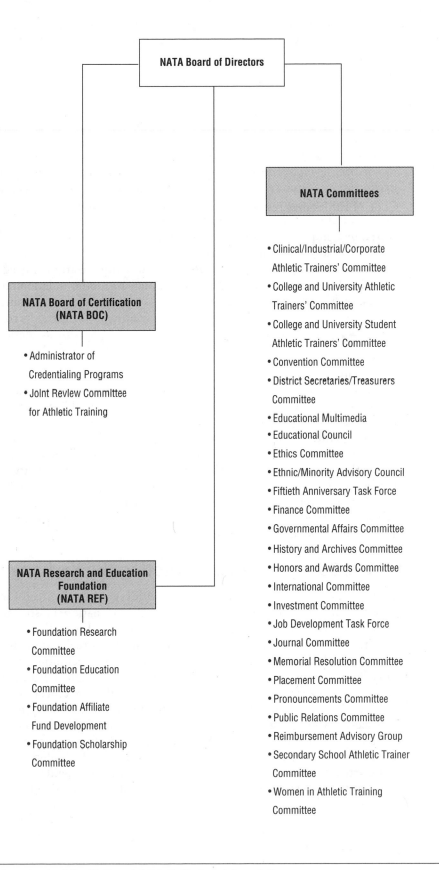

Figure 1.6 Organization chart of the National Athletic Trainers' Association.

To learn about accredited programs, upcoming meetings, membership benefits, publications, placement vacancies, and much more, direct your browser to the National Athletic Trainers' Association Web site at www.nata.org.

state organization; they may serve a group of members from neighboring states through the district level; or they may serve a more global group of members through the national organization. A simple reporting structure maintains coordination of the organization from the state to the national level: State organizations report to the district level, and district organizations report to the national level. Research, scholarship programs, educational programs, and a multitude of committees operate throughout the various levels in the NATA. All levels within the NATA are eligible for financial and administrative assistance if needed. The NATA provides money to state organizations for administrative costs of pursuing licensure, as well as providing money to the Foundation to aid in the pursuit of its research and educational goals.

THE HISTORY OF ATHLETIC TRAINING

Just as familiarity with the early history of the United States helps us understand events that occur today, knowledge of the history of the NATA leads to a better understanding of the profession of athletic training. In the years preceding establishment of the NATA, information regarding the employment and function of the "trainer" was sparse. Not until the early 1950s did athletic trainers develop any organizational structure; then information and communication blossomed. The organization began very small, with only a few athletic trainers across the nation—most of whom worked in the college or university setting. Since then the profession has grown to its current size of more than 22,700 certified and student members worldwide, covering a wide range of jobs in clinics, schools, professional sport, industry, health and fitness organizations, and educational institutions, to name just a few. See figure 1.7 and appendix B for a summary of this chronology.

The 1930s and 1940s: Promoting the Exchange of Ideas

The '30s and '40s marked an awakening with regard to the need for an organization for athletic trainers. The original attempt to establish a national association for athletic trainers was in 1938, at the Drake Relays in Des Moines, Iowa. The athletic trainers working with teams competing at the Drake Relays track meet realized the need for an association of individuals to promote the exchange of ideas and techniques that would be useful in providing athletic training services to athletes. Through the originality of thought and energy of people such as Charles Cramer who sought to establish such an organization, the NATA was founded in 1939. This early organization saw the appointment of a president and secretary-treasurer as well as the establishment of a home office for the association in Iowa City, Iowa. Early on, the NATA published a small, mimeographed monthly newsletter called the *NATA Bulletin*. Members received a copy of the bulletin and were encouraged to write articles for inclusion in future issues. The members paid annual dues of $1.00, which allowed them to receive the bulletin and a membership card. The NATA continued until

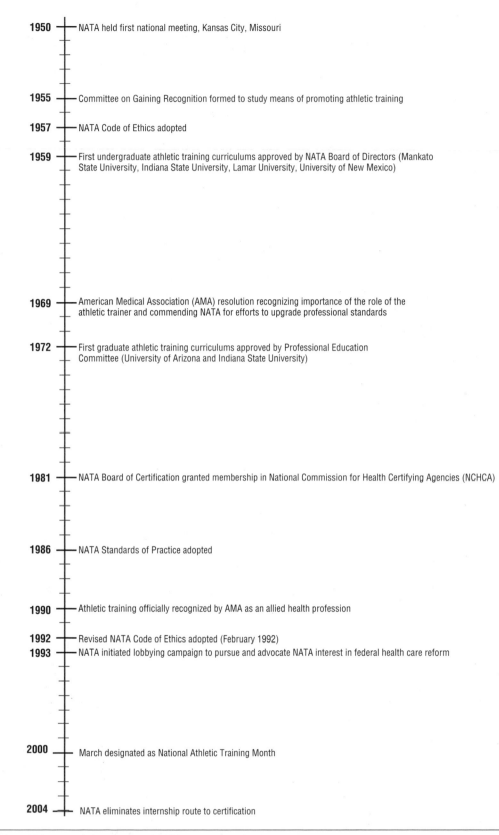

1950 — NATA held first national meeting, Kansas City, Missouri

1955 — Committee on Gaining Recognition formed to study means of promoting athletic training

1957 — NATA Code of Ethics adopted

1959 — First undergraduate athletic training curriculums approved by NATA Board of Directors (Mankato State University, Indiana State University, Lamar University, University of New Mexico)

1969 — American Medical Association (AMA) resolution recognizing importance of the role of the athletic trainer and commending NATA for efforts to upgrade professional standards

1972 — First graduate athletic training curriculums approved by Professional Education Committee (University of Arizona and Indiana State University)

1981 — NATA Board of Certification granted membership in National Commission for Health Certifying Agencies (NCHCA)

1986 — NATA Standards of Practice adopted

1990 — Athletic training officially recognized by AMA as an allied health profession

1992 — Revised NATA Code of Ethics adopted (February 1992)

1993 — NATA initiated lobbying campaign to pursue and advocate NATA interest in federal health care reform

2000 — March designated as National Athletic Training Month

2004 — NATA eliminates internship route to certification

Figure 1.7 A brief history of the National Athletic Trainers' Association.

NATA Governmental Structure

NATA Board of Directors

- President
- District 1
- District 2
- District 3
- District 4
- District 5
- District 6
- District 7
- District 8
- District 9
- District 10

NATA Research and Education Foundation (NATA REF)

- President
- Foundation Research Committee
- Foundation Education Committee
- Foundation Affiliate Fund Development
- Foundation Scholarship Committee

NATA Board of Certification

- President
- Administrator of Credentialing Programs
- Joint Review Committee for Athletic Training

NATA Committees

- Clinical/Industrial/Corporate Athletic Trainers' Committee
- College and University Athletic Trainers' Committee
- College and University Student Athletic Trainers' Committee
- Convention Committee
- District Secretaries/Treasurers Committee
- Educational Multimedia
- Education Council
- Ethics Committee
- Ethnic/Minority Advisory Council
- Fiftieth Anniversary Task Force
- Finance Committee
- Governmental Affairs Committee
- History and Archives Committee
- Honors and Awards Committee
- International Committee
- Investment Committee
- Job Development Task Force
- Journal Committee
- Memorial Resolution Committee
- Placement Committee
- Pronouncements Committee
- Public Relations Committee
- Reimbursement Advisory Group
- Secondary School Athletic Trainer Committee
- Women in Athletic Training Committee

1944, when World War II caused a great strain on the members of the fledgling association. The difficult years of the association from the late 1930s to the mid-1940s saw several accomplishments. The NATA

- established membership classes (1939);
- published the *Trainers Journal* (1941-1942), written for athletic trainers, and the *Athletic Journal*, written for coaches;
- created an insignia and established a certificate (1941);

- established regional divisions of athletic trainers (1942); and
- held national meetings.

Although the early organization failed perhaps due in part to financial and communications difficulties, it appears that many lessons were learned and later applied in the creation of what we know as today's NATA.

The 1950s: Establishing the Organization

Beginning in 1947, more and more schools were employing athletic trainers in their athletic departments, giving a renewed focus to the establishment of the NATA. These athletic trainers often had no formal education to qualify them for their positions. Many had learned the skills and techniques from others in the same field and from physicians working with the sport teams. The new era of the NATA began, and in 1950 the first national meeting was held in Kansas City, Missouri. The various groups of athletic trainers served as regional divisions of the association, providing a strong network throughout the country. In the first five years of this decade the organization achieved success through the financial support of the Cramer Chemical Company, and Charles Cramer was appointed as the first national secretary. The leadership consisted of representatives of each of the 10 "conferences" (now known as districts) who served as members of the board of directors (see figure 1.8). Members were athletic trainers from universities, colleges, junior colleges, and high schools, as well as coaches. Only athletic trainers from accredited universities could serve as the "national director" for a district. This grassroots approach to the development of the NATA allowed every state and every district to share in the decision-making processes of the association.

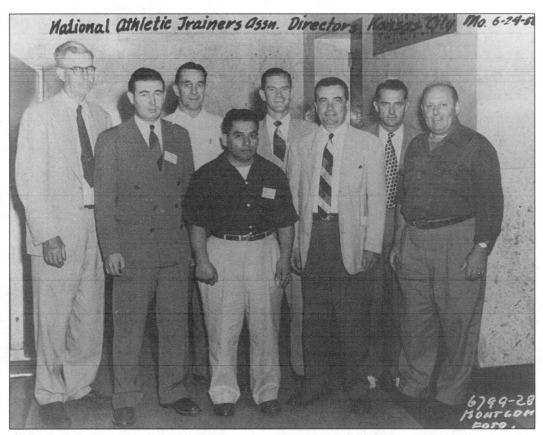

Figure 1.8 National Athletic Trainers' Association Board of Directors, 1950. Pictured left to right are Chuck Cramer, Executive Secretary; Fred Peterson, Wyoming; Al Sawdy, Bowling Green; Frank Medina, Texas; Buck Andel, Georgia; Duke Wyre, Maryland; Joe Glander, Oklahoma; Henry Schmidt, Santa Clara, California. Absent when picture was taken: Frank Kavanaugh, Cornell; Dick Wargo, Connecticut.

Photo courtesy of National Athletic Trainers' Association.

The decade of the '50s was one of considerable growth for the NATA. During the decade, schools began offering undergraduate programs in athletic training (figure 1.9). Outstanding accomplishments of that era included the following:

- The NATA constitution and by-laws were formed (1951).
- The official logo of the NATA was adopted (1952).
- The first nonathletic trainer was accepted as an "honorary member," signifying cooperation between the athletic trainer and other professionals (1953).
- John Cramer replaced Chuck Cramer as the national secretary (1954-1955).
- W.E. "Pinky" Newell was appointed chair of the Committee on Gaining Recognition (the precursor of the Professional Education Committee and Certification Committee) (1955).
- W.E. "Pinky" Newell was appointed as third national secretary (1955-1968).
- *Journal of the National Athletic Trainers' Association* began publication (1956). The mission of the *Journal of Athletic Training* is to enhance communication among professionals interested in the quality of health care for the physically active through education and research in prevention, evaluation, management, and rehabilitation of injuries.
- The NATA Code of Ethics was adopted (1957).
- The first program of undergraduate education of athletic trainers was submitted to and approved by the board of directors (1959).

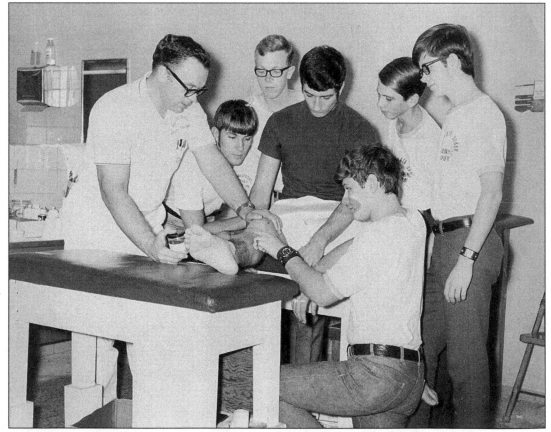

Figure 1.9 Graduates from Minnesota State University Mankato's early undergraduate athletic training program, 1950s.

Photo courtesy of Minnesota State University Mankato.

The *Journal of Athletic Training* is the official publication of the NATA. The tables of contents of previously released issues, as well as upcoming issues, can be found at www.journalofathletictraining.org.

The 1960s: Continuing the Growth

The 1960s allowed a continuation of the organizational start that had occurred in the previous decade. In 1969, the medical profession fully recognized the significance of the NATA when the AMA acknowledged the importance of the role of the athletic trainer and commended the NATA for its role in developing professional standards. Gaining this respect was an important development for athletic training programs and the NATA.

During this era the NATA also accomplished the following:

- Establishment of Helms Hall of Fame for Athletic Trainers (1962)
- Appointment of Jack Rockwell (St. Louis Cardinals professional football club) as executive secretary (1969)
- Establishment of Professional Education and Certification Committees (1969)

The 1970s: Developing Standards for Certification

The decade of the 1970s was marked by a spurt in the growth of the NATA. Committees formed in the '60s were developing standards for certification (first NATA certification examination in July 1970) and educational programs. There was a change in the structure of the association when the 1973 NATA Board of Directors changed the title for the leader of the association from executive secretary to president. Bobby Gunn of the Houston Oilers first served in this post from 1970 to 1974. Educational program development continued through the decade, with a new interest in graduate-level curricula. In 1972 the first graduate athletic training curricula were approved. In 1974, educational interest went beyond curricular issues to continuing education for certified members, and by 1979 the NATA had established continuing education requirements for all certified athletic trainers. In 1975 the 25th annual meeting of the NATA was held in Anaheim, California; here the association adopted official initials for designating the certified athletic trainer (ATC) and, through the generosity of Otho Davis, ATC (head athletic trainer of the Philadelphia Eagles Football Club and then executive director of the NATA), began the first NATA endowment fund.

By the middle of the decade, the attention of certified athletic trainers turned toward state **licensure,** and in 1978 the NATA and the American Physical Therapy Association held joint meetings to discuss licensure of athletic trainers in an attempt to give athletic trainers legal rights of practice. No nationwide cooperation could be established through these meetings, as each state was asked to remain responsible for its own licensure laws. Most states at that time had an act governing the practice of physical therapy; and in some situations, the athletic trainer was potentially in violation of those regulations. The NATA wanted to assist the state organizations of athletic trainers in establishing licensure of its members. This licensure would serve both to protect athletic trainers and to further define the professional role of the association.

To summarize this very busy decade, the NATA in the '70s stimulated more awareness of and attention to the membership, as well as making a strong statement regarding the proper education of the athletic trainer. Less time was spent on the earlier tasks of bringing recognition to the profession or on other organizational tasks as focus shifted toward the members.

The 1980s: Strengthening the NATA's Role

The 1980s brought heightened interest in the certification of the athletic trainer as well as a continued emphasis on education. During this era, the leaders in the areas of education and certification began to sense a disparity between the information being taught within NATA-approved curricula and the information that was tested during the process of certifying the

For more information about NATA's Research and Education Foundation, look at www.natafoundation.org. For information regarding the Education Council, go to www.cewl.com.

student athletic trainer. In the **role delineation study** of 1982, members were surveyed to determine the various duties involved in various positions held by athletic trainers. Role delineation studies conducted by the NATA continue to provide information that aids the association in understanding the skills required of athletic trainers.

In 1982 the National Commission for Health Certifying Agencies granted membership to the NATA, evidencing continued respect on the part of other health professions toward the athletic trainer.

Throughout the '80s, the NATA paid respect to educational leaders in the association through the Sayers "Bud" Miller Distinguished Athletic Training Educator Award. This award, named for a respected educator from Penn State University, honors an individual who has made a significant contribution to professional education of the athletic trainer.

Athletic Training Curriculum Model: Suggested Courses

1959

Anatomy

Physiology

Physiology of exercise

Applied anatomy/Kinesiology

Psychology*

First aid and safety

Nutrition and foods

Remedial exercise

Techniques of athletic training

Advanced techniques of athletic training

Laboratory practices*

Coaching techniques**

Organization and administration of health and physical education

Personal and community hygiene

Laboratory physical science like chemistry or physics*

Additional recommended:

- General physics
- Pharmacology
- Histology
- Pathology

Mid-1970s

Anatomy

Physiology

Physiology of exercise

Applied anatomy/Kinesiology

Psychology*

First aid and safety

Nutrition

Remedial exercise

Basic athletic training

Advanced athletic training

Laboratory or practical experience***

1983-Present Day

Human anatomy

Human physiology

Exercise physiology

Kinesiology/Biomechanics

Psychology

First aid and emergency care

Nutrition

Prevention of athletic injuries/illnesses

Evaluation of athletic injuries/illnesses

Therapeutic modalities

Therapeutic exercise

Instructional techniques

Administration of athletic training programs

Personal/Community health

* Six semester hours (or two courses); ** nine semester hours; *** a minimum of 600 clock hours under the direct supervision of a trainer certified by NATA.

The 1990s: Becoming a Recognized Allied Health Profession

The tremendous growth of the association continued in the 1990s, in terms both of membership (see figure 1.10) and of status in the medical community. Among varied accomplishments during this period was the official recognition of athletic training as an allied health profession by the AMA on June 22, 1990. To the leaders of the NATA, this was a monumental achievement for the young profession of athletic trainers.

Mark Smaha of Washington State University started this decade off by serving the second of his two consecutive terms as president of the NATA (1990-1992). In 1990, Otho Davis resigned after 18 years as NATA Executive Director, and the NATA sought the full-time assistance of Allan Smith, whom it named chief executive officer.

In addition to seeking to promote athletic training and its educational programs, the NATA looked to the AMA's Committee on Allied Health Education and Accreditation (CAHEA) for evaluation of athletic training curricula. This review procedure was accomplished by a joint CAHEA-NATA committee. One of the developments with the greatest impact was the creation of guidelines for schools to follow to assure compliance and give them the best opportunity for program accreditation.

To further raise the bar, the NATA sought to have all college athletic training programs attain the status of an academic major or its equivalent. The NATA recognized that the conventional role of the athletic trainer had changed; athletic trainers now had positions not only in school and team environments but also in clinical and industrial settings. With the change in job opportunities, the educational programs needed to include issues relevant to

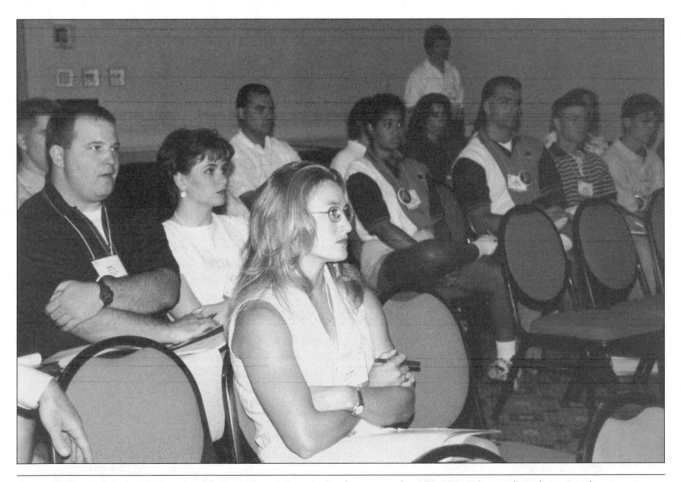

Figure 1.10 Today the National Athletic Trainers' Association has more than 29,000 active and student members.

Photo courtesy of National Athletic Trainers' Association.

those nontraditional settings. Today there are schools that offer specialized degrees in athletic training and sport health care. These programs educate their students in the roles and responsibilities of all aspects of the profession.

During the first two years of the decade, the NATA saw several positive developments. On the educational front, the AMA Council on Medical Education accepted the NATA's guidelines for establishing an athletic training curriculum; in another area, the NATA launched its first public relations campaign. Both developments served to further solidify the professional image of the athletic trainer.

Early in the decade, a protege of the late W.E. "Pinky" Newell was elected the seventh president of the NATA: Denny Miller of Purdue University (1991-1994). As had many other fine leaders, Mr. Miller would go on to serve two consecutive terms at the helm of the association.

A landmark study, sponsored in part by the National Collegiate Athletic Association, examined the practice of drug dispensation in college athletics. It was perhaps not a great surprise at the time that the study indicated a need for closer regulation of medicinal drugs dispensed through college athletic training facilities. This study set off an alarm for many athletic trainers when they realized that some of their "accepted" practices—allowed and sometimes even encouraged by team physicians—were illegal and potentially unsafe. Today's strict regulations are an effect of this report by Laster-Bradley and Berger (1991). By the second year of the decade, research and scholarly publication had become an increasingly prominent goal for the profession. The NATA's Research and Education Foundation was established with the aim of promoting both research and the dissemination of information regarding health care of the physically active.

The association became more active politically as it initiated a lobbying campaign relating to the NATA's interest in federal health care reform. On the home front, the NATA governing board voted on revisions to the Code of Ethics, the membership standards, eligibility requirements and membership sanctions and procedure, and the association by-laws. Later in the decade the NATA was recognized for its excellent code of ethics when it received the Advance America Award of Excellence issued by the American Society of Association Executives. This award served to bring attention and a bit of prestige to the association and began to pave the way toward increased respect for the profession.

Educational issues continued to arise as the AMA dissolved its academic accreditation role and the certifying of athletic training curricula was turned over to the CAAHEP. The NATA Board of Directors, in a proactive step, established the Educational Task Force, charged with studying various perspectives on athletic training education. In an attempt to identify some of the changes in the educational needs of the athletic trainer, the NATABOC published results of the second role delineation survey as the "Role Delineation Matrix"—thus effectively reflecting suggested changes in educational competencies to meet continued changes in job opportunities for athletic trainers.

As a sign of changes to expect, the AMA issued a recommendation that high schools employ an athletic trainer for coverage of sport activities. With the AMA recommendation, the NATA further raised positive awareness regarding athletic trainers and the job they do.

Training and Guiding the Next Generation

As the 1990s ended, the NATA moved forward into the 2000s with a progressive stance. In September 1999, the first woman was named president of the NATA. Ms. Julie Max followed the strong leaders preceding her, with the membership voting her into that office for two

The 1999 Role Delineation Study was the blueprint for NATABOC examinations beginning in 2001. It contains new entry-level standards of practice, content areas of athletic training redefined, an entry-level job analysis, and a review of literature including over 450 publications. To order a copy of the study, go to www.bocatc.org/resources/FAQ/RD.

NATA Research and Education Foundation Goals

1. Advance the knowledge base of the athletic training profession.
2. Encourage research among athletic trainers who can contribute to the athletic training knowledge base.
3. Provide forums for the exchange of ideas pertaining to the athletic training knowledge base.
4. Facilitate the presentation of programs and the production of materials providing learning opportunities about athletic training topics.
5. Provide scholarships for undergraduate and graduate students of athletic training.
6. Plan and implement an ongoing total development program that establishes endowment funds, as well as restricted and unrestricted funds, that will support the research and educational goals of the Foundation.

Courtesy of John Oliver, NATA Foundation Director

---

consecutive terms. In 2004 Mr. Chuck Kimell took the helm as the NATA President, the same year the athletic trainer would no longer be able to become certified through the internship route. From 2004 onward, all athletic training educational programs will be part of at least a bachelor-level sequence with strict guidelines regarding curriculum content. Throughout the decade, the NATA Education Council will continue to refine and develop the competencies by which all athletic trainers are measured, as well as redefining and structuring the clinical education of the athletic trainer. The Foundation will continue its support of national and international research and its emphasis on the education of members as well as of the public on issues of health care. Most certainly, the NATA Foundation will continue to work to enhance health care of the physically active through funding and support of research and education. The role of and respect for the services of the athletic trainer will continue to grow as third party reimbursement begins to take hold. Yet questions regarding the proper name for the profession will continue to surface in an effort to position the NATA and the athletic trainer for a more prominent role in health care of the physically active.

EMPLOYMENT OPPORTUNITIES IN ATHLETIC TRAINING

Where do athletic trainers work? Probably the first thought of most is that the athletic trainer works with sport teams in a college or other school system. Calling this the conventional setting for athletic training employment may not be entirely correct. The NATA conducts periodic surveys of certified members to establish the practice settings as well as the typical job-related duties of the members. These role delineation studies guide athletic training educators in establishing the special skills and knowledge to which the student athletic trainer should be exposed. According to five-year placement records, graduating students find employment in a variety of settings (see table 1.1)—the majority of graduates (20%) taking jobs in clinics, about 10% in schools (colleges and high schools; see figure 1.11), and a small number (<2%) with professional sport teams.

Athletic Training Course Instructors

The instructor of a core-content athletic training course should be a certified member of the NATA. In addition to serving as a course instructor, often this individual is an athletic trainer for the athletic department of the school. Obviously, not all athletic trainers teach, and not all teaching athletic trainers work in the athletic training room. But all athletic trainers have had experience on the field and in the athletic training room, doing all the things that every student athletic trainer is asked to do.

Table 1.1

NATA Accredited Graduate Athletic Training Education Programs
(Graduate Placement Record for Five-Year Period, 1994-1998; Programs and Graduates)

	1994	1995	1996	1997	1998	Totals
Number of programs	13	13	14	12	12 rpt. of 13	–
Number of graduates	154	143	166	122	127	712
Men	73 (47%)	80 (56%)	98 (59%)	53 (43%)	61 (48%)	365 (51%)
Women	81 (53%)	63 (44%)	68 (41%)	69 (57%)	66 (52%)	347 (49%)
Average no. grads	11.8	10.2	11.9	10.2	10.6	–
Athletic training (AT) employment						
% AT employment	131 (85%)	116 (81%)	141 (85%)	101 (83%)	111 (87%)	600 (84%)
Men	62 (85%)	66 (83%)	85 (87%)	41 (77%)	55 (90%)	309 (85%)
Women	69 (85%)	50 (79%)	56 (82%)	60 (87%)	56 (85%)	291 (84%)
Work setting of those employed in AT						
College	38 (25%)	30 (21%)	40 (24%)	36 (30%)	44 (35%)	188 (26%)
Men	16 (22%)	10 (13%)	20 (21%)	14 (26%)	19 (31%)	79 (22%)
Women	22 (27%)	20 (32%)	20 (30%)	22 (32%)	25 (38%)	109 (31%)
High school	15 (10%)	15 (10%)	22 (13%)	16 (13%)	13 (10%)	81 (11%)
Men	7 (10%)	12 (15%)	7 (7%)	9 (17%)	7 (11%)	42 (12%)
Women	8 (10%)	3 (4%)	15 (22%)	7 (10%)	6 (9%)	39 (11%)
Pro sports	4 (2%)	8 (6%)	5 (3%)	1 (1%)	3 (2%)	21 (3%)
Men	4 (5%)	8 (10%)	5 (5%)	1 (2%)	3 (5%)	21 (6%)
Women	0 (0%)	0 (0%)	0 (0%)	0 (0%)	0 (0%)	0 (0%)
Clinics	72 (47%)	60 (42%)	71 (43%)	40 (33%)	50 (39%)	293 (41%)
Men	34 (47%)	33 (41%)	51 (52%)	15 (28%)	25 (41%)	158 (43%)
Women	38 (47%)	27 (43%)	20 (29%)	25 (36%)	25 (38%)	135 (39%)
High school responsibilities	60 (83%)	39 (65%)	55 (78%)	31 (78%)	34 (68%)	219 (75%)
Other	2 (1%)	3 (2%)	3 (2%)	8 (6%)	1 (1%)	17 (2%)
Men	1 (1%)	3 (4%)	2 (2%)	2 (4%)	1 (2%)	9 (2%)
Women	1 (1%)	0 (0%)	1 (1%)	6 (9%)	0 (0%)	8 (2%)
Other employment						
Postgraduate	9 (6%)	8 (6%)	5 (3%)	5 (4%)	2 (2%)	29 (4%)
Other than AT	2 (1%)	1 (1%)	6 (4%)	2 (2%)	2 (2%)	13 (2%)
Unemployed	3 (2%)	0 (0%)	7 (4%)	5 (4%)	3 (2%)	18 (3%)
Unknown	9 (6%)	18 (12%)	7 (4%)	9 (7%)	9 (7%)	52 (7%)
Total	23 (15%)	27 (19%)	25 (15%)	21 (17%)	16 (13%)	112 (16%)

Reprinted from National Athletic Trainers' Association 1999.

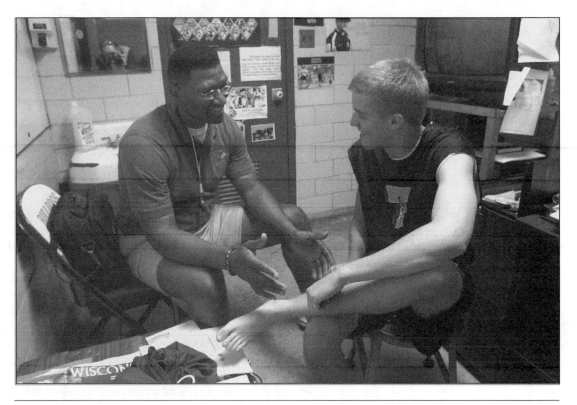

Figure 1.11 About 10% of graduating athletic trainers work in school settings. Some serve as teachers or counselors.

Often the athletic training course instructor has served on the athletic training staff for a school before dedicating increasingly more time to teaching and training students. These instructors can be teaching entry-level students or graduate students, depending on their interests and experiences. These educators are frequently on the cutting edge of the research being done in the profession.

As you may know, student athletic trainers range from those in entry-level undergraduate programs all the way to the doctoral candidates who are choosing to specialize in sports medicine education and research. As the profession grows and the educational needs of the members increase, there will be a need for more and more athletic training educators.

University or College Athletic Trainers

College athletics was the setting in which athletic training first gained recognition, and it remains the case that graduating student athletic trainers often seek positions in college athletics. Colleges generally employ a person to take the leadership role in the health care team; this athletic trainer, usually a full-time employee of the school, carries a title such as head athletic trainer or director of athletic training services. Large colleges and universities often employ several certified athletic trainers to assist with the health care of the intercollegiate teams. In addition to performing daily athletic training duties, college athletic trainers may be asked to teach or to perform other athletic department functions such as coordinating the travel or meals for road games, assisting with the laundry and with equipment distribution, or fulfilling other general duties.

High School Athletic Trainers

Colleges are not the only school settings in which the athletic trainer works with a school sport team. Some high schools employ full-time athletic trainers; other high school athletic trainers serve in a dual capacity, as the athletic trainer and also as a teacher. Occasionally a school system will contract with a sports medicine or physical therapy clinic that employs athletic trainers; in this case the clinic provides the schools of the district with athletic training coverage. Regardless of the contract, these athletic trainers play a critical role in the prevention and care of sport injuries: The absence of such a service could hinder an athlete's chance of obtaining a college athletic scholarship should an injury occur.

The athletic trainer in this setting usually has a team physician who oversees the activities surrounding athletes' medical treatment. This relationship allows the athletic trainer to provide immediate care for the injured athlete and to manage the situation on behalf of the physician.

The Student Athletic Trainer

There are only a few certified athletic trainers who were not formerly student athletic trainers. Most careers begin while the student is in high school or college. The student interested in athletic health care would normally seek out the person or persons providing the athletic training services at that school. Volunteering time as a student athletic trainer is the first step in learning more about the profession and gaining the needed hours toward certification.

High school students fortunate enough to have a full-time athletic trainer at their school can begin observing and learning even before they are able to obtain credit for the experience. But although the high school experience is certainly worthwhile, a student without this early experience is not necessarily disadvantaged by not having the exposure. Regardless of previous experience in athletic training, most colleges accept students into the athletic training program if they meet the established grade point requirements.

In the college setting, the student athletic trainer will undoubtedly have a busy schedule. As students progress in the program they are required to begin accumulating the clinical experience hours. Often students' opportunities and responsibilities with sport teams increase as they gain experience. Ideally, every student athletic trainer will earn the responsibility of working directly with sport teams.

Once the student has fulfilled the NATA requirements of course work, degree, and clinical experience, he or she may apply to take the certification examination. Most often, students take the certification examination at the conclusion of the undergraduate degree; however, a student entering the athletic training program or curriculum late may not be able to accumulate the required 1,500 hours of clinical experience. Without evidence of the required experience, the applicant is not permitted to take the examination for certification.

Graduate School Opportunities

Students who become certified after completion of their bachelor's degree may elect to pursue a master's degree in athletic training or another related field such as exercise physiology, biomechanics, or allied health professions. Many schools contract with an athletic trainer to provide athletic training services for university athletic teams, allowing the student to also pursue an advanced degree. Often, college and universities supplement their full-time staff with these graduate students. But students who wish to pursue an advanced degree in athletic training may do so without serving the school as an athletic trainer. Certified students can often find part-time employment in athletic training in the community.

Athletic Trainers/Coaches

The combination of athletic trainer and coach is not common, mostly because of the somewhat adversarial roles of the two positions (see figure 1.12). Would an athletic trainer and a coach make the same decision regarding the playing status of a key player injured in the final minutes of a critical game? Who would give the injured athlete the needed attention if it was important for the team to have a strategy session?

Clinic Athletic Trainers

Health care clinics also may offer employment opportunities for athletic trainers. These clinics, frequently owned or managed by physical therapists, employ the athletic trainer

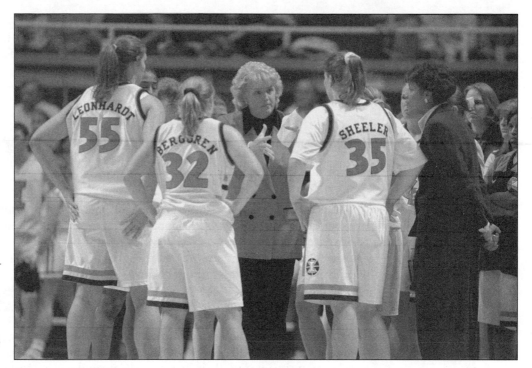

Figure 1.12 An athletic trainer/coach is not a common combination. Performing the duties of both roles is probably not wise. Can you see how the two jobs might conflict?

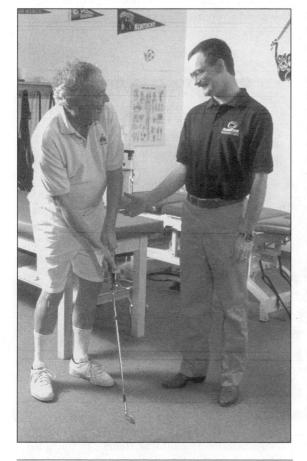

Figure 1.13 Clinics provide athletic trainers with a whole spectrum of injuries and problems as well as a wide variety of individuals and athletes. Many athletic trainers find clinic work exciting and rewarding.

to assist a licensed health care provider in rendering services to the physically active patient (see figure 1.13). In some states, the athletic trainer is allowed to provide services and to bill for those services; other states require the athletic trainer's work to be overseen and countersigned by the licensed physical therapist. The same situation applies when the clinic is owned and operated by a licensed physician; that is, the athletic trainer's services must be supervised and countersigned by the physician. Although this may appear to be a somewhat controlling atmosphere, most athletic trainers employed in the clinical setting are quite happy with the work schedule, the job duties, and the learning opportunities the clinic provides. An athletic trainer considering employment in a clinic should examine the athletic training as well as the physical therapy practice legislation of the particular state to achieve a full understanding of the legal limits of employment. As time progresses, third party reimbursement will continue to be a focus of attention. Third party reimbursement is a step to allow the ATC additional autonomy in the clinic, allowing the ATC to bill for athletic training services in the clinic as well as in more traditional settings.

As mentioned previously, a school system, an individual school, or even a sport team may contract with a sport health care clinic for athletic training coverage. This contract is usually made with the athletic trainer's employer, the clinic, or physician. The employer provides malpractice insurance for the athletic trainer working in an outreach program of health care for the school or team.

Athletic Trainers for Professional Sports

Because of the small size of most professional teams, fewer athletic trainers are employed in this setting than in the others. Some

The Professional Baseball Athletic Trainers Society has online information about the professional baseball athletic trainer, as well as educational material for anyone interested in baseball. Take a look at www.pbats.com.

professional teams, however, utilize students or other certified athletic trainers during camps at which the total team size is much larger than during the regular season. Most athletic trainers working for professional teams were once students too! Many of those individuals spent time as volunteers at the professional level during their vacation periods in the summer months.

Some professional sports, such as tennis, golf, and even rodeo, hire certified athletic trainers to provide evaluation and treatment at major events. The Professional Golfers' Association has a trailer that travels to the sites of major golf tournaments. The trailer houses exercise equipment and treatment facilities as well as a full-time staff to assist the professional golfers with their **musculoskeletal** health care needs (see figure 1.14).

Workplace Athletic Trainers

Industry provides a unique opportunity for the athletic trainer interested in working primarily in a health maintenance capacity. Corporate executives have realized the importance of relaxation time during their hectic workdays and have incorporated regularly scheduled periods for exercise into the workday or the work week. Organizations dedicated to the prevention of cumulative trauma in the workplace have increased corporate attention to the need for frequent, scheduled breaks for exercise and stretching activities. Large corporations

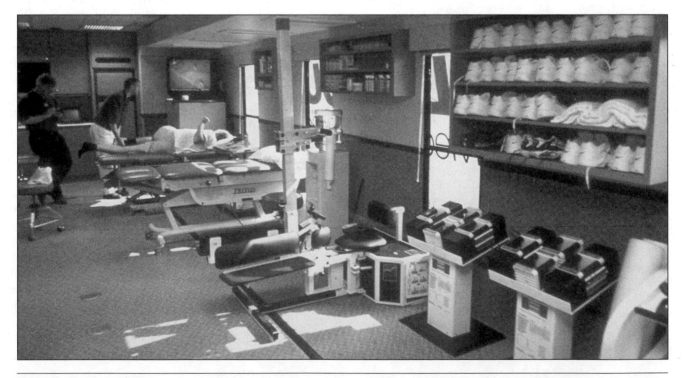

Figure 1.14 Many professional organizations like the Professional Golfers' Association hire athletic trainers to travel to and work at major events.

©PGA Tour

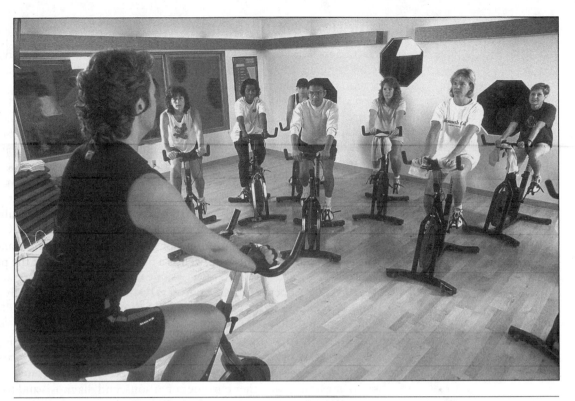

Figure 1.15 Innovative athletic trainers are moving into new areas to practice their craft. Worksite programs are provided to prevent injury and promote wellness at many large corporations such as AC Delco, Microsoft, Dial, Motorola, and Intel.

such as AC Delco, Microsoft, Dial, Motorola, and Intel participate regularly in programs for preventing injury in the workplace (see figure 1.15). A growing number of companies employ athletic trainers or other health care providers to care for both work-related and non-work-related injuries, allowing the employee to manage the injury without having to leave the corporate grounds.

The athletic trainer is not often the first health care professional that companies seek to lead corporate injury-prevention programs, yet the athletic trainer's background is quite well suited to such a position. Athletic trainers who seek opportunities with corporations are often able to work with a physician in the design of programs—not only programs for the prevention and treatment of acute and cumulative trauma on the assembly line, but also exercise programs and fitness routines for administrative-level employees.

Other Potential Opportunities

The potential opportunities for the athletic trainer are without number. Some athletic trainers have established their own corporations; some have obtained medical degrees and now practice as team physicians; and some have started private sports medicine clinics—the list could go on and on. Job opportunities for the athletic trainer may not appear numerous in certain settings, but few people with initiative are ever without employment.

THE SPORTS MEDICINE TEAM

Just as a group of individuals work together to form a sport team, a team of individuals works toward the common goal of health care of the physically active. This sports medicine team includes a variety of individuals from a variety of disciplines.

The Athletic Training Team

Athletic trainers working on a sports medicine team may be categorized according to sport or may be grouped into a total department. For the sake of this discussion we consider the department, rather than the sport team, as the team unit.

Most professional teams and major college programs have more than one athletic trainer on their sports medicine team. Those programs with more than two assistant athletic trainers usually appoint one person to serve as the lead or head athletic trainer. Some programs give this department head another title, most often director. At the college and university level, the head athletic trainer or director of athletic training services has responsibility for a team of trainers. The head trainer reports to the team physician and coaching staff. The team of athletic trainers usually includes any number of certified athletic trainers (full- or part-time people and graduate assistants), as well as a group of student athletic trainers.

Physicians

The typical sports medicine team includes one team physician (either an **allopathic** medical doctor **[MD]** or doctor of **osteopathy [DO]**) who is often a family practice specialist or general medicine practitioner. This individual may be employed full-time by the team or school, or may be hired jointly by the campus medical service and the athletic department. Occasionally the team physician is a local private physician and is paid a retainer for any and all services needed during a set period of time. These services may include, for instance, the diagnosis and treatment of illness and disease, assistance with the treatment of allergies or asthma and other chronic conditions, and diagnosis and treatment of skeletal and neurological trauma.

Many areas of medicine have some interest in the care of the physically active patient. The medical specialty areas, as outlined next, often establish special committees within their medical organizations to study and discuss sports medicine. The list of specialties and organizations may surprise you, but as you learn more about medical care of the physically active you will realize that the medical, dental, and psychological needs of the physically active patient are similar to those of other individuals. Those needs are often magnified by the intense physical demands of athletic participation. Specialists who concentrate on the physically active usually have a good understanding of the physical demands of the sport and also the schedule for the participant's competitive season. Additionally, the highly trained athlete may experience unusual medical problems that must be understood and addressed to allow healthy participation.

Orthopedic Surgeons and Other Specialists

Because of the prevalence of **orthopedic** trauma during sport participation, the orthopedic surgeon is a critical member of the sports medicine team. One or more orthopedic surgeons, like the team physician, may be paid a retainer fee or may receive a fee for services rendered. Sport teams and schools employ few orthopedic specialists full-time.

The orthopedic surgeon, also known as the "orthopod" or the "orthopedist," could be an interested physician from the local medical community or a member of the medical school staff, if the school has a medical school. The orthopedic surgeon's job is to care for injuries to bones and joints. If an athlete has an injury that requires surgery, the orthopod will choose the hospital where the surgery will take place—often because of regulations that each medical facility places on physicians and also because of the equipment available at a particular hospital. A doctor who is allowed to use a facility is said to have "privileges" at that hospital.

Additional physician specialists, such as the dentist, opthamologist, or cardiologist, may be associated with teams or school programs. The number and types of specialists involved often vary with the local interest as well as the philosophy of the sports medicine team and the organization's management. Table 1.2 lists the terms commonly used in athletic medicine to identify particular medical specialists.

Table 1.2
Medical Specialists

Name of specialist	Treatment area	Common consultations
Neurologist, neurosurgeon	Nervous system	Nervous system disturbances, nerve compression syndromes
Orthopedic surgeon	Bones and joints	Sprains, strains, fractures, dislocations, etc.
Cardiologist	Heart	Arrhythmia, heart murmurs
Vascular surgeon	Circulatory system	Thoracic outlet syndrome, other arterial compromise, compartment syndromes
General surgeon	Abdomen and pelvis	Appendicitis, hernia, other internal organ problems
"ENT"	Ear, nose, and throat	Otitis media, hearing disturbance, broken nose or other cases of deviated septum, tonsillitis, etc.
Optometrist	Vision	Corrective lenses, protective lenses
Ophthalmologist	Disease and trauma of eye	Orbital fractures, corneal disease or injury, retinal detachment, etc.
Podiatrist	Foot function	Orthotic fabrication, treatment of bunions, corns, calluses, etc.
Physiatrist	Physical medicine	Muscle strains, general reconditioning and rehabilitation
Dermatologist	Skin	Rashes, allergic reactions, etc.
Gynecologist	Female reproductive system	Menstrual irregularities, other pelvic disorders

Reprinted, by permission, from National Athletic Trainers' Association 1999.

Rehabilitation Specialists

Often an individual is employed by the busy athletic training department to aid in the care and rehabilitation of athletes requiring long periods of absence from team activities. Although certainly within the expertise of the athletic trainer, this rehabilitation duty may be more consistently provided by a clinician who does not have daily duties and travel responsibilities with a sport team. Often the logical choice is the physical therapist. This "rehabilitation specialist" would design and implement treatment and rehabilitation programs for the injured athlete. Having the rehabilitation specialist available even when the team is at practice or away from campus allows more continuous progress toward returning the injured athlete to participation with the team. An additional advantage of the physical therapist in this position is that insurance companies often pay for physical therapy treatments; thus the rehabilitation specialist can generate some income for the athletic department.

Nutritionists

Nutritionists are often employed by the campus medical center or food service but may be called on to supplement the medical staff's attention to the nutritional needs of individual student-athletes or to assist in the management of athletes with eating concerns. The nutritionist may give suggestions to the department that provides training-table service to the athletic teams or, if necessary, may help the athletic trainer in designing a pregame meal for a specific team.

Sport Psychologists

In addition to working with Olympic teams, psychologists specializing in athletics are becoming more involved with sport teams on the college and professional levels. The sport psychologist can be an asset to the noninjured student-athlete in the area of enhancing sport performance or even in dealing with emotional pressures of college life and athletic competition. The injured athlete may seek out the assistance of the sport psychologist in dealing with the emotional difficulties of losing playing status, coping with the injury itself, or going through the resulting rehabilitation program.

Paramedics and Emergency Medical Technicians

Some athletic trainers are also certified as paramedics (EMT-P) or emergency medical technicians (EMT). These people may be able to contribute additional emergency care skills to the sports medicine team, but infrequently will the athletic trainer serve in a dual capacity at an athletic event. More likely, the EMT or paramedic is a member of the ambulance squad hired to cover athletic events, as seen in figure 1.16. These personnel, if assigned to home events, should be familiar with the school's emergency care plan and should discuss any special concerns of their own with the school's athletic training staff. These topics are discussed in detail in chapter 8, "Emergency Care and Medical Management of Athletic Injury."

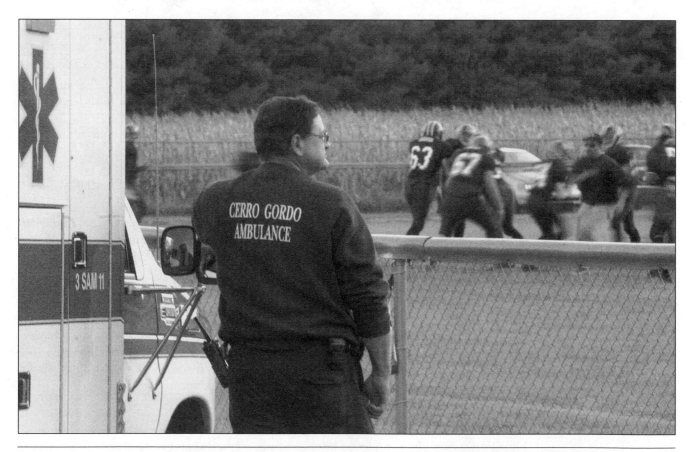

Figure 1.16   Emergency medical technicians are hired to cover a game and will transport injured athletes to a hospital or clinic for further care.

Other Support Staff

As with any team, other staff members contribute to the smooth operation of the athletic training program. The secretarial and insurance personnel are great assets in the management of the medical program, and it is important to regard these individuals as members of the team. The work of administrative staff and insurance personnel not only keeps the athletic department functioning smoothly, but also enables the athletic trainers to concentrate on athletic training concerns.

Coaches and Athletes

Lastly, the coach and the athlete are obviously central to the sports medicine team. The coach can often recognize subtle changes in the athlete's skill performance, academic performance, or general personality that could signal some underlying problem. The coach's critical observation of a decline in performance can save an athlete from exacerbating a small problem. Yet no matter how many individuals there are on the sports medicine team, physically active persons must accept responsibility for their health. Good hygiene, sound nutritional practices, and attention to signs of fatigue or injury are all, ultimately, responsibilities of the individual. Still and all, it is part of the work of the athletic trainer to educate athletes about their bodies and encourage them to take an active role in keeping physically, psychologically, and emotionally healthy (see figure 1.17).

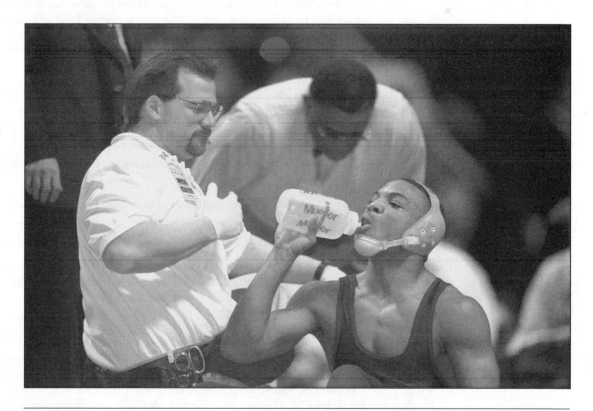

Figure 1.17 Physically active individuals are ultimately responsible for their own health and well-being. However, an athletic trainer can educate and inform these individuals to help keep them safe and active.

SUMMARY

1. *List the characteristics of athletic training that identify it as a profession.*

   The following are the six characteristics of a profession: (1) A profession involves a skill based on theoretical knowledge; (2) a profession involves a skill that requires training and education; (3) the professional must demonstrate competence by passing a test; (4) the professional's integrity is maintained by adherence to a code of conduct; (5) the professional's service is provided for the public good; and (6) the profession is organized. Without debate, athletic training possesses five of these six characteristics. The only one open for discussion is the fifth—provision of the service for the public good. Sociologists would probably agree that service to the physically active does not qualify as service for the public good.

2. *Discuss the five major historical events that shaped the current structure of the NATA.*

   (1) The origin of the association: After an earlier failure, the NATA began in 1950. (2) The start of a profession: The Code of Ethics was adopted in 1957 along with approval of the first undergraduate educational program for athletic trainers. (3) The beginning of medical recognition: In 1969 the AMA recognized the importance of the athletic trainer. (4) The development of standards for certification and continuing education of athletic trainers: The first certification examination for athletic trainers was held in 1970, changing the system from one based on journeyman training to one based on formal education and incorporating minimum-standards evaluation for certification. In 1979 the NATA instituted continuing education for all certified athletic trainers in an attempt to maintain a higher level of competency among its membership. (5) The recognition of the profession: In 1990, the AMA recognized athletic training as an official allied health profession.

3. *Identify the members of a sports medicine team.*

   The sports medicine team always includes the physician, the athletic trainer, the coach, and the athlete. Larger or more advantaged athletic teams may involve additional professionals, including additional medical specialists, nutritionists, sport psychologists, emergency technicians, and support staff.

4. *Identify job opportunities for certified athletic trainers. Explain your ideal job setting.*

   Athletic trainers find employment in a variety of situations—with high school, college, and professional teams; in sports medicine clinics and hospitals; in the workplace; and in educational settings.

5. *Identify the courses at your school that a student interested in athletic training should take.*

   The NATA requires completion of the following courses: health, human anatomy; kinesiology/biomechanics, human physiology, physiology of exercise, basic athletic training, and advanced athletic training.

6. *Explain how the most recent changes in the education of athletic trainers might affect various college and university programs in the United States.*

   As of January 1, 2004, the internship route to certification no longer exists. Candidates wishing to pursue eligibility for the examination via the internship route must have done so before December 31, 2003. This means that colleges and universities throughout the United States must offer a degree program in athletic training if students are to become certified as athletic trainers. If insufficient opportunities exist in current educational institutions, potential athletic training students will be forced to pursue alternate academic plans. Schools and teams that have employed students in the internship route toward NATA certification will be affected by the loss of the pool of student workers. Consequently, schools either will have to reduce their service to sport teams or will have to hire additional part-time and full-time staff to accomplish the same service.

CRITICAL THINKING QUESTIONS

1. You were helping your longtime friend and fellow ATC cover lacrosse practice one afternoon at a local university. You overheard your friend, an assistant ATC at the school, speaking in detail with the soccer coach about the injury status of a lacrosse athlete who was sitting out of practice that day. The athlete, who was sitting on the sideline at the moment, also overheard the conversation, and was very upset with your friend—enough so that he left practice to go find the head ATC at the facility. According to appendix A, which if any part of the NATA Code of Ethics has your friend violated? Do you have any professional responsibilities/obligations in this situation to act? Would you be in violation of any NATA policies if you did nothing? If so, which ones, and what should you do?

2. Athletic training course instructors should be certified members of the NATA, according to your book. What are some of the advantages and disadvantages of having only certified athletic trainers as instructors for core-content classes?

3. Good sport health care in a time of emergency treatment relies on three basic necessities: proper planning and practice, good communication skills, and good working relationships among all staff and support staff. How would you as the head ATC at any level ensure that things ran smoothly during an athletic emergency with each of the following support staff groups? Include any preplanning you would do (practice sessions, letters sent out, meetings, etc.)
   - Paramedics/EMT
   - Orthopedic doctors (team doctors)
   - Student trainers

4. Identify the members of a sport health care team and list their job duties as they pertain to the school's sport teams. As an ATC, what is the importance of maintaining good working relationships with each of the following members?
   - Team physician
   - The athlete
   - Emergency technicians

5. You are in charge of the medical services for your high school. After one year it is clear to you that you have to have some help before the start of the next school year. You decide to go to the athletic director and propose two things: (1) You want to begin seeking reimbursement from your athletes' insurance companies for treatment and rehabilitation you are providing, and (2) you want to hire a full-time assistant to help with the day-to-day sport coverage as well as management of the billing for the insurance reimbursements. Prepare a list of five things you want to be sure to express to the athletic director to support each of your proposed points.

CITED SOURCES

Laster-Bradley, M., and B.A. Berger. 1991. Evaluation of drug distribution systems in university athletic programs: Development of a model of "optimal" distribution system for athletic programs. Unpublished report. Auburn University, Alabama.

Mitchell, G.D. 1973. *A dictionary of sociology.* Chicago, IL: Aldine.

National Athletic Trainers' Association. 2004. *NATA Foundation mission statement.* Dallas: National Athletic Trainers' Association.

ADDITIONAL READINGS

Foster, T. 1995. The father of modern athletic training: William E. "Pinky" Newell. *NATA News*, February, 4-8.

Newell, W.E. 1984. Reflections on athletic training. *Athletic Trainer*, Winter, 256-259, 311.

O'Shea, M.E. 1990. *A history of the national athletic trainers' association*. Greenville, NC: National Athletic Trainers' Association.

Smelser, N.J. 1988. *Handbook of sociology*. Newbury Park, CA: Sage.

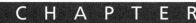
Epidemiology of Athletic Injuries

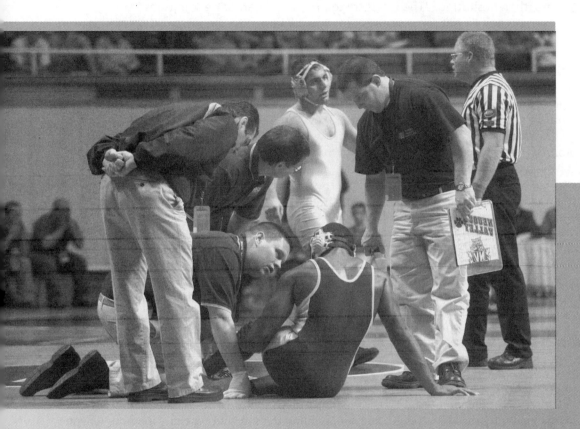

Objectives

After reading this chapter, the student should be able to do the following:

1. Define epidemiology and identify various agencies that collect sports epidemiological data.

2. List the 10 sports the National Athletic Trainers' Association classifies as high-risk sports and explain why it is important for student athletic trainers to have significant exposure to at least one of those sports.

3. Identify conditions that are more common in the preadolescent and the adolescent athlete than in other age groups, and then explain any

effect those conditions might have on the risks of sport participation.

4. Discuss a condition unique to female athletes and explain any effect that condition might have on the risks of sport participation.

5. Support one side of the argument presented in the introduction to the chapter (supposing first that the child, Vincent, is a normal, healthy child; then supposing that Vincent has a heart condition).

Your older sister, knowing you are involved in sports, has called you to get you to settle an argument she and her husband are having. Len, your brother-in-law, wants to get your nephew, Vincent, into the youth soccer league in town. Heidi, your sister, says, "Absolutely no sports!" They want you to settle their monthlong argument.

"Okay," you tell Heidi. "First, what exactly are you worried about?"

"Injuries!" she answers.

"Yes, I assumed that, but what kind of injuries? Like knee, ankle, head, neck. . . . What kind of injury are you afraid about?"

"Well . . . ," Heidi says, then hesitating. "The worst thing probably, head or neck injuries."

"Heidi, give me a few days and I'll get some statistics for you. I'll look into the injury rates for kids playing soccer," you suggest.

"Great! Can you come over for dinner Sunday night and we can talk about what you find out?" she asked enthusiastically.

"Let me call you—I don't know how long this research is going to take!" you say. You're worried about where you will be able to find this kind of information.

Heidi says to her husband, standing over her shoulder, "Okay, Len, the case is closed for now. John will settle this for us, but you have to agree to whatever he says!"

"Don't be ridiculous! I want to hear the stats and then make an informed decision with Vincent, not for Vincent," Len states emphatically.

The pressure is on. You've got to produce the facts. Your sister and her husband are not going to let you in the house again until you come up with some facts and figures so they have enough information to advise their young son.

"Way to go, Einstein," your roommate says after you have told him the story. "Like you aren't totally stressed with midterms next week? When are you gonna find time to research that stuff? Get real."

"Don't worry. We use this book in my sports med class—*Prevention and Management*. I think it has information in one of the chapters," you say as you remember that the midterm in that class is next Monday. "I've got to study that stuff for the exam anyway; this will make the reading more meaningful—maybe I'll remember it better this way!"

Approaches to reducing risks to athletes include understanding injury or illness due to pre-existing medical conditions through the preparticipation physical examination (chapter 3); reducing injury through strength and conditioning training and coaching methods (chapter 4); preventing problems related to facilities and equipment (chapter 6); and preventing injury or reinjury through use of protective bracing or padding (chapter 7). Another approach is to study the types and frequencies of athletic injury. This is an area of research called epidemiology. Epidemiology, or the frequency with which a specific injury or disease occurs, can have significance for designing protective equipment, for establishing or altering rules, and for providing general information to athletes and parents.

From the viewpoint of the athletic trainer, sports epidemiology data help the most by allowing organizers to identify the kinds of health care needed at various practices and competitions. The motto "An ounce of prevention is worth a pound of cure" applies in the use of knowledge gained from epidemiology studies to make a safer environment for play. Epidemiological outcomes point toward risk factors as related to sport participation; these risk factors alert coaches, administrators, and athletic trainers to potential injury situations. The data aid strength and conditioning professionals in developing programs to help reduce the risks, and also serve to alert individuals with increased susceptibility to a particular injury or condition that a particular sport is a high-risk endeavor for them. Additionally the data allow organizers to anticipate injury and take steps toward providing adequate medical coverage. The National Athletic Trainers' Association (NATA) has taken great steps in this use of epidemiological information in detailing its "Recommendations and Guidelines for Appropriate Medical Coverage of Intercollegiate Athletics." This document gives college administrators an excellent resource for determining the number and types of medical care professionals needed at each intercollegiate team practice or competition. In addition, the document lists the many duties and responsibilities of the individual providing medical care for the student-athlete. It is very beneficial for all individuals working with sport teams to review this NATA document (available at www.nata.org/publications/publications.htm) when attempting to determine medical coverage for sport teams. Additional information from the National Collegiate Athletic Association (NCAA) is available on the Web at www1.ncaa.org/membership/ed_outreach/health-safety/care-coverage/index.

RESEARCH IN SPORTS EPIDEMIOLOGY

Sport injury epidemiology is an area of research interest throughout the United States and the entire sport world. Investigators have gathered information on sport and recreational injuries seen in specific health care centers like hospital emergency rooms and health care clinics. Other studies have examined retrospective data on injuries occurring during a particular time period or in a particular sport. Still other investigators collect data from a wide variety of teams over a number of years. The gathering of epidemiological data by each group helps us understand possible relationships between injuries and sports (see figure 2.1); however, not all of the data can be applied to all participants in a particular sport.

Take a minute right now to imagine yourself in charge of the local parks and recreation facilities. Your job is to provide ample opportunities for area residents to participate in physical activities—but you must do it safely. This addition of the element of safety makes provision of recreation and sport activities a little more difficult. Epidemiological data help you understand the risks of participation. If sufficient data could be collected, every injury-producing situation could be known and analyzed so that those interested in engaging in a given activity could take actions to avoid that injury. It might seem impossible that you could have enough information to be able to predict the chances of injury. But with sufficient data,

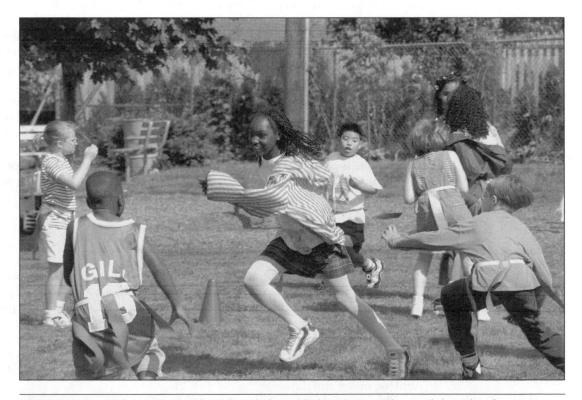

Figure 2.1 Research in sports epidemiology helps athletic trainers understand the risks of participation and prepares them to handle specific injuries and problems.

Exercise Research Associates is a nonprofit research and consulting company that reports on research in health, fitness, sports medicine, and other related sport issues with a focus on epidemiology of sport injuries. For more information go to www.exra.org. In addition, check out the National Library of Medicine at www.nlm.nih.gov. There you'll find health information (Medline) and library services.

much more information can be shared with folks like Len and Heidi who want to provide low-risk physical activities for their children.

Although current data in the literature begin to address the issues of sport and recreational injuries, there is much more information to be gathered. Thankfully, organized efforts to collect long-term statistics are under way; some of the organizations conducting national surveys to collect epidemiological data on sport injuries are identified in table 2.1.

SPORT INJURY SURVEILLANCE SYSTEMS

Although a large number of organizations collect data on injuries during sport participation, those data are not always helpful for understanding injury trends or injury epidemiology. In addition to this type of research, there are numerous studies of injury occurrences in particular regions of the country, at particular levels of participation, or both. Some of the difficulties in reviewing the plethora of literature result from differences in definitions of reportable injuries, limitations from not knowing the population the subjects represent (e.g., in hospital studies in which the number of uninjured athletes is unknown), and limitations imposed by the design of the study. Suppose, for example, that a large metropolitan area has a "fitness weekend" and that there are more than 20 sites throughout the area where people can go to participate in various activities. Some number of individuals participating will undoubtedly get hurt. To obtain accurate data on the frequency of injuries incurred in each of the 20 activities you would need to know (1) how many individuals participated at each location; (2) of these, how many were injured in the activity but continued to participate; (3) how many were injured in the activity and were unable to continue; and (4) how many were injured and did not tell anyone. These are the same factors that epidemiology researchers deal with when attempting to gather sufficient data to issue a statement regarding the frequency of injury.

Nonetheless, collection of any and all injury data is essential to a greater understanding of how to prevent injuries—the goal of gathering information on epidemiology. Data collection is a critical job that must be done with accuracy and in accordance with the guidelines of the organization. All reporters must report on a particular injury in the same way. One of the critical tasks relating to the collection of epidemiological data is establishing what is reportable, how to define the injury, and how to categorize the injury-producing situation. Many of the agencies that collect injury data rely on athletic trainers to provide the needed information from teams they are associated with.

National Athletic Injury Reporting System

The National Athletic Injury Reporting System (NAIRS) is an injury and illness surveillance system that was designed by athletic trainers and other sports medicine personnel to answer the need for a uniform system of reporting injuries and illnesses affecting athletes.

The NAIRS, which originated early in 1974, consisted of a small group of individuals who represented the interests of athletic and sports medicine organizations and were concerned about the increase in litigation surrounding injury resulting from sport participation. Supported by grant money from the NCAA Committee on Competitive Safeguards and Medical Aspects of Sports, NAIRS served as a national collection agency for data on meaningful athletic injury and illness.

This organization was a cornerstone for several groundbreaking developments in sports medicine, including the use of functional codes to categorize injuries, the computerization of injury data, and adaptations allowing customization of injury reports.

Table 2.1

Agencies Involved in Collecting Sport Injury Data

Collection agency	Subjects involved	Comments
National Athletic Injury Reporting System (NAIRS)	College athletes	Wide sampling of college sports.
National Collegiate Athletic Association (NCAA)	College athletes	Multiyear, ongoing survey of NCAA institutions. Covers 16 NCAA sports.
National Athletic Trainers' Association (NATA)	High school athletes	Very complete and specific athletic injury study.
Accident and Injury Reporting System (AIRS)	Professional athletes (through Workers' Compensation Board [WCB])	Electronic reporting of workplace accidents and injuries to the WCB.
National Youth Sports Safety Foundation, Inc. (NYSSF); formerly the National Youth Sports Foundation for the Prevention of Athletic Injuries, Inc.	All youth (compilation of injury data from various sources)	NYSSF serves as an educational resource and clearinghouse for information on safe sport participation for parents, coaches, athletes, health professionals, and program administrators.
Center for Injury Research and Control (CIRCL), University of Pittsburgh Medical Center	Individuals suffering traumatic brain injury and/or spinal cord injury	One of 10 centers in the country to receive official designation by the CDC as an Injury Control Research Center. Gathers retrospective data and produces epidemiological Information through injury records.
National Electronic Injury Surveillance System (NEISS)	General population	NEISS tracks injuries resulting from use of consumer products. Injuries are those treated at 91 selected hospital emergency rooms. NEISS may not accurately represent all recreational injuries.
Centers for Disease Control and Prevention (CDC)	General population	The CDC tracks illnesses and injuries to establish areas of outbreaks (illnesses) or other common trends in epidemiology to attempt to control their occurrence.
Healthy People 2010 (a division of the CDC)	General population	Two major goals are to increase quality and years of healthy life, and to reduce disparities in health among different population groups.
National Football Head and Neck Injury Registry	All levels of football participants	This group collects injury data concerning the head and neck in football and, when appropriate, advocates rule changes to prevent injury.
National Center for Catastrophic Sports Injury Research	High school and college athletes who suffer serious injury or death during participation	This agency collects and analyzes data on injuries in high school and college sports that result in death or permanent severe functional disability. The goal is to recommend ways to prevent such tragedy.

The goal of NAIRS was to obtain reliable, confidential injury reports from all levels of sport teams. The basis of the NAIRS system of injury tracking consisted of functional definitions devised with the intent of ensuring uniform criteria for reportable injuries. Typically the athletic trainer was responsible for reporting the injuries; but further developments allowed schools with no athletic trainer to participate in the system also. To standardize the perception of "an athletic injury," NAIRS has outlined the reportable injuries.

Reportable Injuries As Defined by the National Athletic Injury Reporting System

- Any brain concussion causing cessation of the athlete's participation in order to allow medical observation prior to permitting return to play
- Any dental injury that should receive professional attention
- Any injury or illness that causes cessation of an athlete's customary participation on the day following the day of onset of the problem
- Any injury or illness that requires substantive professional attention before the athlete's return to participation is permitted (i.e., without such attention, the athlete would not have been permitted to return to participation on the next participation day)

National Collegiate Athletic Association Injury Surveillance System (ISS)

The **NCAA** and many college conferences have been collecting injury data on particular teams for a number of years (see figure 2.2). These studies, termed injury/illness surveillance systems, involve collection of injury data over a period of years to allow a longitudinal review of injury patterns and rates in the participating teams. This method of data collection relies on the cooperation and participation of medical care providers in all areas of the country who are working with the target population (age range, level, and sport). For examples of the forms used by the NCAA Injury Surveillance System, see "Weekly Exposure Form—Fall Football" on page 39 and "Individual Injury Form—Fall Football" on pages 40-41.

The NCAA sponsors data gathering from member institutions in 12 intercollegiate sports. The data are analyzed by categories within sports according to the injury being studied. For example, head injuries are analyzed according to sports mandating head protection versus those that do not require helmets or headgear. Data are expressed both as a percentage of all reported injuries in a specific sport and as an injury rate.

National Athletic Trainers' Association High School Injury Study

In 1998, the NATA released the results of a three-year study of 220+ high schools that tracked injuries to athletes in football, boys' and girls' basketball, wrestling, baseball, softball, field hockey, girls' volleyball, and boys' and girls' soccer (Powell and Barber-Foss 1999).

This NATA study, the largest of its kind, not only established injury patterns in each sport but also identified injuries more likely to occur in girls' basketball versus boys' basketball, girls' track versus boys' track, and so on.

In addition, in June of 1998 the NATA issued a call for investigators in the area of youth sport. The organization provided $250,000 for a research project to develop and conduct an epidemiological study to identify injury patterns and at-risk populations among youth sports. The ongoing NATA research conducted under the guidance of the renowned sports medicine and orthopedic specialist, Lyle Micheli, MD, will help to make this study the standard by which all other epidemiological studies are measured.

The National Electronic Injury Surveillance System

The U.S. Consumer Product Safety Commission operates the National Electronic Injury Surveillance System. This agency gathers data nationally on injuries associated with products used in recreational and residential settings. It also attempts to identify reasonable

Weekly EXPOSURE Form—Fall Football
NCAA INJURY SURVEILLANCE SYSTEM

> **EXPOSURE DEFINITION:** An athlete exposure, the unit of risk in the ISS, is defined as one student-athlete participating in one practice or game where he or she is exposed to the possibility of athletics injury.
>
> *Note:* Please be as accurate as possible in reporting number of participants. PRACTICE participants must be included in a majority of the drills. GAME participants must have actual playing time. In most cases, the number of game participants is less than the number of practice participants.

School Code: _____   Week of: _____

(Sunday to Saturday)

PRACTICE

1. This week was part of:

    (1) Preseason (before first regular-season contest)

    (2) Regular season

    (3) Postseason (after final regular-season contest; includes conference, regional and national tournaments)

2. Describe each practice

a. Total # participants (see instructions)	b. Type of practice (check ONE that best describes practice)				c. Type of surface (check ONE that best describes surface)		
Practice	Noncontact	Contact (tackling)	Contact (non-tackling)	Scrimmage*	Artificial turf	Natural turf	Other (e.g., gym floor)
No. 1 _____	_____	_____	_____	_____	_____	_____	_____
No. 2 _____	_____	_____	_____	_____	_____	_____	_____
No. 3 _____	_____	_____	_____	_____	_____	_____	_____
No. 4 _____	_____	_____	_____	_____	_____	_____	_____
No. 5 _____	_____	_____	_____	_____	_____	_____	_____
No. 6 _____	_____	_____	_____	_____	_____	_____	_____
No. 7 _____	_____	_____	_____	_____	_____	_____	_____
No. 8 _____	_____	_____	_____	_____	_____	_____	_____

*(>50 percent practice time devoted to 11-on-11 scrimmaging)

VARSITY GAME

3. Varsity game played?

    (1) No (stop)

    (2) Yes—Home

    (3) Yes—Away

4. Varsity game played on:

    (1) Natural surface

    (2) Artificial surface

5. Number of participants (with actual playing time) in varsity game: _____

6. Number of kickoffs (your team) in game: _____

7. Number of kickoff returns (your team) in game: _____

Reprinted from NCAA Injury Surveillance System.

Individual INJURY Form—Fall Football
NCAA Injury Surveillance System

INJURY DEFINITION: A reportable injury in the ISS is defined as one that:
1. Occurs as a result of participation in an organized intercollegiate practice or contest;
2. Requires medical attention by a team athletics trainer or physician; and
3. Results in any restriction of the athletics participation or performance* for one or more days beyond the day of injury.
4. Any dental injury regardless of time loss.

*See POINTS OF EMPHASIS.

School Code: _____

1. Year (circle one):
   (1) FR   (3) JR   (5) Fifth
   (2) SO   (4) SR

2. Age: _____ years   4. Weight: _____ pounds

3. Height: _____ inches   5. Date of injury: _____
                                            (month/day)

6. Injury occurred during:
   (1) Preseason (before first regular-season contest)
   (2) Regular season
   (3) Postseason (after final regular-season game)
   (99) Other: _____

7. Injury occurred in:
   (1) Competition—varsity (go to next question)
   (2) Not applicable
   (3) Practice (go to question 9)

8. GAME ONLY—Where did this injury occur?
   (1) Home game   (3) Neutral site
   (2) Away game   (99) Other: _____

9. Time of injury:
   Game: (1) 1st qtr.   Practice: (7) first ½ hour
          (2) 2nd qtr.   (8) second ½ hour
          (3) 3rd qtr.   (9) third ½ hour
          (4) 4th qtr.   (10) fourth ½ hour
          (5) Pregame
          (6) Overtime   (99) Other: _____

10. This injury is a:
    (1) New injury
    (2) Recurrence of football injury from previous season
    (3) Recurrence of football injury from current season
    (4) Complication of previous football injury
    (5) Recurrence of other-sport injury
    (6) Recurrence of nonsport injury
    (7) Complication of previous nonfootball injury

11. Has player had unrelated injury recorded this season?
    (1) Yes   (2) No

12. Weather/field conditions:
    (1) No precipitation   (4) Indoor
    (2) Rain   (5) No precipitation/wet field
    (3) Snow

13. How long did this injury keep student-athlete from participating in football? (If end of season, give best estimate.)
    (1) 1-2 days   (5) 22 days or more
    (2) 3-6 days   (6) Catastrophic, nonfatal
    (3) 7-9 days   (7) Fatal
    (4) 10-21 days

14. Injury situation:
    (1) Fundamentals drills   (10) PAT/FG
    (2) Blocking sled   (11) Kickoff
    (3) Rushing play   (12) Punting
    (4) Passing   (13) Punt return
    (5) Pass catching   (14) Fumble recovery
    (6) Pass protection (offense)   (15) Pile up
    (7) Pass rush (defense)   (16) Conditioning, sprints
    (8) Pass defense   (99) Other (specify): _____
    (9) Kickoff return   _____

15. Principal body part injured (for 1-10, complete Head Injury information; for 31 or 32, complete Knee Injury information):
    (1) Head   (22) Upper back
    (2) Eye(s)   (23) Spine
    (3) Ear(s)   (24) Lower back
    (4) Nose   (25) Ribs
    (5) Face   (26) Sternum
    (6) Chin   (27) Stomach
    (7) Jaw (TMJ)   (28) Pelvis, hips, groin
    (8) Mouth   (29) Buttocks
    (9) Teeth   (30) Upper leg
    (10) Tongue   (31) Knee
    (11) Neck   (32) Patella
    (12) Shoulder   (33) Lower leg
    (13) Clavicle   (34) Ankle
    (14) Scapula   (35) Heel/Achilles tendon
    (15) Upper arm   (36) Foot
    (16) Elbow   (37) Toe(s)
    (17) Forearm   (38) Spleen
    (18) Wrist   (39) Kidney
    (19) Hand   (40) External genitalia
    (20) Thumb   (41) Coccyx
    (21) Finger(s)   (99) Other: _____

HEAD INJURY (answer only if response in question 15 was 1-10)

16. This student-athlete was diagnosed as having:
    (1) 1° cerebral concussion. [No loss of consciousness, short posttraumatic amnesia (seconds to one to two minutes).]
    (2) 2° cerebral concussion. [Loss of consciousness (less than five minutes) and amnesia for up to 30 seconds.]
    (3) 3° cerebral concussion. [Loss of consciousness (less than five minutes) and extended amnesia.]
    (4) No cerebral concussion
    (5) Unknown

17. Was a mouthpiece (MP) worn?
    (1) MP worn—dentist fitted
    (2) MP worn—self-fitted
    (3) MP not worn

18. Type eye injury:
    (1) Orbital fracture   (4) Soft tissue
    (2) Cornea   (99) Other: _____
    (3) Ruptured globe

KNEE INJURY (answer only if response in question 15 was 31 or 32)

19. Circle ALL knee structures injured:
    (1) Collateral   (5) Patella and/or patella
    (2) Anterior cruciate   tendon
    (3) Posterior cruciate   (6) None
    (4) Torn cartilage (meniscus)   (99) Other: _____

20. Primary type of injury (circle one):

(1)	Abrasion	(15)	Dislocation (complete)
(2)	Contusion	(16)	Fracture
(3)	Laceration	(17)	Stress fracture
(4)	Puncture wound	(18)	Concussion
(5)	Bursitis	(19)	Heat exhaustion
(6)	Tendinitis	(20)	Heatstroke
(7)	Ligament sprain (incomplete tear)	(21)	Burn
		(22)	Inflammation
(8)	Ligament sprain (complete tear)	(23)	Infection
		(24)	Hemorrhage
(9)	Muscle-tendon strain (incomplete tear)	(25)	Internal injury
		(26)	Nerve injury
		(27)	Blisters
(10)	Muscle-tendon strain (complete tear)	(28)	Boil(s)
		(29)	Hernia
		(30)	Foreign object in body orifice
(11)	Torn cartilage		
(12)	Hyperextension	(31)	Avulsion (tooth)
(13)	AC separation	(99)	Other: _____
(14)	Dislocation (partial)		

21. Did a laceration or wound that resulted in oozing or bleeding occur as a part of this injury?
   (1) Yes   (2) No

22. Did this injury require surgery?
   (1) Yes, in-season
   (2) Yes, postseason
   (3) No

23. Describe the joint surgery:
   (1) Arthrotomy
   (2) Diagnostic arthroscopy
   (3) Operative arthroscopy
   (4) No joint surgery
   (99) Other: _____

24. Injury diagnosis (record single most definitive diagnostic procedure):
   (1) Clinical exam by athletic trainer
   (2) Clinical exam by M.D./D.D.S.
   (3) X-ray
   (4) MRI
   (5) Other imagery technique
   (6) Surgery
   (7) Blood work/lab test
   (99) Other: _____

25. Field surface:
   (1) Natural grass
   (2) Artificial grass
   (3) Non-grass surfaces (e.g., gym floors, etc.)
   (99) Other: _____

26. Injury mechanism:

(1)	Heat illness	(10)	Blocking a kick/punt
(2)	Blocked below waist	(11)	No apparent contact (rotation about planted foot)
(3)	Tackling	(12)	No apparent contact (other)
(4)	Being tackled	(13)	Overuse
(5)	Blocking	(14)	Catching/blocking pass
(6)	Being blocked	(15)	Clipped by offensive lineman in LEGAL clipping zone
(7)	Impact with playing surface	(16)	Clipped
(8)	Stepped on/ fallen on/kicked	(17)	Impact with padded cast
		(99)	Other (specify): _____
(9)	Sprints/running		

27. Position played at time of injury:

Offensive		Defensive	
(1)	End	(10)	Down lineman
(2)	Tackle	(11)	Linebacker
(3)	Guard	(12)	Halfback/cornerback
(4)	Center	(13)	Safety
(5)	Quarterback		Others
(6)	Running back	(20)	Kicker/punter
(7)	Slotback/wing back	(21)	Special teams
		(22)	Nonpositional/conditioning drill
(8)	Flanker/wide receiver	(23)	Long snapper
		(99)	Other: _____

GAME ONLY

28. Was this injury directly related to action that was ruled illegal?
   (1) Yes   (2) No

PRACTICE ONLY

29. Injury occurred in:
   (1) Noncontact (helmet only) practice
   (2) Contact (designated tackling) practice
   (3) Contact (designated non-tackling) practice
   (4) Scrimmage (more than 50 percent of time devoted to 11-on-11 scrimmage) practice
   (99) Other: _____

30. Equipment worn at time of injury:
   (1) Full pads
   (2) Helmets, shoulder pads only
   (3) Helmets only
   (99) Other: _____

31. Injury occurred during:
   (1) Full contact scrimmage (11 on 11)
   (2) Full contact drill (3 or less participants)
   (3) Full contact drill (4 to 9 participants)
   (4) Full contact drill (10 to 16 participants)
   (5) Full contact drill (15 to 21 participants)
   (6) Noncontact drill
   (99) Other: _____

Additional comments (optional) _____

_____

_____

_____

_____

_____

_____

_____

_____

_____

_____

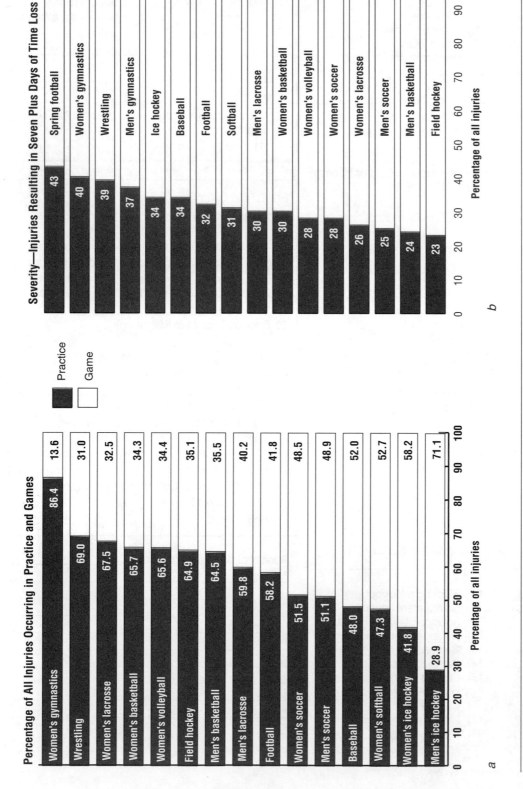

Percentage of All Injuries Occurring in Practice and Games

Sport	Practice	Game
Women's gymnastics	86.4	13.6
Wrestling	69.0	31.0
Women's lacrosse	67.5	32.5
Women's basketball	65.7	34.3
Women's volleyball	65.6	34.4
Field hockey	64.9	35.1
Men's basketball	64.5	35.5
Men's lacrosse	59.8	40.2
Football	58.2	41.8
Women's soccer	51.5	48.5
Men's soccer	51.1	48.9
Baseball	48.0	52.0
Women's softball	47.3	52.7
Women's ice hockey	41.8	58.2
Men's ice hockey	28.9	71.1

a

Severity—Injuries Resulting in Seven Plus Days of Time Loss

Sport	7 or more days time loss	Less than 7 days time loss
Spring football	43	57
Women's gymnastics	40	60
Wrestling	39	61
Men's gymnastics	37	63
Ice hockey	34	66
Baseball	34	66
Football	32	68
Softball	31	69
Men's lacrosse	30	70
Women's basketball	30	70
Women's volleyball	28	72
Women's soccer	28	72
Women's lacrosse	26	74
Men's soccer	25	75
Men's basketball	24	76
Field hockey	23	77

b

Figure 2.2 (a) The percentage of all injuries that occurred in practices and in games through the 2002-2003 season. The few weight-room injuries are not included. It should be noted that these calculations are based only on the absolute number of injuries and do not take exposures into consideration. (b) The percentage of all injuries that caused restricted or missed participation for seven or more days (measure of injury severity) across all sports analyzed in the 1995-1996 season (NCAA 2003).

Reprinted, by permission, from NCAA Injury Surveillance System.

To look at the NCAA's injury data, go to www1.ncaa.org/membership/ed_outreach/health-safety/iss/index.html.

approaches to reducing the frequency and severity of injuries and the occurrence of death. The 91 participating hospitals provide data on over 280,000 case reports per year. This multilevel data collection system includes records from hospital emergency rooms, communication with the injured person, and on-site in-depth investigation of specific cases. Injury trends for products such as fireworks, playground equipment, and all-terrain vehicles are investigated and solutions proposed as part of an attempt to reduce product-related injuries.

As an example, consider the three-wheel all-terrain vehicle. What do you suppose happened to this motorcycle with three wheels? You might suspect that the injury rate associated with this type of motorcycle was high. You're right. Whether people were riding the three-wheeler in an unsafe manner, or whether it was inherently unsafe, too many injuries occurred (as did lawsuits); manufacturers stopped making the product and now offer the more stable four-wheel models. Or, think about the air bag in your car. Initially it was thought that the air bag could reduce injuries in head-on collisions (see figure 2.3). Soon after the auto manufacturers started making air bags standard equipment, it was found that short people and children might actually suffer more harm from the air bag than they would without it. What kind of information would have been needed to determine a relationship in this case? Epidemiological data confirmed that the air bag could be causing some of the injuries seen in car accidents. Epidemiological data have been used in many ways to help keep us safe and to make good products and equipment even better.

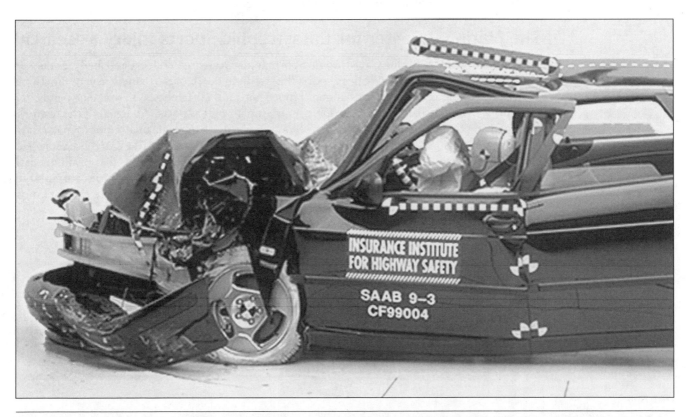

Figure 2.3 Epidemiological data revealed that passengers are safer in cars that have air bags. However, data also showed that harmful injuries occurred more often in smaller adults and children when the air bag was deployed.

Centers for Disease Control and Prevention

The mission of the Centers for Disease Control and Prevention (CDC)/National Center for Injury Prevention and Control (for Sports and Recreational Injuries) is to promote health and quality of life by preventing and controlling disease, injury, and disability. After a long history of work toward its mission, the CDC has evolved into an organization concerned with the prevention of disease through the investigation of causative factors leading to disease, injury, or disability. Although the CDC focuses on disease, it continues to play a role in injury prevention from its unique vantage point. If it is hard to imagine how disease would be related to "injury prevention," suppose you were a wrestler and your team was traveling to a meet at a neighboring school where there was a rumored outbreak of measles, a highly contagious disease. The CDC would be the group to consult on the outbreak because the CDC would be able to track the number of reported cases and determine whether in fact there was an "outbreak." Certainly you would want to contact school officials to be sure there were no cases of measles on the wrestling team; but information from the CDC would be helpful in reducing your team's apprehensions.

The National Football Head and Neck Injury Registry

Started in 1975, the National Football Head and Neck Injury Registry documents head and neck injuries in football participation. The registry solicits information regarding injuries to the head or neck (or both) that meet any of the specifications listed here.

In 1976, the registry presented its initial data to the NCAA. This resulted in rule changes that banned both spearing and the use of the crown of the helmet as the initial point of contact in tackling. The National Federation of High School Athletic Associations implemented similar rule changes. A subsequent decrease in the occurrence rates of both cervical spine fractures and cases of quadriplegia was attributed to these rule changes. In 1976, 34 youngsters were rendered quadriplegic while playing football; in 1984, after the ban on spearing, only 5 players became quadriplegic as a result of engaging in football.

The National Center for Catastrophic Sports Injury Research

The National Center for Catastrophic Sports Injury Research collects and analyzes data on injuries in high school and college sports that result in death or permanent severe functional disability. The center prepares annual reports on football fatalities, permanent paralyzing injuries from football, and catastrophic injuries in all other sports. The goal of the center is to provide the research and analysis to recommend rule changes in an attempt to make sport more safe through coaching techniques and improved equipment. Although these same data may be collected in studies such as the NAIRS or NCAA studies, injuries that result in death or permanent disability are much more easily identified. These types of injuries are certainly at the top of the list of injuries we would want to prevent and thus these are the data most consistently collected.

Specifications of Reportable Head or Neck Injuries

- Injury that required hospitalization for more than 72 hr
- Injury that required surgical intervention
- Injury that involved a fracture or dislocation
- Injury that resulted in permanent paralysis or death

Visit the Healthy People 2010 Web site at www.healthypeople.gov/publications for publications you can download about the goals and objectives of Healthy People 2010.

Healthy People 2010

Healthy People 2010 is a national effort of the Office of Disease Prevention and Health Promotion (committee of the National Health Information Center). The goal of this effort, initiated in 1990, is to reduce injuries and mortality in America. This comprehensive program is organized into 28 focus areas, each with specific supporting objectives. Two major goals of this organization are to increase the quality and years of healthy life and to reduce disparities in health among different population groups. The focus area of Physical Activity and Fitness continues to be a point of emphasis for the Healthy People campaign (U.S. Department of Health and Human Services 2000).

Accident and Injury Reporting System

The Accident and Injury Reporting System is a Canadian system of reporting accidents and injuries to the Workers' Compensation Board (WCB). As in the United States, Canada requires that all injuries and accidents among professional athletes be reported to the WCB because these are considered work-related injuries. Data from the WCB's reporting system can be used to study the epidemiology of injuries in professional athletics.

The National Youth Sports Safety Foundation

Another group interested in youth, the National Youth Sports Safety Foundation, provides current information on sport injury prevention. This organization helps the public learn to evaluate the quality and safety of youth sport programs, learn about sport organizations and the services they provide, and obtain information about guidelines in youth sport participation.

Center for Injury Research and Control

The Center for Injury Research and Control at the University of Pittsburgh Medical Center is an interdisciplinary, comprehensive program involving six schools and 18 departments at the University of Pittsburgh. The center conducts injury-control research, gathers and disseminates information on injuries, provides training for health care professionals, and informs the public and community leaders on injury-control measures. The organization was established in July 1992. In September 1995 it became one of 10 centers in the country to receive official designation by the CDC as an Injury Control Research Center.

The National Youth Sports Safety Foundation, Inc. (NYSSF) is a national nonprofit, educational organization dedicated to reducing the number and severity of injuries youth sustain in sport and fitness activities. For information, event listings, publications, and hot topics, visit the NYSSF at www.nyssf.org.

INJURY TRENDS

Because of the current limitations on injury data collection, data on some sports and many recreational activities are insufficient to provide injury trends. For example, if we were to look at the injury trends for people who run or jog, we might turn to the data collected by hospital emergency rooms. This information would represent only those injured (100% of those seeking attention); it would not allow us to determine the frequency with which an injury occurs among all the people who run or jog. Say there are 100 million people who jog, most of whom never seek medical attention after stepping in a pothole. Suppose further that of the 100 million, 100 went to an emergency room during a particular time period. If the emergency rooms saw only 150 people who had been injured in recreational activities during that same time period, it might appear that running is a very dangerous activity. We must look critically at all injury data to be sure that the data represent the actual occurrence.

It is possible to make several generalizations regarding sport injury by considering the type of sport, type of equipment, type of playing court or field (see figure 2.4), and specific skills related to that activity. Here we'll look briefly at general injury trends for team and individual sports and for projectile and body-movement sports.

Team Sports

Two features of team sports—the very nature of a team and the type of playing field—may affect the risk of participation. Many think that team sports, such as basketball, volleyball, or soccer, pose greater risks for injury than individual sports because of the variety of skill levels on teams. This is often the case in the early years of the athlete's participation, but those factors decrease as maturity, body control, and individual skills increase.

Team sports played on a field and those played on a court pose different problems. The stiffness of the hardwood is thought to contribute to some of the overuse problems in the lower extremity, while the cushion of the natural grass of a field reduces the trauma-producing "stress" reactions.

Unfortunately, not all climates allow the use of natural grass for the playing of field sports. Artificial surfaces or artificial-turf fields are used in areas of the country where grass cannot

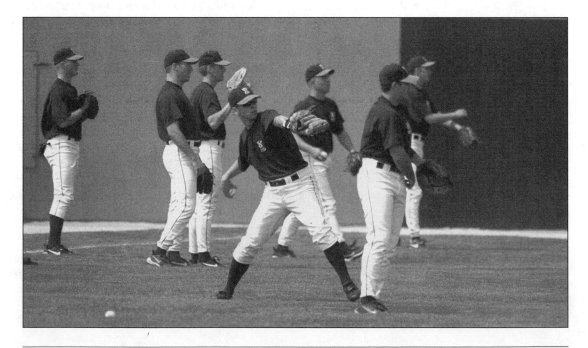

Figure 2.4 The cushion of the natural grass of a field is often credited for reducing the trauma that produces stress-related injuries.

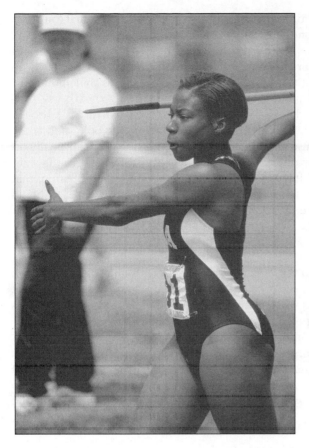

Figure 2.5 It is important to understand the biomechanics of the throwing motions to fully appreciate the stresses that a sport activity places on the area musculature.

be maintained because of weather conditions. The two types of fields, natural grass and artificial turf, produce different stresses on the participant, so that risks of participation depend on the type of field used. It is important for a sport organization to make judgments about the risk of participation on the basis of injury data from the relevant type of field.

Individual Sports

Individual sports, as contrasted to team sports, usually do not pose the potential of injury due to stepping on a teammate's or opponent's foot. Some injuries, obviously, are just as possible in the individual sport as in a team sport, yet this distinction is still useful. We can categorize sports further, on the basis of the skills involved, into projectile versus body-movement sports.

Projectile Sports

Most projectile sports employ a pattern of arm movement. In some projectile sports, athletes use an implement to strike an object; in others, athletes project an object from the hand. Examples of the numerous projectile sports are events in track and field like javelin, shot put, and hammer throw (in which the implement is thrown; see figure 2.5) and sports such as baseball, softball, tennis, and lacrosse (in which the ball is the projectile both as it is thrown and after it is hit). It is important for the sports medicine professional to understand the biomechanics of the throwing/striking motions to fully appreciate the stresses a sport places on the area musculature. Most of the projectile sports involve a preparatory or "cocking" phase, an acceleration phase prior to strike or release, and a follow-through movement that generally entails deceleration of the implement, body part, or both.

Body-Movement Sports

Moving the body as in swimming, running, and gymnastics activities poses problems with overuse; each of these sports also has other specific and unique potentials for injury. The swimmer experiences more injuries of the upper extremities than does the runner, who has mostly lower-extremity problems. Both groups, however, experience low back injury. The gymnast's speed, momentum, and impact pose difficulties in both the upper and the lower extremities. A minor error in technique can often lead to a sudden contact with the floor as the gymnast loses his or her grip on the high bar or uneven parallel bars. Additionally, injuries to the back and neck are not uncommon in the high-contact sport of gymnastics.

HIGH-RISK SPORTS

Epidemiological studies have allowed sports medicine specialists to identify some of the risk factors that lead to athletic injury. Hopefully, most of these known risks have been reduced sufficiently to make the sport safe for participants; however, some risks remain inherent in the sport.

On the basis of a good understanding of the risks involved in sports, the NATA sets sport guidelines for students preparing for certification. The NATA requires that at the time of application, a candidate for certification must verify that at least 25% (200 hours for accredited curriculum or 375 hours for internship applicants) of the required athletic training experience hours credited in fulfilling the Certification Requirements were obtained in actual (on-location) practice or game coverage with one or more of the following sports: football, soccer, hockey, wrestling, basketball, gymnastics, lacrosse, volleyball, rugby, and rodeo. Inclusion of a sport in the NATA's list of sports that provide "acceptable experience" is based primarily on the potential for serious injury as well as the frequency of overall injuries; thus epidemiological information plays a role in the establishment of these NATA guidelines.

High-risk sports are those activities that pose a serious risk to the participant. A broken bat in baseball could cause a serious injury; a high gust of wind during the pole vault could throw the participant off course and cause him or her to land awkwardly or even partially off the mat; bronco riders can lose their grip on the saddle and can be thrown to the ground right under the hooves of the bucking animal. It is easy to think of innumerable other situations that place the participant in serious danger. As you consider what injuries are possible, it should be no wonder that sports in which these situations occur are considered high-risk sports.

Basketball

Basketball, a contact sport according to the NATA, is associated with injuries to the ankle. This, we can assume, relates to the fact that basketball involves jumping, as well as to the fact that the ankle is in a vulnerable position when plantarflexed as in landing from a jump. This vulnerable position, coupled with the potential of landing off balance or on top of another player's foot, greatly increases the risk of significant ankle trauma (see figure 2.6).

The NATA's High School Injury Surveillance Study of 1995 estimated that as many as 38.3% of all injuries involved the ankle and foot (Foster-Welch 1996). In a seven-year study of professional basketball, a reported 18.2% of all injuries were to the ankle. And, in a study by Cohen and Metzl (2000) during the years 1995 to 1998, basketball caused more than 600,000 injuries per year that required emergency care in young athletes. Further, they found that

---

NATA's Classification

The NATA categorizes sports according to both the need for medical coverage as well as the need for a student to gain experience in during his athletic training education. Although similar, these two lists are not identical. The "Appropriate Medial Coverage" list was developed by a NATA task force to determine the highest injury potential sports in an attempt to assist athletic trainers in providing appropriate medical coverage. "NATA Required Sports" is a list of the sports one may use to gain the 25% of the required hours to meet the requirements for certification. This list attempts to ensure all candidates for certification have worked with sports having a high potential for injury. The hours can be gained by working any combination of the sports in that list.

Appropriate Medical Coverage	NATA Required Sports
Basketball (M)	Basketball
Cheerleading	Football
Football	Gymnastics
Gymnastics	Hockey
Ice hockey (M)	Lacrosse
Lacrosse (M)	Rodeo
Rodeo	Rugby
Skiing	Soccer
Soccer (M)	Wrestling
Wrestling	Volleyball

www.bocatc.org/becomeatc/CERT/#BM_SI-MR-TAB3-229

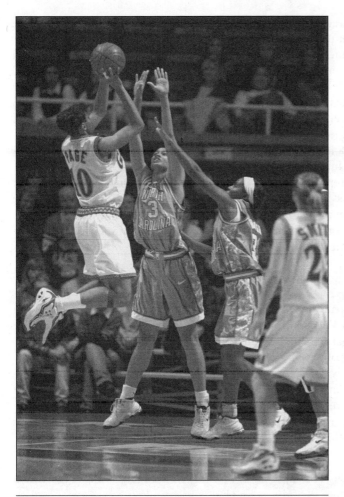

Figure 2.6 As estimated in a NATA study, almost 40% of all injuries in basketball involved the ankle and foot.

ligament sprains were the most common type of basketball-related injury, with the ankle being the most common joint injured (Cohen and Metzl 2000). In another study, Hosea, Carey, and Harrer (2000) followed 11,780 basketball athletes from high schools and colleges in New Jersey. Of all injuries reported, 1,052 (67%) were to the ankle. Of the documented ankle injuries, females had a 25% greater risk of sustaining a Grade I sprain compared to the males in the study. There was no significant difference in the risk for Grade II and III sprains, ankle fractures, or syndesmotic sprains. Results also showed that athletes doubled their risk for sustaining an ankle injury at the collegiate level compared to the high school level.

Second to ankle injuries, injury to the hip, thigh, and leg was seen most frequently in the NATA high school study, accounting for up to 16.6% of all injuries recorded. The injuries falling into this category might range from hamstring strains to thigh contusions to "shinsplints." This wide range of injuries is likely the result of the running and jumping inherent in basketball, coupled with the contact inherent in the competitive event as well as the playing surface.

Although more common, injuries to the ankle and foot typically require less recovery time than the next most frequent injury, the knee injury. Only an approximate 14% of all injuries in professional basketball involved the knee; but knee injury was the cause in 66% of the games missed, while ankle injury accounted for only 18% of the games missed (Henry 1982). The 1995 NATA high school study showed that knee injuries accounted for 10.3% of all injuries experienced by male high school basketball players while 13% of injuries incurred by their female counterparts were injuries to the knee.

The fourth most frequently seen injury in basketball, according to many researchers (Zelisko 1982; Whiteside 1981; Henry 1982), is that involving the hand, wrist, or both. This is probably attributable to the speed of the ball and the athlete's inability to position the hand properly to avoid injury. It appears that injury to the hand, fairly uncommon in comparison to ankle and knee injuries, does not account for many of the games missed (Henry 1982).

It is important to note the increased attention to women's basketball and injury to the knee. Several studies (Moeller and Lamb 1997; Arendt and Dick 1995; Hutchinson and Ireland 1995) indicate a much higher rate of anterior cruciate injury in women basketball players than in their male counterparts. With the success of the Women's National Basketball Association, longitudinal epidemiological studies may be conducted and trends noted.

Cheerleading

Cheerleading is listed by the NATA in terms of the need for medical coverage, yet working as the athletic trainer of a cheerleading squad would not qualify for "contact sport" hours toward certification. Regardless of how it is classified, cheerleading has become a high-impact event associated with organized athletic teams from the elementary school level to the professional level. Cheerleading performances include aspects of gymnastics, dance, tumbling, and pyramid formations. Training for the performances has become a year-round endeavor for many participants, with cheerleading competitions held at times when team support is not needed. Generally, cheerleading has a rather low frequency of injury; yet with the advanced skill levels of the participants, serious injury is quite likely to occur. Many high school and college conferences have issued regulations controlling the types of stunts cheerleaders are allowed to perform in an attempt to reduce the chance of serious injury.

Hutchinson (1997) reported on the frequency of specific types of injuries in high school and collegiate cheerleaders. Although most serious, injuries to the head and neck accounted for only 7% of the total injuries. Mueller and Cantu of the National Center for Catastrophic Sports Injury Research showed that in the 10-year span between 1982 and 1992, only 20 head and neck injuries occurred in cheerleading. Of these 20, 10 occurred during pyramid stunts. Of the 20 injuries, 8 were permanently disabling and, unfortunately, 2 were fatal.

Ankle injuries were the most frequent injury causing loss of time from participation, accounting for 22% of the total injuries. Injuries to the knee, hand, and back occurred less frequently but were fairly often reported as the cause of missed time. One must realize that cheerleaders exhibit gymnastics skills requiring strength, balance, and coordination in one stunt and the next moment are involved in dance or tumbling or a lifting maneuver or pyramid (see figure 2.7). Injury to the nondominant hand of many other athletes may not limit participation, yet in the cheerleader it does.

Football

American football participants span many age and skill levels, from the adolescent playing sandlot or more organized "Pop Warner" football to the adult athlete participating on the college or professional level. Regardless of the skill level, coaches play a critical role in injury prevention through the teaching of proper, safe techniques of blocking and tackling.

Although football is potentially the sport with the highest risk of injury, football injury data are reported inconsistently in the literature. Many studies report injuries in terms of total numbers of injuries or the injuries per 100 players, while others report injury rates in relation to the number of exposures. These various methods of reporting injury statistics make injury-rate analysis very difficult.

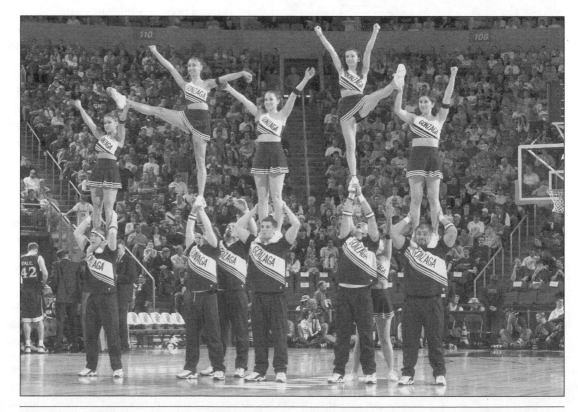

Figure 2.7   Cheerleading performances can include aspects of gymnastics, dance, tumbling, and pyramid formations. Injuries to the ankle occur more frequently than other types of injuries.
© Icon SMI

Head and neck injuries may not be as common in football as in some other sports, yet an injury to the head or neck is potentially much more serious than other, more frequent injuries. Blocking and tackling techniques are critical in the prevention of serious injury, especially to the neck. Axial loading of the spine occurs with the use of improper hitting techniques, and this loading predisposes the spine to serious damage. Flexing the neck forward straightens the cervical spine. Contact to the top of the head in this flexed position causes the axial load where the impact is transferred along the straightened spine. Head injuries or concussions are often the product of the violent nature of the collisions in football and cannot be fully prevented. Recognizing the concussion, as well as consistent grading of the injury, will allow evaluation of further injury information and also make it possible to obtain more accurate injury-rate statistics. In a recent study, Cantu and Mueller (2003) examined brain-related fatalities in American football between 1945 and 1999. The study included incidence and also the cause of death. The authors discovered 497 brain injury-related deaths in the period between 1945 and 1999. The causes of death were traumatic brain injury (TBI) at 69%, cervical spine injuries (16%), and various other injuries (15%); the injuries were experienced predominantly by high school athletes (75%). The most frequent on-field activity involved players tackling or being tackled. The two decades from 1975 through 1994 saw a dramatic reduction in these fatalities. Responsible for the decrease were (1) the 1976 rule change that prohibits initial contact with the head and face during blocking and tackling; and (2) the National Operating Committee on Standards for Athletic Equipment (NOCSAE) helmet standard, which went into effect in colleges in 1978 and in high schools in 1980.

Injuries to the extremities and spine or trunk are not uncommon in football. Involvement of the lower extremity is more frequent than that of the upper extremity, and both of these types of injuries are more common than injuries to the trunk and spine (see table 2.2). This is most probably attributable to the dominant use of the lower extremity in running, blocking, and even tackling. The upper extremity is certainly at risk in throwing and tackling, while injury to the spine might be from overuse (stress fractures and muscle strains) or might consist of acute—and somewhat unusual—trauma (fractures, strains, and sprains).

In studies of injury rates in high school football, the NATA reports that nearly 50% of injuries involve the lower extremity, with the pelvis/hip being involved 17.9% of the time and the ankle (16.6%) and knee (14.6%) being involved almost as frequently (see figure 2.8). The most prevalent injury within the pelvis/hip category is injury to the hamstring muscles. Hamstring strains are not uncommon in any running sport, but football may pose an additional risk for hamstring injury because of the increased load the body must carry (the equipment) or must push (in fighting with an opponent for position or yardage).

Injuries in the upper extremity, according to the NATA, account for approximately 25% of the total injuries recorded in two studies of high school football. Of this 25.35%, injuries to the forearm, wrist, and hand accounted for the majority (15%); injuries to the shoulder and arm (10.35%) were also quite common. The wrist and hand are certainly more prone to injury because of their position on the extremity and the frequent hand-to-body contact involved in the sport. Injury to the shoulder is often seen when the athlete fails to achieve a good tackling position and instinctively reaches out with the arm to make an arm tackle rather than employing the more effective technique of using the body. In the young athlete with a naturally loose shoulder joint, minimal trauma may be sufficient to cause injury. The ligamentous laxity in many adolescent athletes will put additional stress on the muscular support of the joint. With overuse of the muscles, the ligaments are unable to withstand forces of contact, resulting in injury.

National Collegiate Athletic Association ISS data show injury trends in collegiate football to be higher during games than during practices. Although not directly reported in the high school

Table 2.2
Injury Rates in College Football

Area injured	Injuries in practice	Injuries in games
Knee	17%	19%
Thigh	14%	8%
Ankle	13%	18%
Shoulder	12%	13%
Head/Neck	9%	13%
Spine (any level)	7%	6%

Data for 2002-2003 from NCAA Injury Surveillance System from 123 reporting schools.

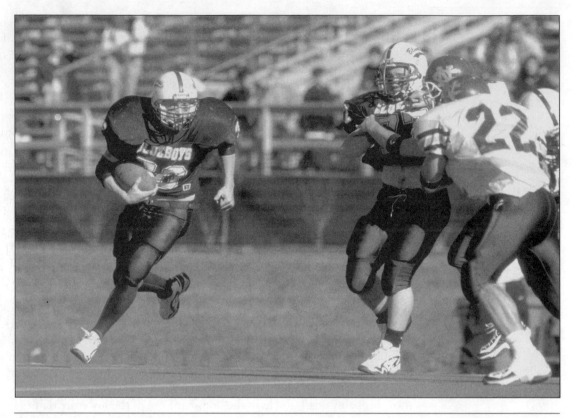

Figure 2.8   According to NATA studies, the most prevalent injuries in football occur in the lower extremity.

study, this fact might seem quite obvious. Additionally, in the 2002-2003 ISS data, injuries to the knee (17%), upper leg (14%), and ankle (12%) were the most common injuries during practice, while injuries sustained during games were more frequent in the knee (20%), ankle (16%), and shoulder (13%). This information is fairly consistent over the past 10 years and perhaps indicates that a slightly different playing technique is being used in games. Along that same line, the ISS data for the past six years show that the most common types of injuries sustained in practice are sprains and strains followed by contusions, while in games, the most common type of injury has consistently been sprains, followed by contusions, with strains being even less common (NCAA 2003).

Gymnastics

Gymnastics combines the stresses of running and jumping and thus involves injuries similar to those incurred in track and field events. Yet gymnastics differs in that events may require extensive use of the upper extremity in weight-bearing maneuvers or in strength and endurance as the gymnast holds on to apparatus during swinging and stunting.

Gymnastics is another sport activity that often takes place in facilities in the neighborhood, in the city gymnasium, or at special clubs. Injury records for the sport are presented in the literature, yet are far from complete.

According to Caine, Caine, and Linder (1996), most injuries occurring in women's gymnastics at all levels (high school, club, and collegiate) involve the lower extremities; injuries to the upper extremity and spine, the next most frequent, are nearly equal to each other in occurrence. In a recent study, Zetaruk (2000) found that women tend to injure their lower extremities (ankles, feet, and knees) more often and men incur more upper-extremity injuries. This finding may be explained by looking at the types of events male gymnasts perform in as compared to those females perform in.

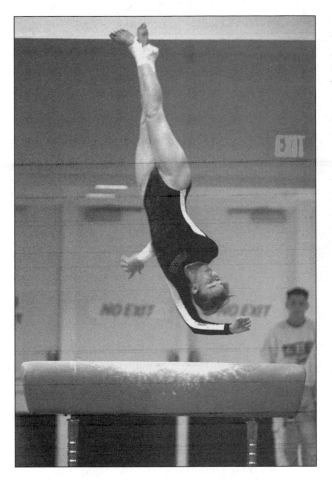

Figure 2.9 In gymnastics, ankle injuries are more frequent than knee joint injuries. Injuries of the upper extremity most frequently involve the elbow in the younger athlete and the shoulder in the older participant.

The typical lower-extremity injuries in gymnastics involve the ankles more than the knee joint (see figure 2.9). Injuries of the upper extremity most frequently involve the elbow in the younger athlete and the shoulder in the older participant. The shoulder is commonly injured in men's gymnastics due to the amount of shoulder strength needed to perform in skills such as the rings and high bar, increased laxity of the joint, and the multidirectional instability of the glenohumeral joint. Bicipital tendinitis, rotator cuff tendinitis, and impingement all occur in the male gymnast (Zetaruk 2000). Injuries to the wrist and fingers are also common in activities requiring the hands for vaulting and catching, as in bar routines. DiFiori et al. (2002) found that taller and older gymnasts experienced more wrist pain compared to their peers.

Problems in the spine most often affect the lower back, regardless of the age of the participant. The extensive flexibility required in performance of the sport tends to localize as stresses in the lower segments of the spine. These conditions are often much more problematic in female gymnasts who are in or are entering menses. The increase in hormone levels has been thought to contribute to the increase in pain in female gymnasts, especially in the later days of their menstrual cycle. Obviously, the menstrual cycle can have an effect on women in any sport, yet the percentage of team members with reports of low back pain is greater in women's gymnastics than in other sports. Zetaruk (2000) reported that 63% of Olympic-level gymnasts have spinal abnormalities. The movements most likely to result in low back injury are chronic repetitive **flexion, extension,** and rotation (Hall 1986). These stresses have been shown to cause spondylolysis, **spondylolisthesis,** posterior element overuse syndrome, atypical Scheuermann's disease, and discogenic low back pain (Zetaruk 2000).

Hockey

In the United States, "hockey" means the winter sport of ice hockey and also the sport of field hockey, usually played in the spring or fall. Both men and women play both sports, but up to now most data have been collected on women in field hockey and on men in ice hockey. The two sports have similarities but also important differences. Similarities include the striking implement (although the sticks are of different construction and striking-surface shapes), the player positions, the offensive and defensive strategies, and the ultimate goal. The major difference is obvious: the playing surface. With the difference in the playing surface comes the difference in velocity of the players.

Ice hockey is often associated with considerable body contact (between opponents and against the boards), while field hockey rules prohibit personal contact. These differences are reflected in the injury rates for the two sports (figure 2.10). The high speed of the game of ice hockey warrants the use of protective equipment for the players, while slower-paced field hockey utilizes protective padding for the goalie and shin guards for others on the team.

Recently field hockey injury statistics have been more available than data on ice hockey due to an increased data collection effort by the NCAA. Although the injury data are fewer, ice hockey is likely to be considered more popular, especially given that in Canada it is considered the national sport. The data on injuries are sparse for several reasons (Caine, Caine, and Linder 1996):

- A lack of compliance by recorders (i.e., trainers, coaches, physiotherapists, and physicians) in reporting ice hockey injuries to a national, standardized reporting system.

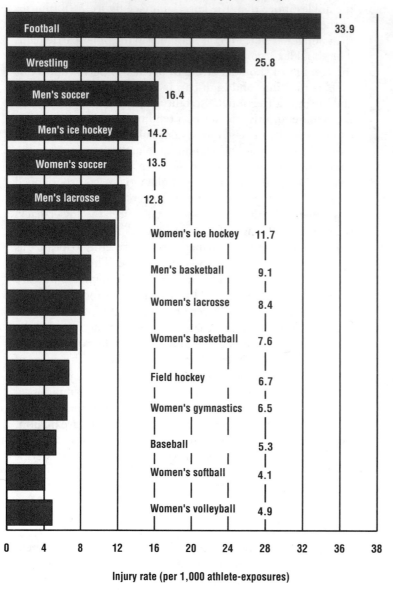

Game Injury Rate Summary (All Sports)

Sport	Injury rate
Football	33.9
Wrestling	25.8
Men's soccer	16.4
Men's ice hockey	14.2
Women's soccer	13.5
Men's lacrosse	12.8
Women's ice hockey	11.7
Men's basketball	9.1
Women's lacrosse	8.4
Women's basketball	7.6
Field hockey	6.7
Women's gymnastics	6.5
Baseball	5.3
Women's softball	4.1
Women's volleyball	4.9

Injury rate (per 1,000 athlete-exposures)

Figure 2.10 The average game injury rate (expressed as injuries per 1,000 athlete-exposures) for all sports analyzed in the ISS in the 2002-03 season. Reprinted with permission from the NCAA.

- A lack of compliance in reporting injury prevalence and incidence; that is, lack of standardization (e.g., use of number of injuries per 1,000 hours of athlete exposure).
- Differences in rules and differing policies with regard to rule enforcement, both within and between different levels of participation.
- Changes in specific rules governing the mandatory use of protective equipment and styles of play over the past two decades.
- Inadequate descriptions of the sample at risk. Most ice hockey injury studies have been reviews of specific injury reports accumulated over a single season. The risk of incurring an ice hockey injury may be inflated artificially.
- Inconsistent definitions used to identify an ice hockey injury.

Because of the difficulties inherent in injury reporting in ice hockey, valid epidemiological data are less available. The kinds of injuries, however, have been identified as contusions, sprains, lacerations, and strains (see figure 2.11). Depending on the study one reads, concussions and fractures appear to be quite common in the sport. One study of junior elite hockey players, conducted over a three-year period, identified strains, lacerations, contusions, and sprains as the most common. This study indicated that the face and shoulder were most often involved, that facial laceration was the most common injury, and that acromioclavicular sprain was the second most common injury (Stuart and Smith 1995).

Much attention in the ice hockey literature has focused on injury to the head and face, the area proposed as the one most frequently injured in ice hockey. The injuries to this area include ocular (eye), dental, facial, scalp, and actual head (concussion) injuries. Differences in the frequency of each type of injury from one study to another may be due in part to the protective headgear and "high sticking" rules enforced within the league of play.

Ice hockey, like football, is not free of catastrophe. Paralysis from **spinal cord lesion** and death from injury to the spinal cord, head, or both have been reported. Hopefully the frequency of these injuries is steadily decreasing as has been the case for football.

Somewhat surprisingly, epidemiological studies focusing on women in ice hockey have surfaced in the literature. These studies, conducted using over 300 recreational players in Canada, showed that the lower extremity was most often injured (31.2%), with more than half of the reported injuries being strains or sprains. As with most sports, more injuries occurred during games than during practices. The reason for the higher incidence of injury during games may be due to the frequency and intensity of practice sessions in the recreational hockey leagues.

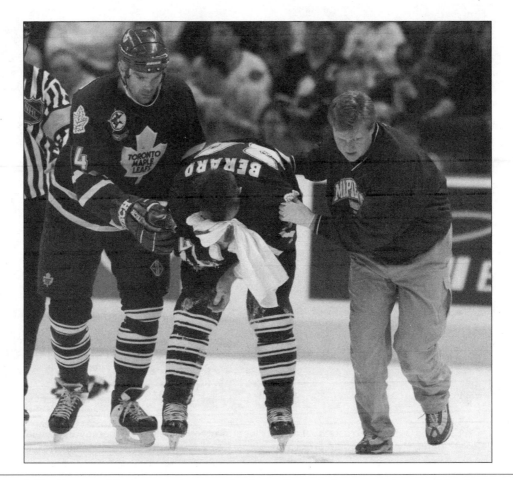

Figure 2.11 Not surprisingly, contusions, sprains, lacerations, strains, concussions, and fractures are quite common in ice hockey.
© Icon SMI

The NCAA has been collecting injury data on women's field hockey (NCAA 2003), surveying over 250 intercollegiate teams over the past two years and 210 to 245 over the previous 14 years. The data indicate that in the 2002-2003 collection year, the most frequent type of injury in practices and games was muscle strain. Sprains were second most common in both settings; tendinitis was the third most common type of injury reported from practice sessions (9% of total), while contusions (15% of total) were more frequent in the game setting. The data over the years from 1997 to 2003 show that the lower extremity was always reported as the most injured anatomical area during practices, while in each of those years injury to the head was predominant in game settings.

Lacrosse

Lacrosse enjoys more popularity in the eastern United States than in the west, yet the sport is certainly gaining popularity throughout this country as has been the case abroad. Because of the infancy of lacrosse on college campuses, few injury data exist. One might assume, on the basis of the characteristics of the sport, that lacrosse players are prone to injuries similar to those affecting the soccer player—with a potential for more frequent injury to the face (because of the height at which the stick is carried and used) and the trunk (because of the rotational stresses placed on the spine during play). Except for the goalie's equipment, the protective equipment for women's lacrosse differs greatly from that for men's: Men wear a helmet as well as protection for the shoulders, chest, and hands, whereas only women goalkeepers wear the helmet (see figure 2.12). This difference points to the importance of looking only at injury data from the same type of team, under similar circumstances of participation. All lacrosse injuries may not be equal.

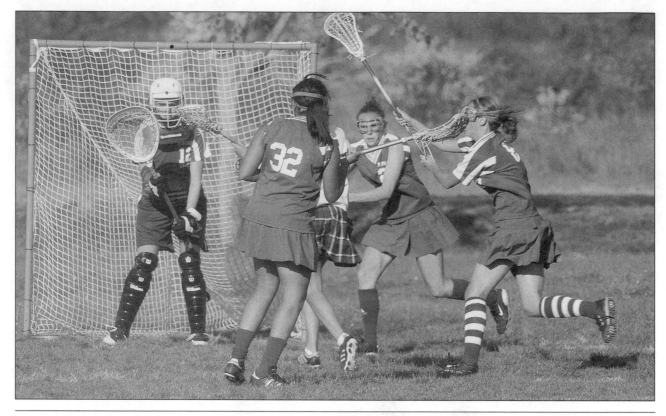

Figure 2.12 Only women lacrosse goalkeepers wear protective helmets, whereas all men lacrosse players wear helmets and also shoulder, chest, and hand protection.

© Dale Garvey

Rugby

Rugby is better supported in other countries (Britain, Australia, New Zealand, and Japan especially) than in the United States. In a report in *Lancet*, Garraway and Macleod (1995) indicate that, except for spinal cord injuries, the frequency and consequences of rugby injuries are not clearly understood (see figure 2.13). To address the issue, these investigators conducted a prospective cohort study involving all the senior rugby clubs in the Scottish Borders. Of the 1,216 eligible players, 1,169 (96%) provided personal details and recorded all 15-a-side matches that they played in the 1993-1994 rugby season. Physiotherapists visited the clubs weekly to check with volunteer linkmen who were appointed to report the circumstances of all new or recurrent injuries occurring in matches or rugby-related training. Results showed that 361 players experienced 584 injuries in 512 injury episodes, 84% of which arose in matches. The period prevalence rate of match injuries was 13.95 (95% confidence interval, 12.64-15.26 per 1,000 playing hours—the equivalent of an injury episode every 1.8 rugby matches). An injury episode took the player away from the game for an average of 39 days; and 28% of injury episodes resulted in absence from employment or school/college work, for an average of 18 days. Rugby injuries, an important source of morbidity in young men, need to be better understood if their frequency and consequences are to be reduced. In this report, the term "morbidity" indicates a loss of time at work or school, rather than a life threatening or life limiting injury. Nonetheless the information appears quite distressing in terms of the epidemiology of rugby injuries here and abroad.

A recent move in the United States toward a rugby union may draw sufficient interest to the sport to result in better rule adherence, stricter referee actions, and strong medical support. Currently, through the work of the American Orthopedic Rugby Football Association (a group of doctors, physical therapists, and other sports medicine professionals), rugby is

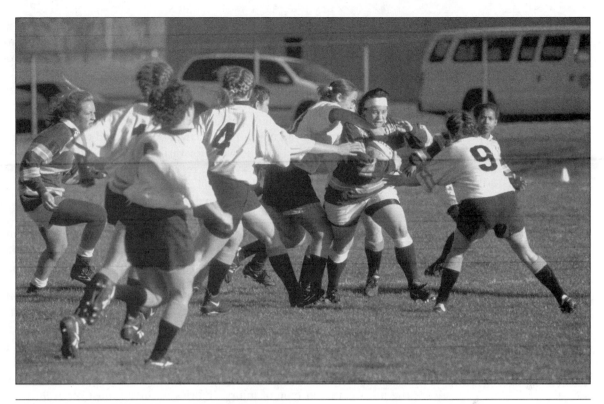

Figure 2.13 Rugby injury rates and patterns are not well understood. Of injuries identified in the literature, head injuries predominate.

obtaining medical expertise to help identify and reduce the injuries associated with rugby football. Members of the association conducted a retrospective study to identify cervical spine injuries between 1970 and 1994. According to the findings, a significantly higher percentage (57.6%) of cervical spine injuries occurred during the scrum phase in U.S. players than in rugby players across the world generally (41%). Interestingly, 48% of those injured in the United States were playing the position of hooker, yet the same position in other nations accounted for only 19% of the reported cases. Also somewhat disconcerting was the relative increase in the frequency of neck injury in the junior-level players (60%) versus the decline seen in the older players (46.4%) in the same time period.

Since 2000, several researchers have focused on the occurrence of injury in various rugby settings. Bathgate et al. (2002) assessed injury patterns and incidence in the Australian Wallabies rugby union players by analyzing data from 1994 to 2000. The results showed that a total of 143 injuries were recorded from 91 matches. The overall injury rate was 69 per 1,000 player hours of game play. However, the injury rates (47/1,000 player hours) before the start of the professional era (1994-1995) were lower than the injury rates (74/1,000 player hours) recorded after the start of the era (1996-2000). Injury rates were also dependent on player position, with the lock position sustaining the highest injury rate among forwards, followed by the number 8 position. The number 10 position was the most injured back, and the least injured position was the halfback. The head was the most commonly injured body site, accounting for 25.1% of total injuries. Of these, 75% were lacerations requiring suturing, 19.4% were concussions, and 5.6% were fractures. The next most injured sites were the knee (14%), thigh (13.6%), and ankle (10.5%). The lower limb was the most commonly injured region (51.7%), followed by head and neck (28.7%) and upper limb (15.4%). Most of these injuries were soft-tissue, closed injuries with joint/ligament sprains/tears being the most common (25.2%). Injuries most often occurred during the tackle phase (either tackling or being tackled). The second half of the game, specifically the third quarter, was when most injuries occurred (40%). This suggests that player fatigue may be a strong influence on injury susceptibility.

Another study was conducted by Gabbett (2000), whose goal was to report the incidence, site, and nature of injuries of 600 players in an amateur rugby league organization over three consecutive seasons. The incidence of injury was 160.6 per 1,000 player-position game hours. The forward position had a significantly higher incidence of injury than backs (182.3/1,000 vs. 142/1,000). The head and neck were the body areas with the greatest injury occurrence, accounting for 40.6 per 1,000 player game hours, while injuries to the face (21.3/1,000), abdomen and thorax (21.3/1,000), and knee (17.8/1,000) were less common. There were no significant differences in the injury rates of the abdomen and thorax, arm and hand, thigh, calf, shoulder, and ankle and foot between forwards and backs. However, forwards sustained more head and neck injuries than backs. In regard to type of injury, muscle hematomas and strains were the most common. The rate of injury in the second half of the game significantly outweighed that of the first half. Additionally, more injuries occurred in the second half of the season than the first.

In another study, Gabbett (2002) investigated the incidence, site, and nature of injuries sustained in amateur rugby league sevens tournaments. Subjects included 168 players competing in three amateur rugby league sevens tournaments, each consisting of several short games (three to four) played on the same day.

The incidence of injury was 283.5 per 1,000 playing hours. Injuries to the lower limb (40%) were more common than injuries to the upper limb (15%). Most injuries occurred at the knee and face (20%), followed by injuries at the ankle and foot and head and neck (15%). Contusions were the most common type of injury, making up 40% of the total. Joint sprains and lacerations followed, making up 30% and 20%, respectively. This differs from the results in the Gabbett (2000) study, which indicated that muscle hematomas and strains were the most common type of injury. Injuries occurred most often during physical collisions and tackles, with no difference noted between being tackled and tackling. An increasing injury incidence was observed over the first (99.2/1,000 hours), second (198.4/1,000 hours), third (347.2/1,000 hours), and fourth (694.4/1,000 hours) games played. In comparison to previously reported injury incidence for conventional amateur rugby league players, amateur rugby league sevens players had a 76.5% higher incidence of injury. This finding, along with the fact that injury increased with the playing of successive matches, suggests that the multi-game nature of amateur rugby league sevens tournaments may increase the players' fatigue and thereby predispose them to injury.

Difficulties in understanding epidemiological data on rugby are related to the number of different types of rugby play. The rugby union, rugby league, and rugby league sevens all pose different risks of injury. Further studies are needed with attention to the type of play to enable full understanding of the sport injury patterns.

Rodeo

Although not widely followed in all areas of the country, rodeo draws participants from all age ranges. With the variety of events, the wide range of ages and abilities, and the variations in individual animals comes the quite variable type of injury experienced by rodeo participants. Serious injury to the head (concussion) or neck (spinal cord injury) certainly occurs, most often when the rider is thrown from the animal (see figure 2.14). Although broken bones, lacerations, and internal organ trauma (punctured lungs, kidney contusion, etc.) occur, overuse injuries are the most common.

Rodeo is a high-injury sport for which there is not much epidemiological information. In addition, data collection in rodeo tends not to be as sophisticated as in other organized sports. The lack of epidemiological data may be due in part to the ability of the participant to "shake off" injuries that would sideline other athletes. If you ever watched a rodeo competition, you may have seen an individual limp to safety after being thrown from his ride. Often participants dismiss knee, leg, and ankle injuries as "just part of the job," and participation continues because the injury does not significantly limit the person's ability to perform. Additionally, the number of people who sustain an injury while practicing for a rodeo event may never be known because the injury is not treated in a hospital or reported to a medical facility.

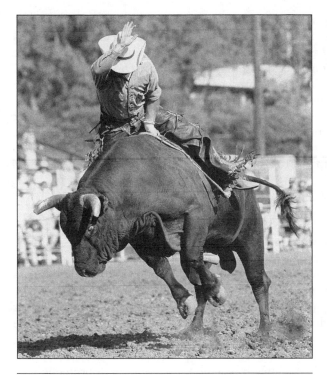

Figure 2.14 In rodeo, concussion and spinal injury occur most often when the rider is thrown from the animal. Broken bones, lacerations, and internal organ trauma (punctured lungs, kidney contusion) also occur.

© Digitalvisiononline.com

In 1996, at the time Caine, Caine, and Linder published their work, only 14 studies involving injuries in rodeo were available. Few comparisons could be drawn between reports because of wide variations in the way in which injuries were tabulated. The rodeo participant, similar to the gymnast, often competes in multiple events within one contest. This creates a difficulty for determining an injury rate. It is wrong in this instance to count the participants on a team and merely say that if x is the number that were injured, the rate of injury is x divided by the number of participants. A more precise way to indicate injury rate would be to report the number of injuries per number of exposures, with participation by one individual in a given event being considered one exposure. Only when rodeo begins to involve health care providers at each contest will injury epidemiological data develop to the point of making a contribution to medical and rodeo literature.

The Justin Boot Company supports the Justin Sportsmedicine Team, a group of athletic trainers, physical therapists, and physicians who cover over 150 sanctioned professional rodeo events throughout the United States. The Justin Sportsmedicine Team operates out of mobile facilities provided by the boot company. These mobile sports medicine centers allow the professionals working with the rodeo participants access to state of the art equipment to help lessen the severity of these athletes' injuries. The Justin Sportsmedicine Team has been collecting injury data since their inception in 1981. Their findings in professional rodeo include the rodeo events in which participants are injured and indicate that bull riding is the event that creates the most injuries by far (over 50% of all reported injuries in all years except two). Bareback riding has consistently been second in the number of injuries, with 23.6%. Next has been saddle bronc riding, which for a five-year span between 1981 and 1985 recorded 18.7% of all injuries but in more recent years (1996-2000) only 13.8% of all injuries.

The site of injury in professional rodeo varies according to event. The Justin data indicate that the major area of injury in calf roping, steer wrestling, and saddle bronc riding, and also among bullfighters/clowns, was the knee. The head and face are the most vulnerable areas for the bull rider, due mostly to the impact with the head or horns of the bull. In bareback riding, the shoulder, elbow, and then the hand are most frequently injured due to the great stress on the control arm. Over all the sports involved, the shoulder was among the top three areas injured.

Skiing

Although not a competitive sport at all levels, skiing poses a great risk to those athletes participating at the college, recreational, Olympic, and professional levels. If one were to use the public media as the source of injury information it might appear that skiing is quite dangerous. But the news media report only on deaths and do not take into consideration the millions of times a skier descends a slope without incident.

In a multiyear report on alpine skiing, a Scottish physician has included detailed information on skiing and snowboarding injuries (www.ski-injury.com/alpine.htm). In this report Dr. Mike Langran remarks on the great decrease in frequency of anterior cruciate ligament

For more information on professional rodeo sports medicine, go to www.msmsinc.com/index.html.

(ACL) injuries since 1970. He suggests that the reduction is due, in part, to improved equipment available, such as improved skis and binding systems. The American College of Sports Medicine (ACSM) reported in 1997 that prior to the changes in equipment, fractures were the most common injury. With the improved designs in equipment, fractures have decreased, but knee ligament injuries have increased in frequency (Ryan and Harvey 1997).

Generally, the more serious injuries occur as a result of collisions. Overall, injuries to the knee are the most frequent problem, followed by sprains of other joints such as the shoulder or thumb. Dislocations hold a high rank in epidemiological studies when one looks at time lost. This should be obvious given the rather lengthy healing and rehabilitation process associated with a dislocation as compared to a sprain or even a fracture.

Soccer

Soccer has grown in popularity in the United States since 1970, yet in Europe the sport has been perhaps the most popular of all team sports. The rise in popularity of the sport, unfortunately, has been paralleled by an increase in injuries.

According to 2002-2003 NCAA injury data, the three most common injury sites for men's soccer players during practice are the upper leg (21%), followed by the ankle at 18% and the knee at 14%; during games, ankle injury is the most frequent (18%), followed by the upper leg at 16% and the knee at 15% of the total injuries reported (see figure 2.15). Injury to the lower extremity is certainly expected in that the sport consists almost exclusively of running and kicking. An interesting factor to note is that many soccer players incur injury to the ankle, yet many do not tolerate the application of tape or bracing for prevention or protection.

The NCAA data indicate that during practice the most common type of injury is strain (36%), followed by sprain (26%) and then contusion (11%); in games, the order changes, with the sprain (31%) being more common than the contusion (25%) and the strain (20%). These data might suggest that the players may become more fatigued during practices, the greater fatigue contributing to the occurrence of muscle injury.

Injuries to the head, spine, and trunk are collectively less frequently observed in soccer. The body-to-body, body-to-ball, and body-to-ground contact is often the cause of these conditions.

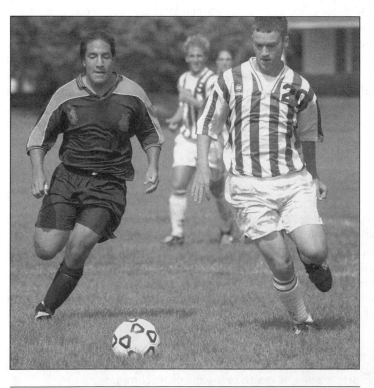

Figure 2.15 Ankle injuries are the most common type of injury for both men and women soccer players, with knee and thigh injuries almost as prevalent.

Injuries to the upper extremities, the feet, and the lower leg are relatively low in occurrence as compared with ankle, knee, and thigh injuries. It may not be surprising that injury rates for the upper extremity as a whole (hands, elbows, shoulders, etc.) account for no more than the total number of injuries just to the lower leg in collegiate male soccer players.

Volleyball

Volleyball, like basketball, has wide popularity and is played by people with a wide range of skill levels. Whether on sand or on a hardwood court, volleyball involves both the upper extremity in hitting and blocking and the lower extremity in the many jumping activities required (see figure 2.16). The range of injuries varies as much as the skill levels of participants. A wide range of organizations participate in volleyball competition, and injury data from some of the less organized teams and clubs are often sparse.

In looking at injury statistics on volleyball at the collegiate level, it is important to realize that there may be differences in injury rates during different times of the year. On the collegiate level, volleyball has developed into a nearly year-round sport. The competitive intercollegiate season is often followed by a somewhat less extensive United States Volleyball

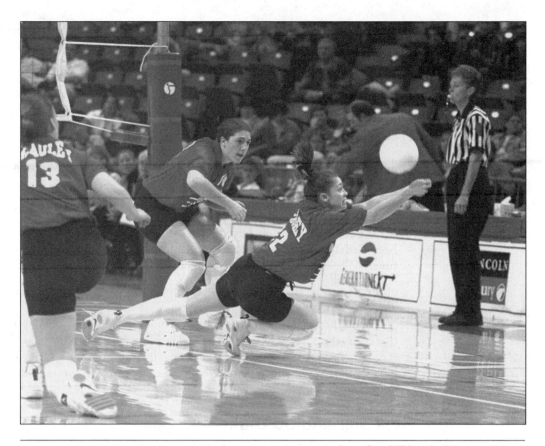

Figure 2.16 In volleyball, the range of injuries varies as much as the skill level of the participants and according to the type of playing surface. Ankle injuries are the most prevalent, followed by finger and hand injuries.

Association season involving players from neighboring colleges as well as some non-university students.

Understanding the seasons of a sport like volleyball allows the athletic trainer to better understand injury patterns. Early-season injury may occur if the athlete is not in optimum physical condition; at the other extreme, late-season injuries and those experienced in the United States Volleyball Association season may be attributable to overuse or fatigue.

The data regarding specific injury rates in volleyball are not as well established as the data on basketball. However, the published data on volleyball injuries show that the more common injuries involve the lower extremity; next most common are upper-extremity injuries and then injuries to the trunk and head (Schafle et al. 1990). Injuries to the ankle are the most common lower-extremity injury in volleyball. These injuries, like jumping injuries in basketball, are often the result of landing off balance or on top of another player's foot. Injuries to the hands and fingers are the next most common and often relate to blocking skills. Injuries involving the knee may be quite prevalent in volleyball owing to the stress of jumping and landing. Injuries to the back and the shoulder joint are fairly common in volleyball and are found much more frequently in the more highly skilled, more explosive players at the college and professional levels (Caine, Caine, and Linder 1996).

Wrestling

The sport of wrestling includes individuals from various ages and skill levels, yet competition is according to weight class. Epidemiological studies vary with respect to the most common injuries, yet most sources agree that shoulder and knee joint sprains are the most frequent problem.

In addition to shoulder and knee joint sprains, reports show that common injuries include chronic bursitis (especially in the anterior knee region), acromioclavicular joint sprain, dermatological conditions (herpes gladiatorum, ringworm, and impetigo), injury to the neck (muscles or brachial plexus), and a condition called "cauliflower ear."

Realize that the professional wrestling often seen on television is not considered in the data on wrestling injuries. Professional wrestling injuries are frequently reported in the media, yet sophisticated studies of injury rates are not well publicized.

OTHER SPORTS

There are several other sports and activities in which an athletic trainer may be involved. Here you'll find information on handball, baseball, softball, track and field, tennis, golf, swimming, in-line skating, and equestrian sports.

Team Handball

Team handball, also known as speedball, combines skills of running, jumping, and throwing on a hardwood court. This sport, although competitive on the Olympic level, is rarely offered as an interscholastic or recreational sport in the United States, making injury data nearly nonexistent.

Throughout Europe, team handball enjoys both recreational and competitive classifications at various age levels, as evidenced in Norway, where team handball includes some 450 senior and approximately 35 junior teams. In studies of those teams, researchers found that injuries in team handball included injury to the elbow (especially in the goalkeeper), ankle, knee, and shoulders.

Baseball and Softball

Baseball and softball are much more similar to each other than the two hockey sports are. Although men and women play both sports, baseball is commonly associated with the male participant; and at the high school and college levels, softball is associated with the female athlete. Both sports enjoy a wide following of athletes; adolescent, high school, and college athletes may all participate. Adults typically play baseball at the amateur-league, semiprofessional, and professional levels, while the adult who plays softball is usually doing so recreationally. There are exceptions to all these statements, though. Women are quite competitive in baseball as well as in softball, and men are certainly highly talented in both fast- and slow-pitch softball leagues throughout the United States and abroad.

Baseball is considered a faster sport in that the velocity of the projectile is greater for the smaller, denser baseball than for the larger, less dense softball. One might assume that the speed of the pitch is far greater in baseball, yet some high-level softball pitchers have recorded speeds of over 60 mph (96.6 km/hr)—certainly not a slow pitch.

Injury rates for these two sports are usually recorded separately, yet it is interesting to note the similarity in the rates of injury reported in two unrelated NCAA studies. A four-year study of baseball showed an injury rate of 2.86 injuries per 1,000 athlete exposures, while a six-year study of softball yielded an injury rate of 2.57 per 1,000 athlete exposures. This remarkable similarity shows that both sports have fairly low rates of injury.

The type of injury most often incurred in either baseball or softball is the abrasion (see figure 2.17). In base running, the player often uses a sliding technique to avoid being called out and frequently ends up with a skin abrasion. In most areas, softball players wear longer pants to protect the legs from abrasions, yet some teams continue to use the less protective shorts as the typical uniform. However, abrasions can occur even through the uniform.

Trauma to the musculoskeletal system typically results in sprains, strains, and sometimes fractures. The upper extremity is almost as likely to be involved as the lower extremity, depending to some extent on the level or type of participation. Upper-extremity injuries most often involve the shoulder and sometimes the elbow joint, especially in pitchers. Repetitive throwing predisposes the athlete to overuse trauma unless the mechanics of the throw are ideal. Younger athletes with poorly developed musculature may incur these overuse injuries more quickly than the stronger, more coordinated adult athlete.

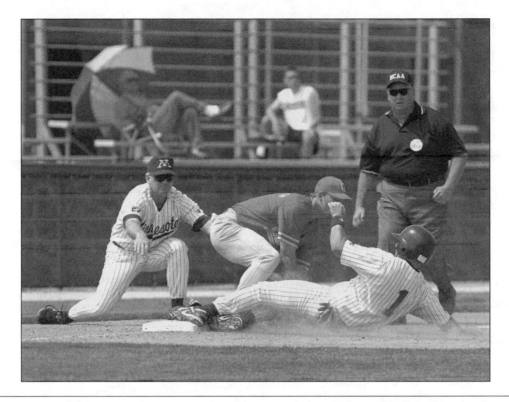

Figure 2.17 Sliding causes the most common injury seen in baseball or softball—a skin abrasion.

In the lower extremity, base running creates a hazard in that stepping on the base or on an opponent's foot may cause ankle or knee sprains. Fielding, especially from the outfield, has the potential of causing hamstring muscle strain because of the sudden burst of speed required to get into position to catch a fly ball, or because of the running and sudden bending required to pick up a fast-moving, bouncing hit.

Baseball and softball, more than most other sports, pose additional risks for position-specific players. The pitcher is prone to overuse injury to the shoulder and elbow, while the catcher in the deep squat may experience knee joint irritation and often elbow strain from throwing in the crouched position.

Track and Field

Throwing events in track include those in which a heavily weighted or difficult-to-throw object is projected primarily through use of the momentum of the body rather than merely through the strength of the arm. Shot put, discus, and hammer are all quite similar in terms of the injuries produced. Generally, the knees and lumbar spine receive most of the stress. The javelin, a much lighter (yet difficult) object to throw, poses much different trauma; the elbow and shoulder are much more frequently affected than with the heavy projectiles.

Body-projectile events in track and field include running and jumping. The predominant injury in both types of activities involves conditions of the leg, ankle, foot, and knee. Stresses from repetitive trauma may be absorbed in any of the structures of the lower extremity. Typically, repetitive-stress syndromes affect areas that have less-than-perfect biomechanics.

The shock absorption that should occur in the feet, ankles, and knees may be poor in one joint, resulting in transmission of the trauma to another area. With the number of foot strikes occurring in a running sport, these forces magnify greatly, and breakdowns occur in the supporting musculoskeletal structures.

Jumping activities, because of the takeoff, flight, and subsequent landing, pose the added risk of joint injuries in the lower extremities and spine (see figure 2.18). Pole vaulters and high jumpers tend to have a higher risk of spinal injuries than horizontal jumpers compet-

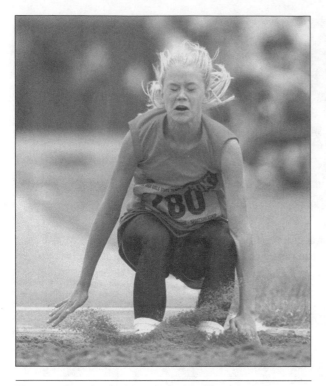

Figure 2.18 Shock absorption should occur in the feet, ankles, and knees but often may be poor in one joint; therefore the trauma is transmitted to the lower extremities and spine.

ing in the long and the triple jump. All jumpers have a high risk of bone and joint pathology at the ankle and knee and of musculotendinous trauma at the knee (patellar tendinitis) and ankle (Achilles tendinitis).

Tennis

Because of the wide popularity of tennis, injury data are difficult to track accurately. Players in private clubs, recreational leagues, and even neighborhood groups may experience injury that goes unrecorded and therefore cannot be included in examination of the risks of participation.

One injury often associated with tennis is "tennis elbow," a strain or inflammation of the muscles attaching to the lateral epicondyle of the humerus. This injury is probably by far the most common one in tennis players and usually relates to backhand skill (see figure 2.19). The wrist extensors, attaching to the lateral **humeral epicondyle,** must accept the stress of contacting the ball. This deceleration mechanism is often the cause of muscle injury at the point of attachment to the lateral epicondyle of the humerus.

Other common injuries in tennis involve the shoulder joint as the player serves, volleys, or overhead smashes the ball. Ankle injury, and the less common knee injury, are also potential risks of a high-speed sport in which the player must engage in considerable lateral movement and changes of direction in order to get into position to return the ball from all parts of the court.

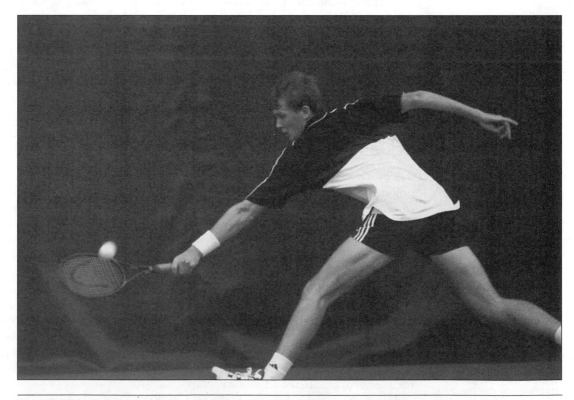

Figure 2.19 A strain or inflammation of the muscles attached to the lateral epicondyle of the humerus is common in tennis players and usually results from the backhand stroke.

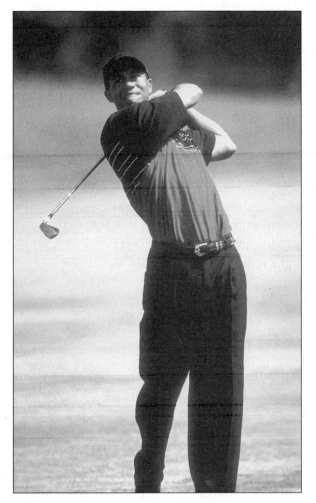

Figure 2.20 Golfers are not immune to injuries. Elbow injuries are common.

Golf

Although it is a projectile sport, golf utilizes the spine more than the upper extremities. The most common injury in the golfer is lumbar spine injury. The pivoting movement around the hips and spine absorbs the force of the golf swing and contributes to injury through repetitive trauma (see figure 2.20).

In a retrospective study, Parziale (2002) conducted an epidemiologic study on 145 golfers who were treated in his program between 1994 and 1997. The majority of subjects were amateur ($n = 138$), male golfers ($n = 116$), with age ranging from 14 to 80 years (mean, 55.7). Low back injuries were the most common diagnosis ($n = 65$), followed by injuries to the shoulder ($n = 20$), elbow ($n = 15$), neck pain ($n = 14$), knee ($n = 12$), and cerebral vascular accident (CVA) or stroke ($n = 11$). This study included such a wide range of ages and skill levels that the data are quite general.

Elbow injuries are not uncommon in golf, especially in less highly skilled players. This injury typically occurs when the golfer contacts the ball "fat," or too close to the ground. The sudden resistance from the solid earth exerts an extremely high load on the swinging extremity, usually the elbow. This injury is typically not an acute, one-time injury, but usually the result of one sudden mis-hit followed by several other impacts of less intensity.

Swimming

The most common problem seen in competitive swimmers involves the shoulder joint (see figure 2.21). Often the trauma is created, or **exacerbated,** by the use of hand paddles in "pulling" workouts. The athlete with ligamentous laxity in the shoulder may experience much more difficulty resulting from the shoulder

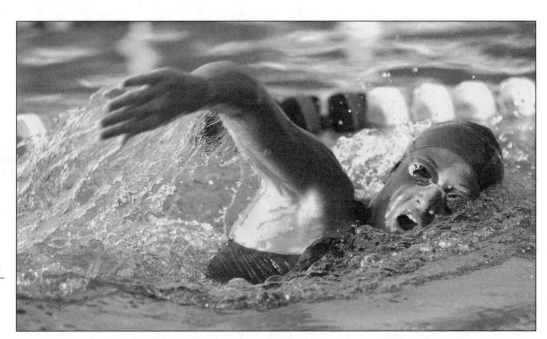

Figure 2.21 Shoulder injuries are the most common type of injury found in swimmers.

activity than other swimmers. Specific exercises and restriction in the use of hand paddles are often necessary.

In addition to overuse injuries to the shoulders, swimming-related injuries or conditions are seen in the muscles of the upper back and neck predominantly. Non-musculoskeletal problems, including conditions of the ear and upper respiratory or **cardiovascular** system, may be related to exercise in the aquatic medium.

In-Line Skating

The sport and recreational activity of in-line skating grew dramatically during the 1990s, and with its rise in popularity came an increased interest in the injuries that occur during participation.

The major injury data on in-line skating have been compiled through the emergency rooms of hospitals. The major sites of injuries treated in emergency rooms include wrist, elbow, face, and ankle; there are also infrequent reports of injuries to the shoulder, head, knee, and trunk. The types of injury encountered in this activity include fractures, dislocations, strains, and of course, skin abrasions.

Equestrian Sports

It is estimated that in athletes under the age of 25, approximately 2,500 equestrian-related injuries require hospital treatment each year in the United States. Although the number of injuries is significant, little research has been conducted in the epidemiology of equestrian sports. In a survey of riders, Christey et al. (1994) found an injury rate of 0.6 per 1,000 riding hours. This survey also showed that sprains or strains were the most common type of injury (41.8%), while lacerations or bruises were almost as frequent (40.0%) and fractures or dislocations (33.3%) were also quite common. Perhaps the most interesting findings from this study were that being female adds an additional risk of injury (odds ratio = 1.81) and that riding English style adds yet more risk of injury (odds ratio = 1.77). Not so surprising is that riders reporting more hours of riding per month also reported more injuries.

When considering equestrian injury, one most likely thinks of injury to the head or neck due to being thrown from the horse. Although the most serious, injuries to the head and neck are not the most common anatomical locations of injury. Given the need for upper body strength in controlling the animal, it is perhaps obvious why injury to the upper limbs is most common.

1996 In-Line Skating Injuries—All Age Groups

Most Frequent Sites of Injury
- Wrist: 24.2% of total injuries
- Forearm: 13.5% of total injuries

Most Frequent Injuries
- Fracture: 40.8% of total injuries
- Strain, sprain: 21.5% of total injuries

Most Frequent Injuries by Type and Site
- Fracture of wrist: 14.4% of total injuries
- Fracture of lower arm: 11.0% of total injuries
- Strain/Sprain of wrist: 8.1% of total injuries

Total injuries in 1996: 102,911.

Reprinted with permission from International Inline Skating Association 1999.

INTRINSIC RISK FACTORS

Just as there are risk factors for specific sports, there are risk factors intrinsic to the individual; four such factors relate to age (development), gender, psychological state, and medical condition. As an athletic trainer, you will need to understand these intrinsic risk factors so that you can provide proper means of prevention.

First, some medical conditions (and their accompanying risk factors) are associated with normal physical growth and development. Therefore, some people are more prone to injury merely because of their level of skeletal maturity. The young skeleton must have the capacity to grow, and this area of growth in the bones (growth plate) is at a higher risk of injury than others. Secondly, some injuries are gender specific, and others tend to affect one sex more than the other. The female athlete is more prone to difficulties if her body fails to start the menstrual cycle or if the cycle suddenly stops. Thirdly, some individuals cope with psychological issues in such a way that their risk of injury can actually increase. You may have noticed times when stress causes you to become quite clumsy or injury prone. The same issue may play a part in any performance. And finally, many persons with existing medical conditions participate in sport and physical activities. Most of those conditions are recognized during the preparticipation physical exam, and steps can be taken to reduce the risks of participation; but some of the problems remain unknown, putting the participant at further risk.

Realize that although the potential risks of sport participation may appear overwhelming, they are not unlike the risks associated with any normal, active lifestyle. What is important is that, if you realize what the risks of sport participation are, you can take precautions to decrease them. As long as we know that the potential for injury exists, we can take the necessary steps to reduce the chance of occurrence. Prevention of athletic injuries, long one of the chief objectives of the athletic trainer, depends on knowledge of the risk factors.

Risk Factors of Normal Growth

Children are becoming more and more involved in competitive, and even elite, athletics. On the international scene one cannot help noticing the stunning performance of Olympic gymnasts who in some cases are barely in their teens. A visit to a local grade school will yield views of highly competitive preteens on the basketball court. Although many youngsters of the preadolescent (11-15 years) ages are merely "participating" on a sport team, many others are truly competitive.

Children's participation in sport is an unequivocal positive, yet some feel that sport for young children can be taken to an extreme with very negative outcomes. Psychological "stress" notwithstanding, sport participation in the preadolescent is certain to produce injury, yet epidemiological studies must take into account the population at risk. This factor becomes extremely difficult to examine because of the vast number of neighborhood, grade school, and church leagues encouraging youngsters to participate.

With the lack of reliable research on the frequency of injury in youth sports, we must turn attention to small studies of types of injuries seen in the pediatrician's office. The concern over contact sports for this young age group has been widespread. The noncontact sports of swimming and gymnastics require considerable repetitive movement and produce a number of injuries. The contact sport of football, on the other hand (when children are playing against others of the same size), produces relatively few injuries.

In general, as mentioned earlier, one of the greatest fears related to allowing or encouraging athletic participation in the skeletally immature child is the risk to the growth plate (see figure 2.22). Several studies have shown a very low percentage of growth plate injuries due to participation in organized sport, while other studies show a much higher number of injuries occurring on the school playground than in sport activities (Zaricznyi et al. 1980).

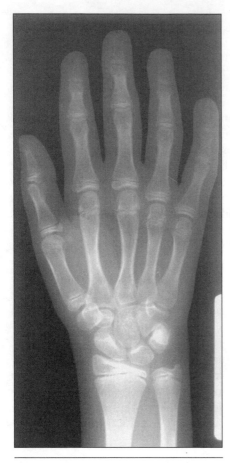

Figure 2.22 A radiograph of a youngster's skeletally immature wrist shows the growth plate.

Courtesy of Arizona School of Health Sciences

Occasionally, orthopedic conditions that affect the preadolescent may be detected early in the child's life and may sometimes preclude athletic participation. These conditions may not surface until after the child begins youth activities. It is important to understand these conditions, perhaps not as much for your ability to recognize or "diagnose" them as to enable you to help the participant and the family understand why competitive participation may not be advisable, and whether and how risks increase as a result of the condition. Such conditions include Legg-Calvé-Perthes disease, osteoid osteoma, and occasionally scoliosis (if severe).

Legg-Calvé-Perthes Disease

Legg-Calvé-Perthes disease is a condition seen in young children, especially boys between the ages of 4 and 12, in which the head of the femur fails to fully form or begins to die. This condition may be secondary to acute or chronic trauma, such as that sustained in sport participation, and is attributed to a decreased blood supply to the bone. The blood supply can become compromised, and over a one- to three-week period the young person perceives hip pain. In approximately 50% of the cases of this condition, surgery is required to repair the femoral head. A young child developing Legg-Calvé-Perthes will have persistent pain in the hip, thigh, and knee and will begin to limp. Such signs would be reason to seek medical attention. If the condition is Legg-Calvé-Perthes, the child's activities must be limited. After the child undergoes surgical repair, however, he or she should be able to participate fully in athletics with no associated risks after the postsurgical healing is complete. Although a participant who has had surgical repair of Legg-Calvé-Perthes should incur no additional risks for injury, he or she should obtain clearance for participation.

Osteoid Osteoma

A bone tumor called **osteoid osteoma** affects the bones of the extremities, most commonly the femur; 90% of the cases occur between 5 and 25 years of age. The condition is a benign bony tumor that resembles sheets of partially calcified bone tissue. The problem is often detected when the patient notices a lump on a bone; but sometimes patients complain of pain at night. Sometimes the bony deposit begins to rub on the overlying muscle, which creates discomfort during or after exercise, and the individual notices the bony lump when rubbing the sore spot. The osteoma must be treated medically prior to continued participation because affected athletes run the risk of associated fracture. After surgical removal of the osteoma and time for healing, participation is permissible and is usually without additional risks. Any bony lump is certainly reason for concern for the participant and the family, and a definitive diagnosis will help greatly in understanding and coping with the problem.

Adolescent Risk Factors

Just as the preadolescent is at risk of orthopedic trauma (see figure 2.23), the adolescent is prone to injury due to the rather common imbalance between muscular strength and bone maturity. It is not uncommon for adolescent athletes to experience a growth spurt of the skeletal system while muscular development and coordination lag behind. This imbalance can lead to bony conditions such as growth plate injury and fractures in the supporting skeletal structure of the spine, called spondylolysis. Although not very common, other skeletal problems seen mainly during the adolescent years are slipped capital femoral **epiphysis** and **osteochondritis dissecans.**

Growth Plate Injury

The concern with growth plate injury is very common in the adolescent athlete, in part because of the increased weight of most adolescent athletes in combination with the still-open growth

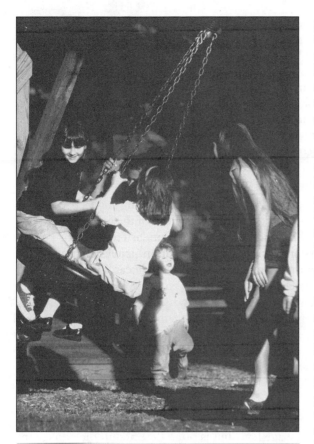

Figure 2.23 A very low percentage of growth plate injuries are due to participation in organized sport. Many more injuries occur on the school playground than in sport activities.

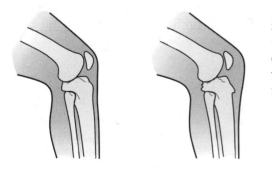

Figure 2.24 Osgood-Schlatter disease.

plate. Since the growth plate—the epiphysis—remains open during the years of bony growth, stress in the area of the open epiphysis can disrupt the fibrous union and alter normal growth of that bone. The epiphysis is easily recognized on radiographs of young athletes; but in addition to the growth plates of long bones, the end plates of the vertebrae are also open and may be at risk in adolescent athletes. Injury to the epiphysis often causes premature closure of the growth plate, leading to a halt in the continued growth of the involved bone while the bone on the uninvolved side continues to develop normally. When this happens in the lower-extremity bones (the tibia or the femur), the result is usually a "leg-length discrepancy." This difference in the lengths of the legs can be significant enough to produce compensatory changes in other joints. A growth plate injury is a very serious condition for the adolescent athlete.

Osgood-Schlatter Disease

Osgood-Schlatter "disease" is actually not a disease but rather a condition in which the point of attachment of the muscles of the front of the thigh, the quadriceps, produces too much force for the bony attachment on the tibia to withstand. When the forces of the muscles are great enough, the bone of the tibia (the tibial tuberosity) can actually be pulled upward and away from the remaining portion of the lower leg bone (the tibia) (see figure 2.24). Usually the individual experiences soreness in the area of the tibial tuberosity, but it usually will not limit performance. If the condition is exacerbated by the person's activity level, the physician may recommend reducing the activities of running and jumping.

Spondylolysis

A condition affecting the spine where a stress fracture first occurs is called spondylolysis. This is a fracture in the area of the **pars interarticularis** (part between the lower and upper articular process on one side of the vertebra) (see figure 2.25). Spondylolysis has been related to early weight bearing during toddlerhood, to athletic participation in sports like football and gymnastics in which lumbar hyperextension is required, and

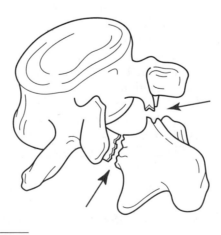
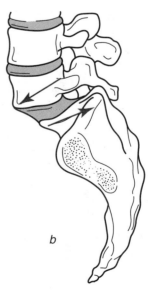

a   *b*

Figure 2.25 *(a)* Spondylolysis showing bilateral fracture of the pars interarticularis (arrows). *(b)* Spondylolisthesis exhibiting slippage (arrows) between the vertebrae.

to an inherent weakness in that particular part of the bone. Regardless of the cause of the fracture, recognition of the condition is necessary to allow an attempt to limit the fracture to one side of the bone and prevent it from becoming bilateral (progressing to spondylolisthesis or forward drift of upper bone on the lower segment).

Fortunately, the adolescent's ligaments are quite strong, and injury to that soft tissue is infrequent. Additionally, the young bone is quite "plastic," and will deform prior to failure and heal very fast if broken. In fact, the adolescent's bone is even capable of correcting poorly aligned fractures, so an injury to the bone may appear quite serious but actually heal quite quickly. There remain, however, a few conditions that adversely affect the adolescent: slipped capital femoral epiphysis, osteochondritis dissecans, and scoliosis. These conditions are not particularly common yet are typically diagnosed in the adolescent patient.

Slipped Capital Femoral Epiphysis

The slipped capital femoral epiphysis (SCFE) is sometimes related to Legg-Calvé-Perthes disease. As the name implies, SCFE is an actual slip or sliding off of the **proximal** growth plate of the femur. This condition is thought to affect young, overweight males but may be found in any body structure and in either gender. In SCFE, the epiphyseal plate weakens during periods of rapid skeletal growth. The stress of the patient's body weight disrupts the attachment of the femoral neck and the femoral epiphysis, with the femoral neck moving upward and forward on the femoral epiphysis. In almost all cases, the slippage must be realigned surgically. Prognosis for sport after successful reduction and fixation of the pseudo-fracture is very good, leaving little risk for further difficulties due to activity level.

Osteochondritis Dissecans

Osteochondritis dissecans is a fracture of the articular surface of the bones. As with the other conditions, osteochondritis may affect any age level but is often detected in the adolescent. The most common sites of osteochondritis are the hip, knee, and elbow joint. The condition presents itself more frequently in the active adolescent; some think that sport activity actually could be the etiology or cause of the problem. Prognosis following osteochondritis is not as good as for some other conditions, merely due to the type of injury. When the articular surface (hyaline cartilage) is injured, healing is limited and the site of injury seldom returns to its preinjury state. Quite often, patients with osteochondritis dissecans require further treatment as the joint surface becomes more significantly involved.

Gender-Specific Concerns

Although most injuries affect men and women relatively equally (given participation at equal skill levels), women are predisposed to additional problems. Female athletes may become amenorrheic (have absence of menstrual periods) because of low body weight, which is frequently the result of intensive training (see figure 2.26). This might seem good to some young women, but along with the amenorrhea comes premature bone loss or osteoporosis. When the calcium of the bone is lost in this premature osteoporosis, the likelihood of fractures increases. In addition to intensive training as a cause of this problem, disordered eating can precipitate the condition. Athletes consciously attempting to maintain a low body weight may develop disordered eating habits like bulimia or anorexia nervosa, which can trigger the onset of amenorrhea. This combination of symptoms (disordered eating, amenorrhea, and loss of bone density with subsequent fractures) is called the "female triad," and affected athletes should receive proper nutritional, psychological, and medical counseling. It is a very serious cascade of events that can easily be prevented.

Psychological Risk Factors and Trauma

Obviously with the number of youngsters participating in sport, there must be a balance between the benefits of participation and the risks of physical and psychological injury. To minimize the chance that the athlete will participate in sport to satisfy a parent, sport for the

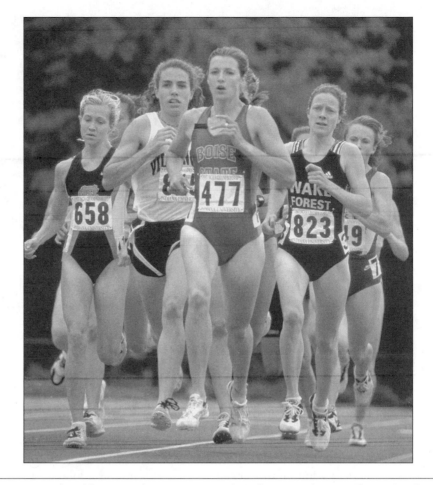

Figure 2.26 Female athletes may become amenorrheic (have an absence of menstrual periods) as a result of having a low body weight. Amenorrhea may then cause premature bone loss and an increased likelihood of fractures.

preadolescent should remain a matter of the child's motivation; the choice of sport and of the intensity with which it is enjoyed should remain in the control of the athlete. Guidance in exercise modification to protect the child from physical injury should be the role of the adult.

The continued debate over psychological trauma to the competitive preadolescent cannot be fully resolved. Simon and Martens (1979) reported a survey on children's anxiety in relation to participation in various activities. Surprisingly, participation on sport teams like football and baseball produced a lower level of anxiety in the children than did taking an academic test. The authors reported that sports with more individual performance requirements produced more anxiety than the academic test, yet still much less anxiety than that associated with the performance of a solo in band. Stress or anxiety concerning sport participation, as measured by the subjects' heart rates, proved to be much lower than many would have predicted.

Researchers have conducted studies to evaluate the correlation between psychological or emotional stress and the frequency of injury. As you would probably guess, the relationship is very strong. Just as students tend to get sick during periods of high stress (perhaps at exam time), the athlete tends to "break down" during periods of high emotional stress (see figure 2.27).

Certainly there is a dichotomy with respect to an athlete's level of arousal, or stress. An individual might be overly concerned and anxious about an upcoming event and perform quite well. On another day, the same performer might be totally relaxed and feeling quite "detached" and run the best race of his or her life. For most competitors, too much anxiety creates fear.

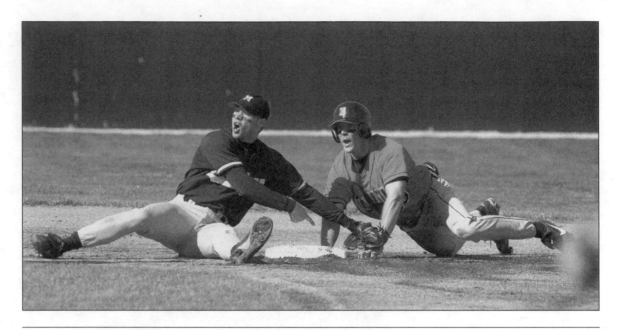

Figure 2.27   Just as students tend to get sick during periods of high stress like exam time, athletes tend to "break down" during periods of high emotional stress.

Fear is a negative emotion that usually interferes with performance. Outside **stressors** may serve to compound the anxiety athletes feel, causing them to focus not on the task at hand but on external problems. A healthy mind helps to build a healthy body. Finding a way to release the external and internal stresses can improve the chances of remaining injury free.

Physical injury has been shown to be the cause of psychological or emotional stress. In addition to fears about what may lie ahead following an injury, athletes may fear the loss of association with team members or the loss of status with the team (e.g., starting position). Whatever reason there might be, the stress is quite real and potentially destructive to the athlete's complete, speedy recovery. The coach, athletic trainer, and athlete must realize this difficulty and, in working with the sport psychologist, formulate a plan to overcome the fears and set logical and attainable goals for recovery and return to the team.

Throughout sport participation, injury management, and rehabilitation, the people involved with the health care of the physically active should be aware of signs of psychological strain. If one observes unusual personality traits, sudden changes in personality, or other causes of concern for psychological health, the athlete should be referred to an appropriate mental health professional for further assessment and care.

Risk Factors Associated With Medical Conditions

Most people take good health for granted; some, however, are challenged by chronic illnesses or other medical conditions that may limit their involvement in physical activity. Individuals usually participate quite well despite their medical conditions. It is important to understand these conditions so that the athlete trainer, the medical staff, and the coach may work together in reducing the risks associated with participation of a person who has such a medical condition.

Scoliosis

Idiopathic scoliosis, or curvature of the spine from unknown causation, affects many more children than any other single condition. **Scoliosis** is defined as a lateral curvature of the spine, although the condition actually is a complex three-dimensional deformity that involves all planes (see figure 2.28). The risk of athletic participation in patients with scoliosis depends on the extent of the spinal curve. With mild or moderate curves, the athlete may have normal

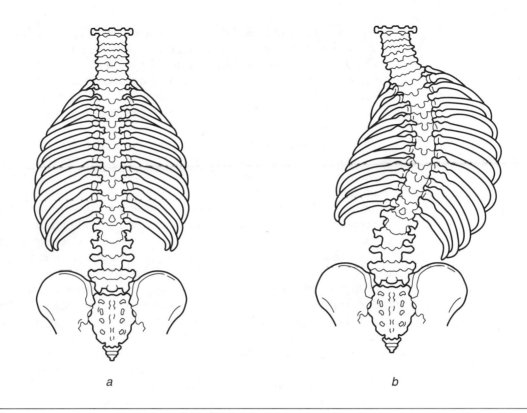

Figure 2.28 *(a)* Normal spine and *(b)* scoliotic spine.

exercise tolerance and no additional risks of participation. Patients with more extreme curves (over 80°) may experience shortness of breath and increased heart rate. This cardiopulmonary difficulty is thought to be a result of the change in interior dimensions of the chest, which in turn is a result of the rotation associated with scoliosis.

The most common risk for the athlete with moderate to severe scoliosis is muscle discomfort that is not proportional to exercise intensity. Obtaining the highest scores in sports such as gymnastics and diving depends on the athlete's erect, elongated posture; and scoliotic athletes in these sports may experience more muscle discomfort than others performing the same exercises. The presence of hip pain associated with scoliosis has also been reported with some level of correlative significance (Saji, Upadhyay, and Leong 1995).

Leg-Length Difference

A small difference in the length of the legs is not uncommon, yet when the difference is severe the patient demonstrates an abnormal gait pattern (a limp). In addition, the athlete with a significant leg-length discrepancy may experience shin, knee, hip, and low back problems because of the uneven weight bearing through the lower extremity.

Most often the athlete with a leg-length difference can be treated with a shoe insert or other elevation of the shoe. Recognizing the difference in leg length is important in understanding risks of lower-extremity injuries associated with conditioning and sport participation, since the most common risk related to leg-length inequality is the development of discomfort and muscle pain around the knee, hip, and back.

Epilepsy

It may not seem surprising that children with epilepsy are unlikely to be involved in sport participation. In a 1996 study designed to assess the social and physical activity of patients with epilepsy, Steinhoff et al. (1996) concluded that persons with epilepsy manifest a considerable lack of physical fitness that might have an important impact on their general health and quality of life.

Epilepsy is a neurological disorder characterized by seizures. It is estimated to affect 1% of the U.S. population, or 3 million people. Absence seizures (**petit mal**) occur primarily in children and are characterized by brief lapses in consciousness during which the person appears to be staring into space. The child does not fall, and recovery is rapid. Convulsive seizures (grand mal) are more severe, lasting from 1 to 7 min and involving loss of consciousness and motor control. The person falls and the body goes rigid, with jerking and twitching of the extremities.

Although the mechanisms of epilepsy are not well understood, the seizures are known to result from the misfiring of neurons in the brain. Instead of transmitting electrical impulses in an orderly manner, epileptic neurons fire all at once, creating a storm that disrupts normal brain function.

In most cases, epilepsy can be controlled by **anticonvulsant** medication. Many patients with epilepsy experience an aura, or a signal that a seizure may occur. Unfortunately, the aura is not always followed immediately by the seizure; the seizure may occur hours later. In any case, most adults with epilepsy are able to control their seizures with medication or are able to predict an occurrence and get into a safe environment.

Athletes with controlled epilepsy should not be restricted from athletic participation. In the event that a seizure does occur with an athlete, someone needs to move objects out of the way of the twitching and jerking movements. If the seizure appears to last for more than about 3 min, or if one seizure appears to be followed by another within a minute or two, medical help should be obtained. If the epilepsy is well understood and controlled, there should be no additional risks for participation in physical activity. Children with known epilepsy should receive medical permission to participate; then close monitoring should be provided and exercise and activity encouraged. It is possible for a seizure to happen at any time during physical activity, just as it may happen at any time during daily activities. Because the most common risks for participants with epilepsy are injury to themselves during the seizure and cessation of breathing or heartbeat, it is important to be able to clear the area around the patient having a seizure, as well as to ensure that all those who are supervising the participant have up-to-date knowledge of emergency airway management and cardiopulmonary resuscitation.

Diabetes

It is well known that patients with diabetes can function very well in athletics if they exercise great care in monitoring their food intake and activity level. Diabetes mellitus is a condition in which the pancreas either stops producing insulin or fails to produce sufficient amounts of the hormone for the body's needs. The lack of insulin causes poor absorption of glucose in the cells (which need glucose for energy) and in the liver (which is the storage site for glucose). The glucose in the body, rather than being absorbed, circulates in the blood.

Depending on age at onset of diabetes, patients may or may not be dependent on insulin. Typically, type I diabetes has its onset in the early years and is thus called juvenile-onset diabetes. Individuals with this condition are typically dependent on insulin because the pancreas production is very low if present at all. In type I diabetes, the body is unable to use glucose because of the lack of insulin and, in an effort to obtain energy for activity, utilizes fat. This can lead to the medical emergency called "diabetic coma."

Type II diabetes typically affects people over the age of 40, and patients usually do not depend on insulin; thus it is termed adult-onset diabetes or insulin-independent diabetes. This type of diabetes, generally related to diet, affects people who overeat. The overeating produces an excess of glucose in the blood, and the pancreas cannot produce as much insulin as is needed. As people age, the function of the pancreas decreases, and this exacerbates adult-onset diabetes.

Methods of testing the blood allow patients with diabetes to control the condition through adjusting insulin doses and carbohydrate intake in accordance with their activity level (see figure 2.29). The risks of diabetes are still present, regardless of advances in technology. The key to reducing the risks of diabetes-related difficulties is a combination of careful monitoring of the diet, exercise, and insulin doses.

The most common risk for the athlete with type I diabetes is hypoglycemia (low blood sugar) during exercise. The athlete must understand the effect of exercise in lowering blood

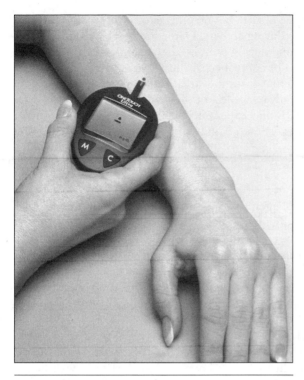

Figure 2.29 People can control diabetes by adjusting insulin doses and glucose intake in sync with their physical activity.

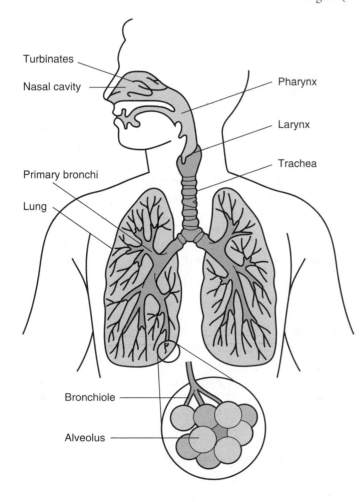

Turbinates

Nasal cavity

Pharynx

Larynx

Trachea

Primary bronchi

Lung

Bronchiole

Alveolus

glucose and must make appropriate adjustments in insulin administration. In the case of hypoglycemia, the patient may not have anticipated the amount of exercise and may have administered too much insulin.

Sport participation for people with diabetes is certainly not contraindicated, yet these athletes must inform the coach and the athletic trainer of the condition so that these personnel are aware of the situation should a problem develop. The athlete must also communicate with the physician regarding the level of activity to be undertaken. Adjustments in insulin dosage will be made and problems prevented. All people with diabetes must also realize that insulin needs will change during periods of illness such as influenza, or when other common health problems occur. Communication with the physician will help the patient to understand the changes in diet and insulin administration that are needed during these periods of stress.

Asthma

Asthma is a chronic respiratory condition that affects the bronchial walls. The athlete with asthma can inhale, but may find it difficult to fully exhale the air. Air becomes trapped in the bronchioles of the lungs, and air exchange is diminished (see figure 2.30); cyanosis (blue coloration of the lips and face) can result from the lack of oxygen in the tissues. In most cases an asthma attack can be stopped by medication. Most asthma is triggered by an allergen (allergy-producing substance), but some asthma is induced by exercise **(exercise-induced asthma).** The greatest risk for participants with asthma is the inability to catch their breath after exertion.

Individuals with asthma who wish to participate in athletics must understand their condition and prevent episodes by using the prescribed medications, usually taken as pills, liquids, or inhalants. If asthma attacks are infrequent, the physician may prescribe a **bronchodilator** to be used once an attack has started. With the proper therapy, the risks of participation to the patient with asthma are quite controllable and should not cause withdrawal from the sport.

Exercise-Induced Bronchoconstriction

People with exercise-induced bronchoconstriction (EIB) have asthma-like symptoms that occur only as a result of exercise. How common EIB is remains unclear, but it appears to affect 15% to 20% of the general population (Voy 1986; O'Donnell and Fling 1993; Rupp, Guill, and Brudno 1992). Studies have indicated that nearly 11% of Olympic-caliber athletes (Voy 1986), 31% of a group of healthy military personnel (O'Donnell and Fling 1993), and 29% of middle school and high school athletes (Rupp, Guill, and Brudno 1992) showed symptoms of EIB.

Figure 2.30 Oxygen exchange happens at the terminal ends of the bronchiole tree of the lung. In asthma, air becomes trapped in the bronchioles of the lungs, and air exchange is diminished.

Several theories exist regarding the cause of EIB, but no one factor is thought to be solely responsible for the constriction of airways during activity. Detection of EIB requires evaluation of the athlete's lung capacity at rest and during exercise to determine the extent of the bronchiole constriction. The condition can be controlled by the use of bronchodilators prior to the onset of exercise. This is quite different from the situation for persons with chronic asthma, who often must take medication daily regardless of their activity level. Just as for the participant who has asthma, those with EIB may experience feelings of shortness of breath or an inability to catch their breath after exertion, yet the symptoms can be well controlled by medication.

Marfan Syndrome

Marfan syndrome is a disorder of the collagen that gives tissues, including blood vessels and heart valves, their strength. Perhaps the first public knowledge that Marfan syndrome could occur in an athlete was in 1986 when Flo Hyman died during a volleyball tournament in Japan. This tall female Olympian collapsed and died at the age of 31 as a result of a ruptured aortic aneurysm. Although Marfan affects all collagen (ligaments, tendons, etc.), the heart structures most prone to being affected are the **aortic** and **mitral valves** and the aorta itself. Individuals with Marfan are characteristically tall and thin, with long fingers and toes.

The greatest risk to the person with Marfan is rupture or dissection (splitting) of the aorta. An athlete with Marfan has a much higher risk of aortic rupture than nonathletic Marfan patients. The reason may be the increased heart rate and power of the heart in a well-conditioned, athletic individual. For this reason it is very important for individuals with Marfan to receive medical permission before engaging in competitive physical activities.

Congenital Heart Abnormalities

Most **congenital** heart abnormalities are discovered well before the child joins an athletic team. **Stenosis** of the aorta or aortic or pulmonary valves, as well as defects in the ventricular or atrial walls, is usually recognized and treated prior to adolescence. Sometimes during the preparticipation physical examination, the physician notes a heart murmur. The sound of the murmur indicates its significance, and murmurs that indicate problems may be evaluated further. Often the murmur detected in a physical exam is insignificant and will require absolutely no extra precautions.

Myocarditis

Myocarditis or inflammation of the heart muscle is a rather rare condition, but it may affect athletes. Some infections or other diseases can damage the heart muscle, with the patient noticing only mild chest pain or shortness of breath and an increased heart rate. In the participating athlete, these symptoms may become more obvious, necessitating rest and treatment. Because the condition makes participants feel tired during exertion, they are at risk of further damage to the heart if forced to continue exertion. Whenever a participant exhibits undue fatigue, it is advisable to monitor the pulse rate and blood pressure.

Cardiomyopathy

Cardiomyopathy, or damage to the heart muscle, may be nutritional or hypertrophic. Nutritional cardiomyopathy usually results from a nutritional deficiency (vitamins and minerals), or from poisoning by dangerous substances or even chronic alcoholism.

Hypertrophic cardiomyopathy occurs in some individuals who are born with defective cells in the walls of the heart. In response to the defect, the heart muscle enlarges (becomes hypertrophic); in very extreme cases, this may actually decrease the amount of blood leaving the heart. Cardiomyopathy may be treated with drugs, but athletes with this condition must be monitored very closely to avoid heart failure. The greatest risk for the person with cardiomyopathy is overexertion, which obviously is common in high-level athletic participation.

Absence of One of a Paired Set of Organs

Although there are no current regulations against participation by people who have only one of the organs of a paired set, it is interesting to consider the physician's view on contact sport participation for an athlete with only one kidney. In a 1995 survey of physicians, 54% of the respondents indicated that they would allow full participation after appropriate counseling (Anderson 1995). When the scenario was changed so that the athlete was the physician's son or daughter, however, only 41% answered in the same way. Although sport participation is not medically prohibited, the risks to the athlete with only one of a paired set of organs must be clearly understood. Unfortunately, most young people have an attitude of invulnerability that clouds evaluation of the situation.

Visual Impairments

Having only one eye that functions relatively normally is similar to the situation of having only one of a paired set of organs. Participation in contact athletics when one eye is visually impaired is not recommended. Although eye protection can be provided, the change in depth perception with monocular vision may pose risks to the athlete and other players. One could certainly find a number of athletes currently participating quite well with a significant visual deficiency in one eye (see figure 2.31). Potential effects of injury to the unaffected eye should be discussed with the athlete and the family; and if the athlete is permitted to play, appropriate eye protection should be required.

Athletes who are visually impaired obviously encounter increased risks of injury. Adapted sports give such athletes opportunity to use their typically well-developed auditory pathways to achieve success in the sport. You may see athletes with visual impairment playing a game like baseball in local parks. You might watch in fear that the athletes will hurt themselves as they run bases after hitting the ball. This risk, however, appears to be minimal because of the lack of muscle guarding associated with anticipated danger. You sometimes hear of a motorist who walked away from a terrible accident because he or she was not aware that a collision was about to happen. This same concept explains why a direct collision between two athletes who are visually impaired allows both to walk away uninjured.

Communicable Disease

Unfortunately, diseases can be transmitted through the air or by bodily contact. Many sport competitions attract spectators whose presence may increase the risk of communicable disease transmission through the air, especially in closed environments. According to Ehresmann et al. (1995), an outbreak of measles that occurred at an International Special Olympics competition was traced to an infected spectator sitting in the stands above the athlete's entrance at opening ceremonies. Sixteen other individuals were infected as a result of that and subsequent exposures during the competition. This case, although unusual, is an example of the potential of transmission of an airborne virus.

Disease transmission due to contact is more common in sport participation because of the frequency of bodily contact among participants, as well as between participants and the equipment. It should be no surprise that the wrestling room is an excellent breeding ground for herpes, ringworm, and impetigo, causing a contact **dermatitis** that is spread from one infected individual to the next vulnerable victim who comes into contact with the same area on the mat. Nor should we be surprised to learn that the camaraderie that teammates display through bodily contact can be a cause of the spread of hepatitis, chicken pox, and other diseases.

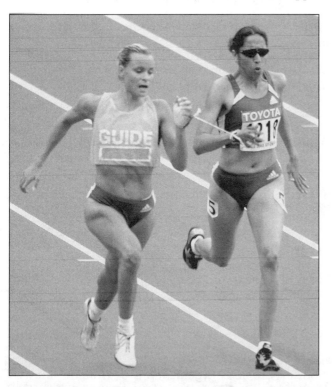

Figure 2.31 Athletes who are visually impaired may need a bit of assistance but do achieve success in their sport.
© Icon SMI

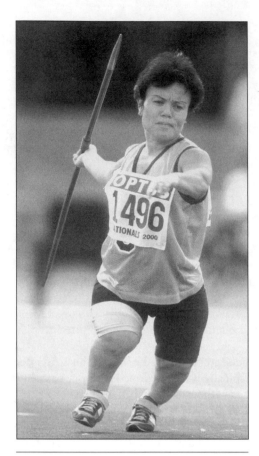

Figure 2.32 For athletes who are disabled, most studies report injury trends similar to those for the general athletic population.

© Sport The Library

Although a risk of contracting communicable diseases comes with sport participation, the risk is no greater than that associated with any other community function such as kindergarten or nursery school. Touch is a form of communication and thus a method of communicating disease as well. Teaching and practicing frequent hand washing may be the most important steps we can take in preventing the transmission of viruses and bacteria.

Special Risks for Athletes With Disabilities

Although it may seem that athletes with disabilities incur risks unlike those for able-bodied athletes, this is not entirely true. According to Harmer (Caine, Caine, and Linder 1996) most studies have reported injury trends among this group that are similar to those for the general athletic population (see figure 2.32). These studies do, however, note various conditions unique to participants in sports for persons who are disabled, including pressure sores, carpal tunnel syndrome, and urinary tract and bladder infections in athletes in wheelchairs. The following surmises are based on the few available studies of the epidemiology of sport participation for athletes who are disabled:

- Skiing is a low-risk undertaking for persons who are disabled, whether they are competing (2 injuries/1,000 skier days) or learning (3.5 injuries/1,000 skier days).
- The risk of injury for competitive athletes of various disability groups is not high (9.45 per 1,000 athlete exposures), but does vary according to sport.
- Special Olympians have an extremely low risk of injury while engaged in competition (0.4 injuries/1,000 hours of exposure).

In looking at injury trends associated with specific disabilities, Harmer (1996) reports that

- a majority of athletes in wheelchairs will sustain one or more injuries in training or competition, with the risk related to the sport undertaken;
- athletes with cerebral palsy seem to have a smaller percentage of injuries than athletes with other disabilities;
- the percentage of Special Olympians (as a group) needing treatment for illness or injury at competitions is lower than that for any other disability group (approximately 10%); and
- a high percentage of soccer players with amputations sustain injuries, but few are even of moderate severity.

Athletes With Spinal Cord Injury

As indicated by Harmer (1996), athletes with spinal cord injury (SCI) have the highest injury rate among those athletes who are disabled. This may be a reflection of the number of SCI

For a plethora of sport training and athletic competition resources for persons with disability, go to www.sportquest.com/resources/disabled.cfm. You'll find links to such organizations as United States Association of Blind Athletes, United States of America Deaf Sports Federation, United States Cerebral Palsy Athletic Association, and Wheelchair Sports, USA.

athletes with highly functional upper extremities. Certainly, depending on the level of the spinal cord lesion, these athletes are capable of varying degrees of upper-body strength. With such abilities, SCI athletes have the opportunity to participate in a number of adapted sports. It is important to understand that athletes with a spinal cord lesion may be unable to cool their bodies through the normal heat-dissipation method of perspiration. Assisting the body's heat-dissipation mechanisms through use of light sprays of water creates cooling effects from evaporation and proves to be quite effective.

Injury to the spinal cord causes loss of motor function as well as loss of sensation below the area of injury. Athletes with impaired sensation to one or more parts of the body may sustain an injury without being aware of it. This is especially important in relation to preventing excessive bleeding following a contusion or other musculoskeletal injury. When a sensory-deprived limb is injured, the medical professional must closely observe the extremity for signs of bleeding, swelling, or deformity. For example, observation following an injury to the lower extremity may aid in preventing compartment syndromes associated with bleeding into a confined area such as the lower leg.

Some of these same patients may have a loss of sensation internally, for example, inside the pelvis or abdomen. It is important for the health care provider to recognize signs of abdominal (peritoneal) irritation. Increase in resting heart rate, change in blood pressure, and changes in the patient's emotional level can all be subtle signs of trouble. When one is working with SCI patients, understanding the warning signs of internal distress is essential in order to avoid a sudden emergency due to neglected conditions like appendicitis.

As Harmer (1996) suggests, injury data for athletes with a disability are severely lacking. More attention to the tracking of injuries per exposure (number of times an individual participates) could shed much more light on this overlooked area. As more and more activities and competitions are introduced for this population, equal attention must be given to medical supervision and injury tracking.

SUMMARY

1. *Define epidemiology and identify various agencies that collect sports epidemiological data.*

   Epidemiology is the study of the frequency with which a specific injury or disease occurs. The various agencies collecting sports epidemiological information include the following:
   - National Athletic Injury Reporting System (NAIRS) collects a wide sampling of injury data on college sports.
   - National Collegiate Athletic Association (NCAA) has an ongoing survey of NCAA institutions covering 16 NCAA sports.
   - National Athletic Trainers' Association (NATA) has conducted a very complete and specific athletic injury study on high school athletics.
   - Accident and Injury Reporting System (AIRS) reports workplace accidents and injuries to the Workers' Compensation Board. This covers professional athletes.
   - The National Youth Sports Safety Foundation, Inc. (NYSSF) provides an educational resource and clearinghouse for information on safe sport participation for parents, coaches, athletes, health professionals, and program administrators for all youth sports.
   - Center for Injury Research and Control (CIRCL), University of Pittsburgh Medical Center, is one of 10 centers in the country to receive official designation as an Injury Control Research Center by the CDC. They gather retrospective data and produce epidemiological information through injury records of individuals experiencing TBI and spinal cord injury.
   - National Electronic Injury Surveillance System (NEISS) tracks injuries resulting from use of consumer products. Injuries are those treated at one of 91 selected hospital emergency rooms.

2. *List the 10 sports that the NATA classifies as high-risk sports and explain why it is important for student athletic trainers to have significant exposure to at least one of those sports.*

   The following are the 10 sports classified as high-risk sports by the NATA:
   - Football
   - Basketball
   - Gymnastics
   - Hockey
   - Lacrosse
   - Rodeo
   - Rugby
   - Soccer
   - Volleyball
   - Wrestling

3. *Identify conditions that are more common in the preadolescent and the adolescent athlete than in other age groups, and then explain any effect those conditions might have on the risks of sport participation.*

   The rapid bone growth that the adolescent experiences makes injuries to bones much more damaging when incurred by the preadolescent or adolescent. When an injury to the bone occurs during the years prior to the end of the growth spurt, irreversible changes can take place that have the potential of lifelong effects. The following injuries and conditions are often seen in this age range and should be well understood to allow early detection and treatment when possible.
   - Legg-Calvé-Perthes disease
   - Osteoid osteoma
   - Growth plate injury
   - Osgood-Schlatter "disease"
   - Slipped capital femoral epiphysis
   - Osteochondritis

4. *Discuss a condition unique to female athletes and explain any effect that condition might have on the risks of sport participation.*

   Female athletes may become amenorrheic (have absence of menstrual period) due to a low body weight, which often is the result of intensive training. Along with the amenorrhea comes premature bone loss or osteoporosis. When the calcium of the bone is lost in premature osteoporosis, there is an increased likelihood of fractures. In addition to intensive training as the cause of this problem, disordered eating can precipitate the condition. Female athletes consciously attempting to maintain a low body weight may develop disordered eating habits like bulimia or anorexia nervosa, which can trigger the onset of amenorrhea.

5. *Support one side of the argument presented in the introduction to the chapter. First suppose that the child, Vincent, is a normal, healthy child; then suppose that Vincent has a heart condition.*

   If Vincent is a normal, healthy child, there are positive social and psychological effects to support participation in sport. However, with participation comes an increased risk of injury. If Vincent has a heart condition, moderate activity may strengthen his heart, and sport participation will have positive social and psychological effects; but the increased demand on his heart may lead to further tissue damage. Also, with participation, Vincent may have an increased risk of injury secondary to cardiac insufficiency.

CRITICAL THINKING QUESTIONS

1. Johnny is playing soccer as a freshman for your high school varsity team. During the second half he is kicked in the shin by a larger opponent who was clearly winding up for a long downfield pass of the ball. The opponent struck Johnny's shin in the distal third of the anterior tibia just below his shin guard. Johnny is unable to continue playing due to the intense pain and immediate swelling in the area of contact.

   a. Please describe what factors you as the certified athletic trainer will take into consideration on initial evaluation of an athlete suffering this type of trauma who clearly has not completed his growth spurt.

   b. What are the associated complications for the athlete who sustains this type of injury?

2. As the high school's certified athletic trainer you notice that one of your female cross country players has lost more weight than commonly occurs over a season. She also appears to be more withdrawn and tired than normal. Her coach comes to you with concerns about what might be going on, as the athlete was overheard mentioning to teammates that she had stopped menstruating. What are your thoughts about what might be occurring? Please describe the pathology as well as its signs, symptoms, and health complications for the athlete. What is your plan of action for dealing with this situation?

3. A school board member comes to you, the certified athletic trainer for your school, questioning you regarding the participation of two of the school's athletes. It was noted on the preparticipation physical exam forms that one of the athlete has diabetes and the other has a history of epileptic seizures. This school board member is concerned as to the legal complications of allowing these students to participate. Please write your response to these concerns. Start by describing the two conditions. Then mention any reasons why or situations in which either of the students should not participate. What are the reasons they should participate? What special accommodations will you, as the certified athletic trainer (ATC), and the athletic department/school have to make if you do recommend that the students be allowed to participate?

4. Describe the goals of the National Athletic Injury Report System (NAIRS), the National Collegiate Athletic Association Injury Surveillance System, and the National Athletic Trainers' Association study. What are the advantages and disadvantages of sport injury surveillance systems in general? Who is primarily relied on for data collection?

5. Based on the injury surveillance studies mentioned in your text, please list and describe the most common injuries associated with each of the following sports:

   - Soccer
   - Gymnastics
   - Football
   - Basketball
   - Baseball

6. The school athletic director comes to you, the certified athletic trainer, questioning the participation of one of the school's athletes. It was noted on the nurse's physical forms that the athlete is on the girls' volleyball team and is known to have sight in only one eye. The athletic director is concerned about the legal complications of allowing this student to participate. Please write a statement of your response to these concerns. Start by describing the complications, if any, of being able to see with only one eye in relation to a sport such as volleyball. Then list any reasons the student should not participate, including any current legal regulations. List any reasons she should be allowed to participate. What special accommodations will you as the ATC make if you

feel the student should participate? Identify any recommendations you might make to the athletic director in regard to your decision to allow the athlete to participate. What are the arguments the student-athlete and parents may present in defense of allowing the athlete to participate?

CITED SOURCES

Anderson, C.R. 1995. Solitary kidney and sports participation. *Arch Fam Med* 4(10): 885-888.

Arendt, E., and R. Dick. 1995. Knee injury patterns among men and women in collegiate basketball and soccer. *Am J Spts Med* 23(6): 694-701.

Bathgate, A., et al. 2002. A prospective study of injuries to elite Australian rugby union players. *Br J Spts Med* 36: 265-269.

Caine, D.J., C.G. Caine, and K.J. Linder, eds. 1996. *Epidemiology of sports injuries.* Champaign, IL: Human Kinetics.

Cantu, R.C., and F.O. Mueller. 2003. Brain injury-related fatalities in American football, 1945-1999. *Neurosurgery* 52: 846-853.

Christey, G.L., D.E. Nelson, et al. 1994. Horseback riding injuries among children and young adults. *J Fam Pract* 39(2): 148-152.

Cohen, R., and J. Metzl. 2000. Sports-specific concerns in the young athlete: Basketball. *Ped Emerg Care* 16(6): 462-486.

DiFiori, J.P., J.C. Puffer, A. Bassil, and F. Dorey. 2002. Wrist pain, distal radial physeal injury, and ulnar variance in young gymnasts: Does a relationship exist? *Am Orthop Soc Spts Med* 30(6): 879-886.

Ehresmann, K.R., C.W. Hedberg, M.B. Grimm, C.A. Norton, K.L. MacDonald, and M.T. Osterholm. 1995. An outbreak of measles at an international sporting event with airborne transmission in a domed stadium. *J Infect Dis* 171(3): 679-683.

Foster-Welch, T. 1996. NATA releases results from high school injury study. *NATA News*, April, 16-23.

Gabbett, T. 2000. Incidence, site, and nature of injuries in amateur rugby league over three consecutive seasons. *Br J Spts Med* 34: 98-103.

Gabbett, T. 2002. Incidence of injury in amateur rugby league sevens. *Br J Spts Med* 36: 23-26.

Garraway, W.M., and D.A.D. Macleod. 1995. Epidemiology of rugby football injuries. *Lancet* 345: 1485-1487.

Hall, S.J. 1986. Mechanical contribution to lumbar stress injuries in females. *Med Sci Spts Exerc* 18(6): 599-602.

Harmer, P. 1996. Disability Sports. In *Epidemiology of sports injuries.* Caine, D.J., C.G. Caine, and K.J. Linder, eds. Champaign, IL: Human Kinetics.

Henry, J.H. 1982. Injury rates in pro basketball. *Am J Spts Med* 1: 16-18.

Hosea, T., C. Carey, and M. Harrer. 2000. The gender issue: Epidemiology of ankle injuries in athletes who participate in basketball. *Clin Orthop* 327: 45-49.

Hutchinson, M.R. 1997. Cheerleading injuries: Patterns, prevention, case reports. *Phys Sptsmed* 25(9): 89-91. www.physsportsmed.com/issues/1997/09sep/hutch.htm (accessed June 15, 2004).

Hutchinson, M.R., and M.L. Ireland. 1995. Knee injuries in female athletes. *Spts Med* 19(4): 287-302.

Moeller, J.L., and M.M. Lamb. 1997. Anterior cruciate ligament injuries in female athletes: Why are women more susceptible? *Phys Sptsmed* 25(4): 41-42. www.physsportsmed.com/issues/1997/04apr/moeller.htm (accessed June 15, 2004).

National Collegiate Athletic Association. 2003 NCAA injury surveillance system. www1.ncaa.org/membership/ed_outreach/health-safety/iss/index.html (accessed June 15, 2004).

O'Donnell, A.E., and J. Fling. 1993. Exercise-induced airflow obstruction in a healthy military population. *Chest* 103(3): 742-744.

Parziale, J.R. 2002. Healthy swing: A golf rehabilitation model. *Am J Phys Med Rehab* 81: 498-501.

Powell, J.W., and K.D. Barber-Foss. 1999. Injury patterns in selected high school sports: A review of the 1995-1997 seasons. *JATA* 34(3): 277-284.

Rupp, N.T., M.F. Guill, and D.S. Brudno. 1992. Unrecognized exercise-induced bronchospasm in adolescent athletes. *Am J Dis Child* 146(8): 941-944.

Ryan, S.W., and J. Harvey. 1997. ACSM current comment: Skiing injuries. www.acsm.org/pdf/skiing.pdf (accessed June 15, 2004).

Saji, M.J., S.S. Upadhyay, and J.C. Leong. 1995. Increased femoral neck-shaft angles in adolescent idiopathic scoliosis. *Spine* 20(3): 303-311.

Schafle, M.D., R.K. Requa, W.L. Patton, et al. 1990. Injuries in the 1987 National Amateur Volleyball Tournament. *Am J Spts Med* 18(6): 624-631.

Simon, J., and R. Martens. 1979. Children's anxiety in sport and nonsport evaluative activities. *J Spts Psych* 1(1): 160-169.

Steinhoff, B.J., K. Neususs, H. Thegeder, and C.D. Reimers. 1996. Leisure time activity and physical fitness in patients with epilepsy. *Epilepsia* 37(12): 1221-1227.

Stuart, M.J., and A. Smith. 1995. Injuries in junior A ice hockey. A three-year prospective study. *Am J Spts Med* 23(4): 458-461.

U.S. Department of Health and Human Services. 2000. *Healthy people 2010.* www.health.gov/Partnerships/Media/hlthcomm.htm (accessed June 15, 2004).

Voy, R.O. 1986. The US Olympic Committee experience with exercise-induced bronchospasm, 1984. *Med Spts Exerc* 18(3): 328-330.

Whiteside, J.A. 1981. Fracture and refracture in intercollegiate athletes: An 11 year experience. *Am J Spts Med* 9(6): 369-377.

Zaricznyi, B., T.A. Shattuck, R.V. Mast, R.V. Robertson, and G. D'Elia. 1980. Sports related injuries in school age children. *Am J Spts Med* 8(5): 318-323.

Zelisko, J.A. 1982. Compilation of men's and women's pro basketball injuries. *Am J Spts Med* 10: 297-299.

Zetaruk, M.N. 2000. The young gymnast. *Ped Adol Spts Inj* 19(4): 757-780.

ADDITIONAL READINGS

Amadio, P.C. 1990. Epidemiology of hand and wrist injuries in sports. *Hand Clin* 6: 370.

Backx, F.J., H.J. Beijer, E. Bol, and W.B. Erich. 1991. Injuries in high-risk persons and high-risk sports. A longitudinal study of 1818 school children. *Am J Spts Med* 2(19): 124-130.

Boyer, J., N. Amin, R. Taddonio, and A.J. Dozor. 1996. Evidence of airway obstruction in children with idiopathic scoliosis. *Chest* 109(6): 1532-1535.

Brkich, M. 1995. Infectious waste disposal plan of the high school athletic trainers. *J Athl Trng* 30(3): 208-209.

Brown, E.W., and C.F. Branta. 1988. *Competitive sports for children and youth: An overview of research and issues.* Champaign, IL: Human Kinetics.

Cahill, B.R. 1997. Current concepts review: Osteochondritis dissecans. *JBSJ* (Am) 79(3): 471-472.

Chandy, T.A. 1985. Secondary school athletic injuries in boys and girls: 3 yr. comparison. *Phys Sptsmed* 13: 106-111.

Cohen, F., and J. Durham. 1993. The challenge of AIDS for health care workers. In *Women, children and HIV/AIDS,* 286-297. New York: Springer.

Connolly, P.J., H.P. Von Shroeder, G.E. Johnson, and J.P. Kostuik. 1995. Adolescent idiopathic scoliosis: Long-term effect of instrumentation extending to the lumbar spine. *JBJS* (Am) 77(8): 1210-1216.

Daniels, N. 1992. HIV infected professions, patient rights and the "switching dilemma." *JAMA* 267(10): 1368-1370.

Dryden, D.M., L.H. Francescutti, B.H. Rowe, J.C. Spence, and D.C. Voaklander. 2000. Epidemiology of women's recreational ice hockey injuries. *Med Sci Spts Exerc* 32(8): 1378-1383.

Dryden, D.M., L.H. Francescutti, B.H. Rowe, J.C. Spence, and D.C. Voaklander. 2000. Personal risk factors associated with injury among female recreational ice hockey players. *J Sci Med Spt* 3(2): 140-149.

DuRant, R.H. 1992. Findings from pre-participation physicals and athletic injuries. *Am J Dis Child* 146(1): 85-91.

Durham, J., and F. Cohen. 1991. *The person with AIDS: Nursing perspectives,* 2nd ed. New York: Springer.

Eiland, G., and D. Ridley. 1996. Dermatological problems in the athlete. *J Orthop Spts Phys Ther* 23(6): 388-402.

Emmerson, R.J. 1993. Basketball knee injury and the ACL. *Clin Spts Med* 12(2): 317-328.

Fredericson, M. 1996. Common injuries in runners: Diagnosis, rehabilitation and prevention. *Spts Med* 21(1): 49-72.

Gersoff, W.K., and W.G. Clancy. 1988. Diagnosis of acute and chronic anterior cruciate ligament tears. *Clin Spts Med* 7(4): 727-738.

Gill, T.J., and L.J. Micheli. 1996. The immature athlete: Common injuries and overuse syndromes of the elbow and wrist. *Clin Spts Med* 15(2): 401-423.

Gray, J. 1985. Survey of injury to the ACL of knee in female basketball players. *Int J Spts Med* 6: 314-316.

Griffin, L.Y. 1992. The female as a sports participant. *J Med Assoc Georgia* 81(6): 285-287.

Hilibrand, A.S., A.G. Urquhart, G.P. Graziano, and R.N. Hensinger. 1995. Acute spondylolytic spondylolisthesis: Risk of progression and neurological complications. *JBJS* (Am) 77(2): 190-196.

Ho, C.P. 1995. Sports and occupational injuries of the elbow: MR imaging findings. *Am J Roentgenol* 164(6): 1465-1471.

Hogue, R.E. 1970. Principles for the prevention of sports injuries in the eight to seventeen year old age group. *Progress Phys Ther* 1(2): 118-123.

Hollister, D., M. Godfrey, L. Sakai, and R. Pyeritz. 1990. Immunohistologic abnormalities of the microfibrillar-fiber system in the Marfan syndrome. *New Eng J Med* 323: 152-159.

Ikata, T., S. Katoh, T. Morita, and M. Murase. 1996. Pathogenesis of sports-related spondylolisthesis in adolescents: Radiographic and magnetic resonance imaging study. *Am J Spts Med* 24(1): 94-98.

Keller, C.S., F.R. Noyes, and C.R. Buncher. 1997. The medical aspects of soccer injury epidemiology. *Am J Spts Med* 15(3): 230-237.

Kirk, A.A. 1979. Dunk lacerations. *JAMA* 242(5): 415.

Korniewicz, D., M. Kirwin, and E. Larson. 1991. Do your gloves fit the task? *Am J Nurs* 91: 38-40.

LaLanne, E. 1986. *Fitness after 50*. Lexington, MA: Stephen Greene Press.

Lee, B., M. Godfrey, E. Vitale, H. Hori, M. Mattei, M. Sarfarazi, P. Tsipouras, F. Ramirez, and P. Hollister. 1991. Linkage of Marfan syndrome and a phenotypically related disorder to two different fibrillin genes. *Nature* 352: 330-334.

Malina, R.M. 1988. *Young athletes: Biological, psychological, and educational perspectives*. Champaign, IL: Human Kinetics.

McClain, L.G. 1989. Sports injuries in a high school. *Pediatrics* 84(3): 446-450.

McDermott, E.P. 1993. Basketball injuries to the foot and ankle. *Clin Spts Med* 12(2): 373-393.

McKusick, V.A. 1991. The defect in Marfan syndrome. *Nature* 352: 279-281.

McNabb, K., and M. Keller. 1991. Nurses' risk taking regarding HIV transmission in the workplace. *West J Nurs Res* 13(6): 732-745.

Meyers, M.C., J.R. Elledge, J.C. Sterling, and H. Tolson. 1990. Injuries in intercollegiate rodeo athletes. *Am J Spts Med* 18(1): 87-91.

Micheli, L.J. 1995. Sports injuries in children and adolescents: Questions and controversies. *Clin Spts Med* 14(3): 727-745.

Micheli, L.J., and R. Wood. 1995. Back pain in young athletes: Significant differences from adults in causes and patterns. *Arch Ped Adol Med* 149(1): 15-18.

Miyake, R., T. Ikata, S. Katoh, and T. Morita. 1996. Morphologic analysis of the facet joint in the immature lumbrosacral spine with special reference to spondylolysis. *Spine* 21(7): 783-789.

Molnar, T.J. 1993. Overuse injuries of the knee in basketball. *Clin Spts Med* 12(2): 349-362.

Montepare, W.J., R.L. Pelletier, and R.M. Stark. 1996. Ice hockey. In *Epidemiology of sports injuries*. Caine, D.J., C.G. Caine, and K.J. Linder, eds. Champaign, IL: Human Kinetics.

Morita, T., T. Ikata, S. Katoh, and R. Miyake. 1995. Lumbar spondylolysis in children and adolescents. *JBJS* (Br) 77(4): 620-625.

Moyer, R.A. 1993. Injuries of the posterior cruciate ligament. *Clin Spts Med* 12(2): 307-315.

Muschik, M., H. Hahnel, P.N. Robinson, C. Perka, and C. Muschik. 1996. Competitive sports and the progression of spondylolisthesis. *J Ped Orthop* 16(3): 364-369.

Nachemson, A.L., and L.E. Peterson. 1995. Effectiveness of treatment with a brace in girls who have adolescent idiopathic scoliosis. *JBJS* (Am) 77(6): 815-822.

National Athletic Trainers' Association. 1995. Blood-borne pathogens: Guidelines for athletic trainers. *J Athl Trng* 30(3): 203-204.

National Intercollegiate Athletic Association. 2003. *Sport specific injury data* [PDF files]. www1.ncaa.org/membership/ed_outreach/health-safety/iss/Reports2002-03 (accessed June 15, 2004).

Newell, R.L. 1995. Spondylolysis: An historical review. *Spine* 20(17): 1950-1956.

Obedian, R.S., and R.P. Grelsamer. 1997. Osteochondritis dissecans of the distal femur and patella. *Clin Spts Med* 16(1): 157-174.

Ohmori, K., Y. Ishida, T. Takatsu, H. Inoue, and K. Suzuki. 1995. Vertebral slip in lumbar spondylolysis and spondylolisthesis: Long-term follow-up of 22 adult patients. *JBJS* (Br) 77(5): 771-773.

Patten, R.M. 1995. Overuse syndromes and injuries involving the elbow: MR imaging findings. *Am J Roentgenol* 164(5): 1205-1211.

Payne, W.K. III, and J.W. Ogilvie. 1996. Back pain in children and adolescents. *Ped Clin North Am* 43(4): 899-917.

Peterson, L.E., and A.L. Nachemson. 1995. Predication of progression of the curve in girls who have adolescent idiopathic scoliosis of moderate severity. *JBJS* (Am) 77(6): 823-827.

Pettrone, F.A., and E. Ricciardelli. 1987. Gymnastic injuries: The Virginia experience. *Am J Spts Med* 15(1): 59-62.

Pyeritz, R.E. 1986. The Marfan syndrome. *Am Fam Physician* 34: 83-94.

Ramirez, N., C.E. Johnston, and R.H. Browne. 1997. The prevalence of back pain in children who have idiopathic scoliosis. *JBJS* (Am) 79(3): 364-368.

Rettig, A.C., R. Ryan, K.D. Shelbourne, R. McCarroll, F. Johnson Jr., and S.K. Ahlfeld. 1989. Metacarpal fractures in the athlete. *Am J Spts Med* 17(4): 567-572.

Robinson, D.M., and M.J. McMaster. 1996. Juvenile idiopathic scoliosis: Curve patterns and prognosis in one hundred and nine patients. *JBJS* (Am) 78(8): 1140-1148.

Rosenberg, M. 1977. *Sixty plus and fit again.* New York: Evans.

Ryan, A.J. 1973. Technological advances in sports medicine and in the reduction of sports injuries. *Exerc Spts Sci Rev* 1: 285-312.

Saal, J.A. 1991. Common American football injuries. *Spts Med* 12(2): 132-147.

Saperstein, A.L., and S.J. Nicholas. 1996. Pediatric and adolescent sports medicine. *Ped Clin North Am* 43(5): 1013-1033.

Schneiderman, G.A., R.F. McLain, M.F. Hambly, and S.L. Nielsen. 1995. The pars defect as a pain source: A histologic study. *Spine* 20(16): 1761-1764.

Sickles, R.T., and J.A. Lombardo. 1993. The adolescent basketball player. *Clin Spts Med* 12(2): 207-219.

Silloway, K.A., R.E. McLaughlin, R.C. Edlich, and R.F. Edlich. 1985. Clavicular fractures and acromioclavicular joint dislocations in lacrosse: Preventable injuries. *J Emerg Med* 3(2): 117-121.

Skaggs, D.L., and G.S. Bassett. 1996. Adolescent idiopathic scoliosis: An update. *Am Fam Physician* 53(7): 2327-2335.

Sponseller, P.D. 1996. Evaluating the child with back pain. *Am Fam Physician* 54(6): 1933-1941.

Stirling, A.J., D. Howel, P.A. Millner, S. Sadiq, D. Sharples, and R.A. Dickson. 1996. Late-onset idiopathic scoliosis in children six to fourteen years old: A cross-sectional prevalence study. *JBJS* (Am) 78(9): 1330-1336.

Thorton, M.L. 1974. Pediatric concerns about competitive preadolescent sports. *JAMA* 227(4): 418-419.

Upadhyay, S.S., A.B. Mullaji, K.D. Luk, and J.C. Leong. 1995. Relation of spinal and thoracic cage deformities and their flexibilities with altered pulmonary functions in adolescent idiopathic scoliosis. *Spine* 20(22): 2415-2420.

White, T.P. 1993. *The wellness guide to lifelong fitness.* New York: Rebus of Random House.

Williamson, L.R., and J.P. Albright. 1996. Bilateral osteochondritis dissecans of the elbow in a female pitcher. *J Fam Pract* 43(5): 489-493.

Wilmore, J.H., and D.L. Costill. 1994. *Physiology of sport and exercise.* Champaign, IL: Human Kinetics.

Wilson, R.L., and L.D. McGinty. 1993. Common hand and wrist injuries in basketball players. *Clin Spts Med* 12(2): 265-291.

Wood, J.B., R.A. Klassen, and H.A. Peterson. 1995. Osteochondritis dissecans of the femoral head in children and adolescents: A report of 17 cases. *J Ped Orthop* 15(3): 313-316.

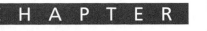

CHAPTER 3

The Preparticipation Physical Examination

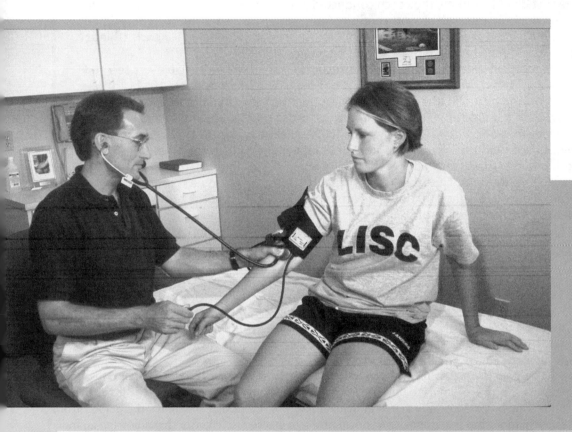

Objectives

After reading this chapter, the student should be able to do the following:

1. Discuss the importance of a preparticipation physical examination for sport team members or for someone beginning a fitness program.

2. Discuss how knowledge of preexisting conditions may help in the medical care of the athlete or physically active individual.

3. Present the two main ways to conduct a physical examination for an athletic team, and list the advantages and disadvantages of each.

4. List the types of examinations to be included in the preparticipation physical examination, and identify the members of the medical team needed to conduct these exams in a group physical.

5. Compare and contrast aspects of the group physical and the individualized examination.

6. Identify problematic areas in conducting a group physical and list ways in which those situations may be managed.

A scholarship student-athlete, Jose, was involved in an auto accident during the summer and incurred a herniated lumbar disc. During the preparticipation physical examination, the physician asked about injuries, but Jose "forgot" to mention the accident and the resulting back problem. He'd been taking it easy since the accident, and his back was good enough to do most normal daily activities.

"Whew, that was lucky," Jose thought silently. "Nobody questioned my back, so I'm not going to say a word about it unless I have to." And as it was, no indication of back problems was observed, and the doctor signed off on Jose's physical.

The next day, the first day of football, the coach conducted "physical testing" to see how well the returning players had done in their off-season conditioning program. The testing included timed shuttle run, vertical jump, bench press, and squat tests. All four tests were scheduled for each athlete, and each athlete had to finish all testing before joining the team on the field.

Jose finished the shuttle run with the same minor difficulties many of the other players seemed to be having. He considered that pretty good, since he'd not been able to work out in the last three weeks. Then he moved to the next test, the vertical jump. During the vertical jump, Jose experienced a "twinge" in the low back but elected to continue in the testing. On the final jump he really had to explode, and he knew at that point that his back wasn't 100% quite yet.

"Remember, guys, Coach won't let you on the field until I give him your scores on *all* the tests," shouted the strength coach as players milled around talking about their summers.

"Almost there . . . ," Jose thought, "just the strength tests, then I'll go get some treatment for my back." Jose's back became increasingly "stiff" until he attempted his final lift in the squat rack, when suddenly he experienced the feeling of his back "going out" and his legs collapsed under him. Not only did Jose not finish the testing; he was unable to practice and ended up missing most of the season.

Whenever one works with a group of physically active individuals, it is wise to know the medical conditions existing prior to the first day of participation. In the scenario just presented, why do you suppose the physician failed to note Jose's back condition? Who is now responsible for Jose's medical treatment? How could you change the preparticipation physical examination to alter the course of events in the case of this scholarship athlete?

The goal in establishing a **preparticipation physical examination (PPE)** policy is to control the risk of injury before it occurs (see figure 3.1). No one wants to learn that an athlete or other physically active individual has a problem that precludes the person from participation. But working with a known problem is ultimately better than allowing an individual to potentially suffer serious injury or permanent impairment because he or she has been allowed to play.

Another consideration in evaluating athletes for participation is the type of sport in which they intend to participate. Needless to say, some conditions may not pose a problem in particular sports but would be a firm contraindication to participation in others. For example, an athlete found to have spinal stenosis, a narrowing of the spinal canal, may be fine for participation in swimming but could be restricted from participation in a contact sport such as football. The American Academy of Pediatrics has published recommendations for the classification of sports in terms of contact to help in the evaluation of an athlete's relative risk of participation. See "Classification of Sports by Contact," which shows the American Academy of Pediatrics summary of contact/collision status of various sports.

THE ESSENTIAL ELEMENTS OF THE PREPARTICIPATION PHYSICAL EXAMINATION

For athletes, the National Collegiate Athletic Association (NCAA) has established guidelines for all member institutions to follow regarding the preparticipation physical examination (PPE). Additionally, many states have established their own policies for providing the high

Classification of Sports by Contact

Contact or Collision

Basketball	Ice hockey[b]	Ski jumping
Boxing[a]	Lacrosse	Soccer
Diving	Martial arts	Team handball
Field hockey	Rodeo	Water polo
Football (tackle)	Rugby	Wrestling

Limited Contact

Baseball	Football (flag)	Snowboarding[e]
Bicycling	Gymnastics	Softball
Cheerleading	Handball	Squash
Canoeing or kayaking (white-water)	Horseback riding	Ultimate Frisbee
Fencing	Racquetball	Volleyball
Field events (high jump, pole vault)	Skating (ice, in-line, roller)	Windsurfing and surfing
Floor hockey	Skiing (cross country, downhill, water)	
	Skateboarding	

Noncontact

Archery	Field events (discus, javelin, shot put)	Sailing
Badminton		Scuba diving
Bodybuilding	Golf	Swimming
Canoeing or kayaking (flat water)	Orienteering[d]	Table tennis
Crew or rowing	Power lifting	Tennis
Curling	Racewalking	Track
Dancing (ballet, modern, jazz)[c]	Riflery	Weightlifting
	Rope jumping	
	Running	

[a] Participation not recommended by the American Academy of Pediatrics.

[b] The American Academy of Pediatrics recommends limiting the amount of body checking allowed for hockey players 15 years and younger to reduce injuries.

[c] Dancing has been further classified into ballet, modern, and jazz since previous statement was published.

[d] A race (contest) in which competitors use a map and compass to find their way through unfamiliar territory.

[e] Snowboarding has been added since previous statement was published.

From American Academy of Pediatrics 2001.

school PPE of student-athletes. These NCAA and state regulations have been written to ensure consistent treatment of athletes from the early years of interscholastic sport to the final years of collegiate participation. Many states require a yearly physical examination for all student-athletes. This means that each student-athlete must undergo a thorough physical exam each school year of participation in sport. The NCAA, as well as some states (Arizona, for example), requires only a "one-time physical examination," meaning that the athlete must have a thorough physical examination prior to the first year of participation at a particular school. During subsequent (sequential) years of participation, the athlete is required to have an abbreviated physical based on interim medical history as supplied by the athlete or the athlete's family (or both) and the team's medical staff.

NCAA medical policies can be found at www.ncaa.org/library/sports_sciences/sports_med_handbook/2003-04/index.html. Choose from the list of Medical Guidelines. Or contact the NCAA for written materials.

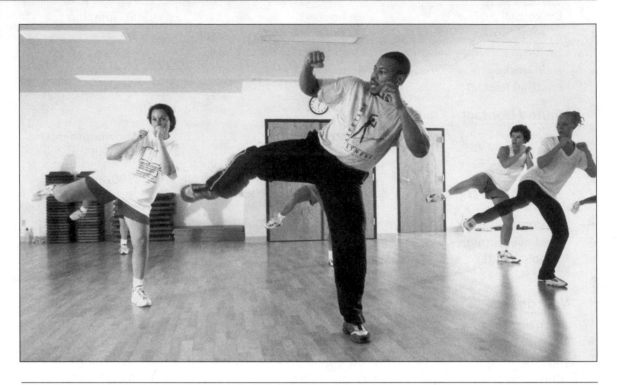

Figure 3.1 Prior to the start of any strenuous physical activity, individuals should undergo a physical examination.

People wishing to participate on teams or in athletic clubs, or in any strenuous physical activity, should undergo a physical examination prior to the start of participation. Those who participate in school sports may be allowed to provide a copy of the signed school physical examination form as evidence of the current health status. For example, the National Youth Sports Program (NYSP) offers structured recreational activities for young people in many metropolitan areas. An individual who plays on the junior high school team and wishes to participate in NYSP may be allowed to bring a copy of the completed junior high sport physical to fulfill the PPE requirement of the youth sport program. What would you suggest if you were in charge of a master's swim team and a 47-year-old swimmer brought a copy of his most recent annual physical provided by his family physician? Would you accept this physical as evidence that there is no reason to restrict this person from strenuous activity? What would you want to be sure was included in this physical examination?

It is important that all individuals participating in organized physical activities undergo an examination to ascertain that they have no additional risks from strenuous exercise. Regardless of the level of participation, able-bodied participants as well as those who are disabled should have their health status checked. This evaluation can vary considerably, but should include several essential components (see table 3.1), each of which we will consider later in this chapter. Before beginning any physical examination, the patient will be required to provide certain types of information for administrative purposes as well as for the physician's review.

NCAA Guidelines 1B: Medical Evaluations, Immunizations, and Records

Preparticipation Medical Evaluation

A preparticipation medical evaluation should be required upon a student-athlete's entrance into the institution's intercollegiate athletics program. This initial evaluation should include a comprehensive health history; an immunization history as defined by current Centers for Disease Control and Prevention guidelines; and a relevant physical exam, part of which should include an orthopedic evaluation. Subsequent to the initial medical evaluation, an updated history should be performed annually. Further PPEs are not believed to be necessary unless warranted by the updated history.

The American Heart Association has modified its 1996 recommendation for a cardiovascular screening every two years for collegiate athletes (American Heart Association 1996). The revision recommends cardiovascular screening as a part of the physical exam required upon a student-athlete's entrance into the intercollegiate athletics program (American Heart Association 1998). In subsequent years, an interim history and blood pressure measurement should be taken. Important changes in medical status or abnormalities may require more formal cardiovascular evaluation.

Medical Records

Student-athletes have a responsibility to report any changes in their health to the team's health care provider. Medical records should be maintained during the student-athlete's collegiate career and should include the following:

1. A record of injuries, illnesses, pregnancies, and operations, whether they occurred during the competitive season or the off-season.
2. Referrals for and feedback from consultation, treatment, or rehabilitation.
3. Subsequent care and clearances.
4. A comprehensive entry-year health status questionnaire and an updated health status questionnaire each year thereafter. The health history should include, at a minimum, questions concerning
   - chronic illness, recent acute illness, previous hospitalization and surgery;
   - allergies, including hypersensitivity to drugs, foods, and insect bites or stings;
   - medicines taken on a regular basis;
   - recent conditioning status;
   - previous and current injuries to the musculoskeletal system;
   - previous concussion or loss of consciousness;
   - syncope or near syncope with exercise;
   - symptoms of exercise-induced **bronchospasm;**
   - loss of paired-organ function (eye, kidney, or testicle);
   - history of a heat-related illness;
   - cardiac symptoms, history of cardiac disease;
   - family history of sudden death in a family member under the age of 50 from nontraumatic causes or from Marfan syndrome;
   - menstrual history; and
   - possible exposure to tuberculosis.
5. Immunizations. It is recommended that student-athletes be immunized for
   - measles, mumps, rubella;
   - hepatitis B; and
   - diphtheria and tetanus (and boosters when appropriate).
6. Written permission, signed by the student-athlete, that authorizes the release of medical information to others. Such permission should specify all persons to whom the student-athlete intends the information to be released. The consent also should specify whether all or only some of the information may be released.

(continued)

Follow-Up or Exit Examination

Pregnant student-athletes or those who have sustained a significant injury or illness during the sport season should be given a follow-up examination to reestablish "playability" before resuming participation in a particular sport. This is especially relevant if the event occurred before the student-athlete left the institution for summer break. Clearance for individuals to return to activity is solely the responsibility of the team physician or that physician's designated representative. An exit evaluation at the conclusion of that student-athlete's participation also is recommended.

Reprinted from NCAA 1999.

Table 3.1
Essential Components of a Preparticipation Physical Examination

Examination classification	Specific examinations used	Purpose of evaluation
Physical measures	Height, weight, body composition	Data collection, baseline for future reference.
Cardiovascular	Blood pressure, heart rate, electro-cardiogram (ECG), exercise ECG	Heart health at rest and with stress, cardiac problems.
Visual screening	Vision test and visual tracking examination	Visual acuity and need for correction.
Blood tests	Complete blood count Hemoglobin/Hematocrit	Acute problems, infections. Look for anemia.
For older athletes (40+)	Lipid profile	Evaluate cholesterol levels.
For black athletes only	Sickle cell	Presence of sickle trait/cell.
Urinalysis (UA)	UA using dipstick Laboratory evaluation of UA	Protein, sugar, or blood in urine. Infections, blood, protein, sugar, or other problems.
Ear, nose, and throat	Clinical evaluation with specialized equipment (otoscope)	Evaluate inner ear, eardrum; nasal septum position, polyps, general health of tonsils.
Heart and lung evaluation	Clinical evaluation	Cardiac and pulmonary health, aortic abnormalities, asthma, etc.
Internal examination	Clinical evaluation	Check for hernia, evaluation of organ systems.
Orthopedic examination	Clinical evaluation	Check bones and joints for laxity or other pathology.
Neurological examination	Clinical evaluation, electroencephalogram	Evaluate nervous system, observe brain waves.
Dental examination	Clinical evaluation	Note dental caries, bridges, other appliances for records.
Flexibility measures	Various tests depending on objective	For research and/or baseline data.

HEALTH STATUS INFORMATION

Entering the individual's personal information into the medical information database is the first step in conducting the PPE. The patient's legal name, date of birth, and some identifying number (social security or other identification number) are essential for the proper recording of medical information and the results from subsequent examinations. Other information collected during this time includes the following:

- Signatures on any legal forms that may be required for participation. If the athlete is not of legal age, the parent or guardian's signature must be obtained, usually prior to or at the physical examination.

- Address and telephone information.

- Emergency contact information: name and phone number of the individual to be notified in the event of an emergency, accident, or other medical need.

- Health insurance information.

- Health status information.

Background information regarding the individual's health status can also be termed the medical history. This health status information is critical to the examining physician's ability to anticipate and understand the need for special examinations and laboratory tests. Medical information can be obtained through simple questionnaires and forms that can be distributed before or at the physical exam and collected at check-in. (For examples of forms, see "Health Status Questionnaire" on pp. 94–96 and "PAR-Q & You" on p. 97.)

Medical experts agree that the medical history is the cornerstone of the examination process, potentially capable of identifying an athlete's medical problems without further physical examination. As the single most important aspect of the examination, the medical history form should be well thought out and reviewed before it is printed for inclusion in the examination process.

The medical history questionnaire is a document of questions to be answered by the individual being tested, or by a parent or legal guardian if the person is under 18 years of age. The questions should draw out information without putting too many words into the person's mouth. Rather than asking, "Have you ever sprained your ankle badly?" ask, "Have you ever had to miss a practice or game due to an ankle injury?"

The medical history form should include questions such as the following:

- Have you been medically advised not to participate in any sport? If so, what was the reason for such advice?

- Have you been hospitalized or under a physician's care in the past 12 months? At any time in your life? If so, what was the reason for such care?

- Have you undergone any surgery? If so, what was the reason for the surgery and the approximate date of operation?

- Have you had any inoculations or childhood diseases? If so, what and approximately when?

- Have you ever experienced convulsions or seizures? If so, what were understood to be the precipitating factors, if any, and when did they occur?

- Is there a history of heart disease or sudden death in any member of the family? If so, in whom and at what age was the diagnosis or the sudden death?

- Have you had frequent shortness of breath, syncope, or heat intolerance? If so, identify symptoms and indicate approximate date of last episode.

- Have you experienced a loss of consciousness? If so, what was the nature of the events preceding the period of unconsciousness and what treatment did you receive, if any?

- Have you had a fracture of any bone or dislocation of any joint? If so, describe the injury.

Health Status Questionnaire

Instructions

Complete each question accurately. All information provided is confidential if you choose to submit this form to your fitness instructor.

Part 1. Information about the individual

1. _____
   Social Security number   Date

2. _____
   Legal name   Nickname

3. _____
   Mailing address   Home phone

   _____
                                                             Business phone

4. EI_____
   Personal physician   Phone

   _____
   Address

5. EI _____
   Person to contact in emergency   Phone

6. Gender (circle one): Female Male (RF)

7. RF Date of birth: _____
                     Month   Day   Year

8. Number of hours worked per week: Less than 20   20-40   41-60   Over 60

9. SLA More than 25% of time spent on job (circle all that apply)

   Sitting at desk   Lifting or carrying loads   Standing   Walking   Driving

Part 2. Medical history

10. RF Circle any who died of heart attack before age 50:

    Father   Mother   Brother   Sister   Grandparent

11. Date of

    Last medical physical exam: _____
                                      Year

    Last physical fitness test: _____
                                      Year

12. Circle operations you have had:

    Back SLA   Heart MC   Kidney SLA   Eyes SLA   Joint SLA   Neck SLA

    Ears SLA   Hernia MC   Lung SLA   Other _____

13. Please circle any of the following for which you have been diagnosed or treated by a physician or health professional:

Alcoholism SEP	Diabetes SEP	Kidney problem MC
Anemia, sickle cell SEP	Emphysema SEP	Mental illness SEP
Anemia, other SEP	Epilepsy SEP	Neck strain SLA
Asthma SEP	Eye problems SLA	Obesity RF
Back strain SLA	Gout SLA	Phlebitis MC
Bleeding trait SEP	Hearing loss SLA	Rheumatoid arthritis SLA
Bronchitis, chronic SEP	Heart problem MC	Stroke MC
Cancer SEP	High blood pressure RF	Thyroid problem SEP
Cirrhosis, liver MC	Hypoglycemia SEP	Ulcer SEP
Concussion MC	Hyperlipidemia RF	Other _____
Congenital defect SEP	Infectious mononucleosis MC	

14. Circle all medicine taken in last 6 months:

Blood thinner MC	Epilepsy medication SEP	Nitroglycerin MC
Diabetic SEP	Heart rhythm medication MC	Other _____
Digitalis MC	High blood pressure medication MC	
Diuretic MC	Insulin MC	

15. Any of these health symptoms that occurs frequently is the basis for medical attention. Circle the number indicating how often you have each of the following:

5 = Very often   4 = Fairly often   3 = Sometimes   2 = Infrequently   1 = Practically never

a. Cough up blood MCg.
   1   2   3   4   5

b. Abdominal pain MC
   1   2   3   4   5

c. Low back pain MC
   1   2   3   4   5

d. Leg pain MC
   1   2   3   4   5

e. Arm or shoulder pain MC
   1   2   3   4   5

f. Chest pain RF MC
   1   2   3   4   5

Swollen joints MC
   1   2   3   4   5

h. Feel faint MC
   1   2   3   4   5

i. Dizziness MC
   1   2   3   4   5

j. Breathless with slight exertion MC
   1   2   3   4   5

k. Palpitation or fast heart beat MC
   1   2   3   4   5

l. Unusual fatigue with normal activity MC
   1   2   3   4   5

Part 3. Health-related behavior

16. RF Do you now smoke?   Yes   No

17. RF If you are a smoker, indicate number smoked per day:

Cigarettes: 40 or more   20-39   10-19   1-9

Cigars or pipes only: 5 or more or any inhaled   Less than 5, none inhaled

(continued)

Health Status Questionnaire (continued)

18. RF Do you exercise regularly?   Yes   No

19. How many days per week do you accumulate 30 minutes of moderate activity?

    0 1 2 3 4 5 6 7   days per week

20. How many days per week do you normally spend at least 20 minutes in vigorous exercise?

    0 1 2 3 4 5 6 7   days per week

21. Can you walk 4 miles briskly without fatigue?   Yes   No

22. Can you jog 3 miles continuously at a moderate pace without discomfort?   Yes   No

23. Weight now: _____ lb   One year ago: _____ lb   Age 21: _____ lb

Part 4. Health-related attitudes

24. RF These are traits that have been associated with coronary-prone behavior. Circle the number that corresponds to how you feel:

6 = Strongly agree	5 = Moderately agree	4 = Slightly agree	3 = Slightly disagree	2 = Moderately disagree	1 = Strongly disagree

I am an impatient, time-conscious, hard-driving individual.

    1 2 3 4 5 6

25. List everything not already included on this questionnaire that might cause you problems in a fitness test or fitness program:

Code for Health Status Questionnaire

The following code will help you evaluate the information in the Health Status Questionnaire.

EI = Emergency Information—must be readily available.

MC = Medical Clearance needed—do not allow exercise without physician's permission.

SEP = Special Emergency Procedures needed—do not let participant exercise alone; make sure the person's exercise partner knows what to do in case of an emergency.

RF = Risk Factor for CHD (educational materials and workshops needed).

SLA = Special or Limited Activities may be needed—you may need to include or exclude specific exercises.

OTHER (not marked) = Personal information that may be helpful for files or research.

Reprinted from Howley and Franks 1997.

Physical Activity Readiness
Questionnaire - PAR-Q
(revised 2002)

PAR-Q & YOU

(A Questionnaire for People Aged 15 to 69)

Regular physical activity is fun and healthy, and increasingly more people are starting to become more active every day. Being more active is very safe for most people. However, some people should check with their doctor before they start becoming much more physically active.

If you are planning to become much more physically active than you are now, start by answering the seven questions in the box below. If you are between the ages of 15 and 69, the PAR-Q will tell you if you should check with your doctor before you start. If you are over 69 years of age, and you are not used to being very active, check with your doctor.

Common sense is your best guide when you answer these questions. Please read the questions carefully and answer each one honestly: check YES or NO.

YES	NO	
❏	❏	**1. Has your doctor ever said that you have a heart condition <u>and</u> that you should only do physical activity recommended by a doctor?**
❏	❏	**2. Do you feel pain in your chest when you do physical activity?**
❏	❏	**3. In the past month, have you had chest pain when you were not doing physical activity?**
❏	❏	**4. Do you lose your balance because of dizziness or do you ever lose consciousness?**
❏	❏	**5. Do you have a bone or joint problem (for example, back, knee or hip) that could be made worse by a change in your physical activity?**
❏	❏	**6. Is your doctor currently prescribing drugs (for example, water pills) for your blood pressure or heart condition?**
❏	❏	**7. Do you know of <u>any other reason</u> why you should not do physical activity?**

If

you

answered

YES to one or more questions

Talk with your doctor by phone or in person BEFORE you start becoming much more physically active or BEFORE you have a fitness appraisal. Tell your doctor about the PAR-Q and which questions you answered YES.

- You may be able to do any activity you want — as long as you start slowly and build up gradually. Or, you may need to restrict your activities to those which are safe for you. Talk with your doctor about the kinds of activities you wish to participate in and follow his/her advice.
- Find out which community programs are safe and helpful for you.

NO to all questions

If you answered NO honestly to <u>all</u> PAR-Q questions, you can be reasonably sure that you can:

- start becoming much more physically active – begin slowly and build up gradually. This is the safest and easiest way to go.
- take part in a fitness appraisal – this is an excellent way to determine your basic fitness so that you can plan the best way for you to live actively. It is also highly recommended that you have your blood pressure evaluated. If your reading is over 144/94, talk with your doctor before you start becoming much more physically active.

DELAY BECOMING MUCH MORE ACTIVE:

- if you are not feeling well because of a temporary illness such as a cold or a fever – wait until you feel better; or
- if you are or may be pregnant – talk to your doctor before you start becoming more active.

PLEASE NOTE: If your health changes so that you then answer YES to any of the above questions, tell your fitness or health professional. Ask whether you should change your physical activity plan.

<u>Informed Use of the PAR-Q:</u> The Canadian Society for Exercise Physiology, Health Canada, and their agents assume no liability for persons who undertake physical activity, and if in doubt after completing this questionnaire, consult your doctor prior to physical activity.

No changes permitted. You are encouraged to photocopy the PAR-Q but only if you use the entire form.

NOTE: If the PAR-Q is being given to a person before he or she participates in a physical activity program or a fitness appraisal, this section may be used for legal or administrative purposes.

"I have read, understood and completed this questionnaire. Any questions I had were answered to my full satisfaction."

NAME _____

SIGNATURE _____ DATE _____

SIGNATURE OF PARENT _____ WITNESS _____
or GUARDIAN (for participants under the age of majority)

Note: This physical activity clearance is valid for a maximum of 12 months from the date it is completed and becomes invalid if your condition changes so that you would answer YES to any of the seven questions.

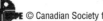 © Canadian Society for Exercise Physiology

Supported by: ■◆■ Health Santé
Canada Canada

- Do you take any medication on a regular basis? If so, what is (are) the name(s) of the medication and what are the reasons for use?
- Do you have allergies such as hives, asthma, or reaction to bee stings? If so, what?
- Have you experienced frequent chest pains or palpitations? If so, what was the approximate date of the last episode and what is the frequency of occurrence?
- Have you had a recent history of fatigue and undue tiredness? If so, when did it begin, or how long have you noticed the symptoms?
- Do you have a history of fainting? If so, under what circumstances?

All information obtained during the medical history must be reviewed during the PPE and thereafter if necessary. Subtle information obtained from the individual on the medical history may be as important as the physical examination findings in the remaining portion of the evaluation.

THE PHYSICAL COMPONENTS OF THE PREPARTICIPATION PHYSICAL EXAMINATION

As indicated in table 3.1, the physical testing of the athlete should include examination of all the major systems of the body—heart and lungs, abdomen, musculoskeletal system, ear/nose/throat, and eyes and vision—as well as physical measurements and laboratory tests.

Height and Weight

Height and weight measurements are a part of every physical examination, regardless of the athletic involvement of the patient. This information on any patient can signal conditions that may otherwise be overlooked. In addition, height and weight information on athletes allows one to notice changes in these statistics that may help in understanding some types of injuries. For example, consider Sara, a junior on the cross country team, who has complaints of pain in her lower back. In looking back at her PPE records, you note that Sara's weight was 23 lb (10.4 kg) less last year. Could this change in physical size play any role in the pain? Without the records, this clue might have been overlooked.

Blood Pressure and Pulse Rate

Elevated blood pressure (hypertension) or increased pulse rate may be a warning of a current medical condition in the athlete. Should the blood pressure reading recorded in the physical examination be elevated from "normal" (120/80 mmHg for teenagers and young adults), changes in weight should be evaluated, as well as the possibility that drugs or other medications are the cause of the hypertension. For the general population of adults, blood pressure below 140/90 mmHg is considered normal, and a pressure above 160/100 mmHg is considered too high. Elevated blood pressure during the physical examination should be reevaluated to ensure that the initial reading was not merely due to the patient's anxiety about the examination. To ensure that the measurement is valid (that it is correct), a series of repeat readings should be taken over the next several days at various hours during the day. To ensure reliability, it is important that the same clinician perform all of the follow-up pressures. After three to five measurements have been collected, the blood pressure is usually quite consistent, and this should be the reading used for evaluation (see table 3.2).

An unexplained elevated blood pressure could signify the use of anabolic steroids, since one of the side effects of steroid use is hypertension. Should the athlete's blood pressure be elevated and remain elevated during repeat measures, further investigation into the cause should include evaluation of changes in the athlete's weight, physical appearance, and performance increases. Usually the suspicion of steroid use is heightened as a combination of signs is observed.

Table 3.2
Blood Pressure Ranges

Category	Systolic (mmHg)		Diastolic (mmHg)	Follow-up recommended
Optimal*	Less than 120	and	Less than 80	Recheck in 2 years
Normal	Less than 130	and	Less than 85	Recheck in 2 years
High normal	130-139	or	85-89	Recheck in 1 year
Hypertension:				
Stage 1 (mild)	140-159	or	90-99	Confirm within 2 months
Stage 2 (moderate)	160-179	or	100-109	Evaluate within 1 month
Stage 3 (severe)	180 or higher	or	110 or higher	Evaluate immediately or within 1 week depending on clinical situation

*Unusually low readings should be evaluated for clinical significance.

Normal Value for Resting Heart Rate

- Newborn infants: 100 to 160 beats per minute
- Children 1 to 10 years: 70 to 120 beats per minute
- Children over 10 and adults: 60 to 100 beats per minute
- Well-trained athletes: 40 to 60 beats per minute

Blood Tests

It is not always necessary to do a blood test; such testing may not provide significant information if the patient is in good health. However, if an individual has been ill, the physician may order this test to help explain unusual symptoms or suspicious information contained in the medical history. It is customary to obtain a routine complete blood count (**CBC**) or **hemoglobin/hematocrit** (Hb/Hct), or both, during the physical examination on individuals new to a program.

Red blood cells (RBCs), called erythrocytes, contain hemoglobin, which is bright red because of the iron it contains. About 60% to 70% of the iron in your body is in the hemoglobin in your blood. The percentage of RBCs in the blood is called the hematocrit. The primary function of the RBCs is to carry oxygen to the cells.

Minimally, each new participant should have an evaluation of Hb/Hct to check for iron-poor blood, or anemia. In addition to evaluating people new to the club or team, it may be desirable to evaluate female and endurance athletes each year because of the prevalence of iron deficiencies in these groups. For example, consider John, a 31-year-old male who had been participating in a local running club for the past several years. In the last two years his interests had changed from the shorter-distance 10K race to the longer marathon and the ultramarathon (100 miles [161 km]). Last year his success at Leadville, an ultramarathon event, had caused John to increase his running in preparation for the upcoming season. During the PPE for the running club, this athlete admitted to the physician that he had had several cases of tendon injuries during the last year, as well as a feeling of fatigue with normal workouts. John had convinced himself that the fatigue was a direct result of the tendon problems.

The physician ordered a CBC with Hb/Hct to fully evaluate the oxygen-carrying capacity of John's blood. The Hb/Hct was slightly below the norm for John's age and gender, and the findings indicated a progressive form of iron deficiency anemia. In questioning John about other aspects of his life that could contribute to the blood-work findings, the physician discovered that John had been a vegetarian for the past two years and had been on nonsteroidal anti-inflammatory drugs (NSAIDs) off and on for the past year and a half. It was finally found that John lacked iron in his body and that this low iron level was the cause of his blood test results. Both the NSAIDs and the vegetarian diet could have contributed to the problem. The physician made several dietary suggestions for John and asked him to schedule a follow-up visit for another blood test in four months (the life span of the RBC is 120 days, so changes would not show up before that time). John left the PPE with mixed emotions; he felt a bit of sadness that he would need to cut back on his ultra-distance training but also relieved to know that something he was doing (and thus something he could change) was what was jeopardizing his health.

Because of the prevalence of sickle cell anemia in the black population, a special test of the blood, the sickle cell test, is important for black individuals (see figure 3.2). The sickle cell is an unusually shaped RBC (erythrocyte) that, if present, may become trapped and unable to exit the capillary wall because of its shape. Athletes with sickle cell anemia or sickle cell trait are at risk of complications during exertion. Close monitoring of athletes with the sickle cell is necessary during participation, and education and counseling play a critical role in helping the person understand the condition.

Urinalysis

During the physical examination, urine may be collected for use in detecting some medical conditions as well as for random drug testing. Athletes must be informed of the reason the **urinalysis** is being done if it is for drug-testing purposes, and in this case legal consent must be obtained; but the routine urinalysis for medical evaluation requires no legal permission. Findings of the urinalysis may indicate urinary tract infection, dehydration, diabetes, or kidney pathology. Urinary tract infection is indicated by an excessive number and by the type of white blood cells in the urine. The urine specific gravity is an indication of the level of hydration and could signal impending difficulties with heat tolerance if the patient is not well hydrated. Diabetes will be suspected if the level of sugars (glucose) in the urine is elevated to between 80 and 120 mg/100 ml. Red blood cells found in the urine may be an indication of kidney disorders and would warrant further testing.

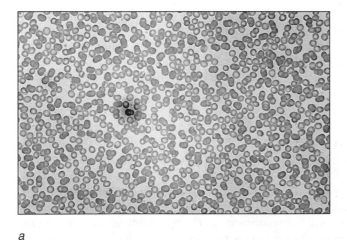

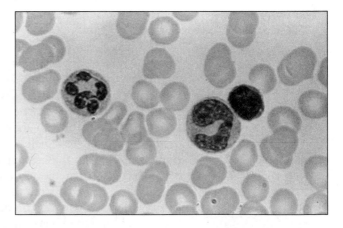

a

b

Figure 3.2   *(a)* Normal red blood cells and *(b)* abnormal sickle cells.

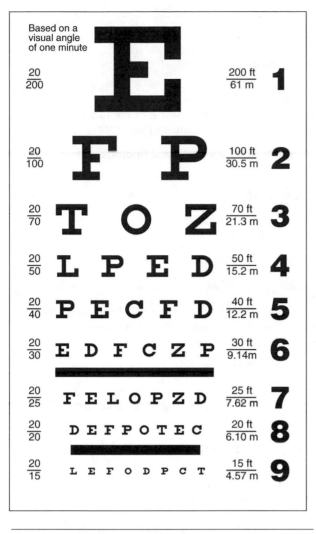

Based on a
visual angle
of one minute

$\frac{20}{200}$	E	$\frac{200\ ft}{61\ m}$ 1
$\frac{20}{100}$	F P	$\frac{100\ ft}{30.5\ m}$ 2
$\frac{20}{70}$	T O Z	$\frac{70\ ft}{21.3\ m}$ 3
$\frac{20}{50}$	L P E D	$\frac{50\ ft}{15.2\ m}$ 4
$\frac{20}{40}$	P E C F D	$\frac{40\ ft}{12.2\ m}$ 5
$\frac{20}{30}$	E D F C Z P	$\frac{30\ ft}{9.14m}$ 6
$\frac{20}{25}$	F E L O P Z D	$\frac{25\ ft}{7.62\ m}$ 7
$\frac{20}{20}$	D E F P O T E C	$\frac{20\ ft}{6.10\ m}$ 8
$\frac{20}{15}$	L E F O D P C T	$\frac{15\ ft}{4.57\ m}$ 9

Figure 3.3   Snellen Eye Chart.

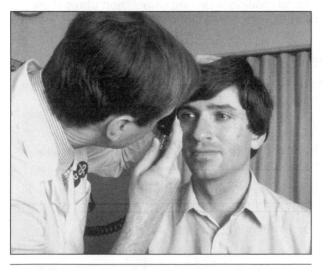

Figure 3.4   The physician performs a general medical examination that includes dental, heart and lung, abdomen and pelvis, ear/nose/throat, and musculoskeletal examinations.

© Bruce Coleman, Inc.

Visual Acuity

Changes in the individual's vision could certainly affect performance. A quick and simple visual acuity test using the Snellen Eye Chart can provide the sports medicine staff with enough information to determine whether further evaluation might be warranted (see figure 3.3). In the evaluation of visual acuity using the Snellen Eye Chart, the patient must read the chart from the chart-specified distance (usually 20 ft [6.1 m]), and the area of the testing should be well lighted.

General Medical Examination

The general medical examination includes dental, heart and lung, abdomen and pelvis, ear/nose/throat (**ENT**), and musculoskeletal examinations. Trained physicians must perform these examinations, and frequently specialists are used in lieu of the general practitioner (see figure 3.4).

The reasons for evaluation of these areas include detection of pathology as well as the establishment of normative data for the athlete. For example, a young athlete with an **undescended testicle** may experience no trouble with the condition yet, but if he were struck in the groin during practice or competition, this otherwise undiscovered finding could be a cause for great concern.

Other Testing

Some of the special evaluations to be conducted include, but are not limited to, the items listed in table 3.3. Any physician can perform testing in any of the evaluation areas if a specialist is not available or willing to serve in that capacity.

Specific Tests for Individuals With Disabilities

When providing PPEs for persons with disabilities, it may be necessary to perform additional medical tests to clarify the existing pathologies involved. Depending on the type of disability, more in-depth clinical evaluation may be necessary. Most importantly, laboratory testing (blood tests and urinalysis) should be delayed until all other aspects of the physical examination have been completed. After the clinical examination is complete, the physician will be more prepared to order the particular special tests that may be needed. In the PPE of a participant who is physically challenged, it is critical to consider the events or activities that the person will be participating in. There is no reason to withhold an athlete with a disability from participation if the sport does not create additional risks.

FITNESS OR PERFORMANCE TESTING

Some teams conduct fitness testing or performance testing as part of the PPE. Other groups use performance testing to serve as a baseline for exercise prescription. It should be an

Table 3.3
Special Evaluations

Specialist and area of examination	Specific target of examination
Optometrist or ophthalmologist	
Examination of the eyes	Evaluate visual acuity, use of eyeglasses or contact lenses; examine the sclerae for the presence of jaundice.
Examination of the optic disc and retina if examination environment allows	Look for the presence of any abnormal findings.
Ear, nose, and throat specialist	
Examination of the ears	Determine the presence of acute or chronic infection, perforation of the eardrum, and gross hearing loss.
Examination of the nose	Assess the presence of deformity that may affect endurance.
Orthopedic surgeon	
Examination of the skin	Determine the presence of infection; scars of previous surgery or trauma; jaundice; and purpura (to be performed by all examiners).
Assessment of the neck	Determine range of motion and the presence of pain associated with such motion.
Assessment of the back	Determine range of motion and abnormal curvature of the spine.
Examination of the extremities	Determine abnormal mobility or immobility, deformity, instability, muscle weakness or atrophy, surgical scars, and varicosities.
Neurological examination	Assess balance and coordination and presence of abnormal reflexes.
Cardiac specialist or general/family practitioner	
Examination of chest contour	Pay attention to conditions causing constriction of the chest such as scoliosis.
Auscultation and percussion of the lungs	Listen for signs of airway obstruction, wheezing, or abnormal congestion.
Assessment of the heart	Pay attention to the presence of murmurs, noting rhythm and rate before and after exercise.
General surgeon or general/family practitioner	
Assessment of the abdomen	Look for possible presence of hepatomegaly, splenomegaly, or abnormal masses.
Examination of the testes	Determine the presence and descent of both testes, abnormal masses or configurations, or hernia.
Assessment of physiological maturation	Determine normal growth and development.

For an example of an orthopedic screening tool from the American Academy of Family Physicians, go to www.aafp.org/afp/20000501/2696.html.

individual organizer's decision what performance tests, if any, to include in the physical exam, yet special attention should be given to older athletes. The American College of Sports Medicine recommends that all men over the age of 40 and all women over 50 be evaluated with a graded exercise test (with a physician present) before being allowed to enter into high-intensity exercise (see figure 3.5). This test is also recommended prior to participation for any patient with a high risk of heart disease. Complete fitness evaluations are often performed when a new member joins a fitness facility or when someone hires a personal trainer (see "Fitness Evaluation Form" on p. 104).

Less stressful measurements of physical abilities, such as the sit-and-reach test for hamstring and low back flexibility (see figure 3.6), can be easily included in the examination, whereas it may be necessary to schedule a cardiovascular fitness evaluation (graded exercise test) for another time, after the other portions of the PPE have been performed. One can establish the number and types of fitness tests on the basis of the time allowed for each individual going through the PPE. Certainly you do not want to include tests that will substantially affect the length of time needed in the physical exam unless you have done prior planning and allotted sufficient time.

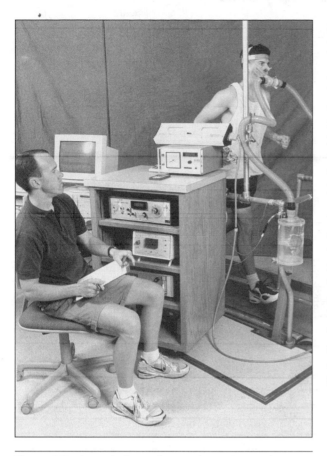

Figure 3.5 A graded exercise test is used to evaluate cardiorespiratory function and is administered using a bench, cycle ergometer, or treadmill.

PREPARTICIPATION PHYSICAL EXAMINATION RESULTS

Results from the physical examination will assist in the decision-making process through which the physician allows, or more precisely, finds no reason to limit, the patient's participation in the desired activity. One must be careful not to assume that a participant who is cleared for participation in one activity will automatically be suited for a more strenuous event or sport. As an example, consider Jason, who was born with spina bifida, a condition in which the vertebrae fail to fully form around the spinal cord. In Jason's case, the condition caused some muscle weakness in the lower extremities. Jason was able to walk and could even run short distances but would fatigue quite quickly, and with the fatigue came a loss of muscle coordination. The family's physician evaluated Jason for the local bowling team and signed the form stating that there was no reason to limit this athlete's participation on that team. After the season, Jason asked his parents if he could participate in the Athletes with Disabilities Soccer League. Since Jason had done so well on the bowling team, his parents gave their permission.

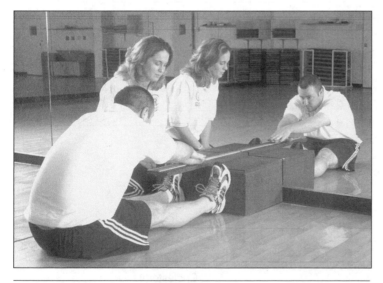

Figure 3.6 Sit-and-reach tests provide evaluators with information regarding an individual's flexibility.

For information regarding fitness testing, visit the American College of Sports Medicine's Web site at www.acsm.org.

Fitness Evaluation Form

Date ____ / ____ / ____

Member name _____ Membership number _____

Member address _____ City _____ State _____ (Zip) _____ Member phone number _____

Physician's name _____

Physician's address _____ City _____ State _____ (Zip) _____ Physician's phone number _____

VI. General physiological information   Birthdate ____ / ____ / ____   1. Age ____   2. Sex M ☐ F ☐
3. Risk category _____ 4. Height _____ ft. _____ in. 5. Weight _____ 6. RHR _____
7. RBP _____ 8. Predicted Max HR _____ 9. Medications _____
10. Exercise history _____

II. Cardiovascular assessment

1. RHR supine _____
2. RBP supine _____
3. RBP standing _____
4. Predicted heart rate

Max _____
90% _____
80% _____
70% _____

5. HVHR _____
Protocol _____
Equipment _____
Max HR _____ Max BP _____ / _____
Max met _____

Stage	Time	Speed	KPM	Grade	HR	BP	DP	ST	Comments
		1							
	1	2							
		3							
	1								
2	2								
	3								
	1								
3	2								
	3								
	1								
4	2								
	3								
	1								
5	2								
	3								
R	1								
e	3								
s	6								
t	9								

III. Lung capacity
1. Vital capacity ___ / ___ % Pred.
2. FEV ___ / ___ % Pred.

IV. Flexibility
1. Sit and reach ___ ___ ___ in.

V. Muscular strength and endurance
1. Grip _____ / _____ / _____   KgR _____ / _____ / _____ KgL
2. Trunk curl/sit-up _____ # _____ Time
3. _____

VI. Body composition

A. Skinfolds   1   2   Avg.
1. Chest   _____ _____ _____
2. Subscapula   _____ _____ _____
3. Suprailiac   _____ _____ _____
4. Umbilical   _____ _____ _____
5. Tricep   _____ _____ _____
6. Ant. thigh   _____ _____ _____
            Total skinfolds _____

C. Girths
1. Neck _____   6. Thigh ____ R ____ L
2. Shoulder _____   7. Calf ____ R ____ L
3. Chest _____   8. Bicep ____ R ____ L
4. Waist _____   9. Forearm ____ R ____ L
5. Hips _____

B. Body fat
1. Percent fat _____ %
2. Fat wt. _____ lb
3. Lean wt. _____ lb
4. Ideal percent fat _____ %
5. Ideal wt. _____ lb

VII. Blood chemistry
1. Cholesterol _____
2. Chol./HDL _____
3. LDL/HDL _____
4. Triglycerides _____
5. Glucose _____
6. Hematocrit _____

Note. RHR = resting heart rate; MET = unit of metabolic measurement; HVHR = hyperventilating heart rate; FEV = forced expiratory volume; HR = heart rate; BP = blood pressure; DP = double produce; ST = S-T segment; KgR = kilogram right hand; KgL = kilogram left hand. The law varies from state to state. No form should be adopted or used by any program without individualized legal advice.

Reprinted from Club Corporation of America 1995.

Jason was delighted, but the joy was short-lived; the coach told him that he would not be allowed to play until he had had the proper PPE for youth soccer. "No, son, I cannot accept the physical from your bowling league—soccer is a much different sport." Unfortunately, as Jason had feared, the physician would not clear him to play soccer.

Why wouldn't Jason be allowed to play soccer if he was physically able to participate on the bowling team? The answer relates to the purpose of the PPE, which in turn relates to the most difficult decision—that of approval for participation. The Preparticipation Physical Evaluation Task Force (Smith et al. 1997) has identified three categories of clearance: (1) unrestricted clearance, (2) clearance after completion of further evaluation or **rehabilitation,** and (3) not cleared for certain types of sports or, in extreme cases, any sports. Table 3.4 shows example clearances for some common conditions.

Each PPE form must clearly state the sport or activity in which the athlete is to participate. The coach and the athlete must realize that the permission applies only to the sport(s) or activities indicated.

Most physicians and organizations attempt to counsel the participant in finding a safe sport—and also attempt to provide the rehabilitation or medical assistance needed to allow the athlete some level of involvement with the team.

Medical Referral

In all cases of restricted clearance for activity, the underlying reason for limiting the athlete should be fully evaluated, even in cases in which the athlete is allowed full participation but only if supervised. One should not only refer the individual to a medical provider, but if possible should also make the appointment for the participant. Usually the referring party will receive notification of the evaluation and treatment rendered by the consultant. This information, an important part of the athlete's medical information, should be obtained, discussed, understood, and retained in the individual's medical records. Later follow-up with the same specialist is frequently necessary to allow the practitioner to follow the person's progress.

Activity Clearance With Supervision

Occasionally a participant will have some medical condition that is currently under control but warrants supervision. In such instances, the physician may permit the individual to participate

Table 3.4
Common Medical Conditions Limiting Sport Participation

Condition	Clearance decision	Recommendation
High blood pressure	Pass	Monitor blood pressure (BP) for several days. If BP fails to stabilize, refer for evaluation.
Anterior cruciate insufficiency	Defer for evaluation	Establish baseline strength; fully evaluate joint stability.
Spinal disc pathology	Defer for evaluation	Refer to specialist for magnetic resonance imaging (MRI), etc. to establish health of disc. Refer to rehab for evaluation and strengthening.
Sickle cell anemia	Fail	Counsel athlete regarding high risks of athletics. Encourage toward alternative involvement (manager position).
Absence of one of a paired organ	Pass with limitations	Athlete must be allowed to participate in sport only where there is little to no risk of injury to the healthy organ. If some risk does exist, legal counsel must be involved to establish consent to play.
Diabetes	Pass	Staff and students involved with this athlete must be educated on the warning signs of diabetic emergencies. Athlete should be closely monitored for blood sugar levels.

in the indicated activity or sport under the stipulation that he or she have the supervision of a medical or other trained person. This merely indicates that in sports in which the coach or other supervisors are not always present, the athlete is not allowed to participate. Conditions such as asthma, bronchitis, diabetes, epilepsy, bleeding trait, colitis, and other treatable ailments may require this type of supervision.

Disqualification of an Athlete

The team physician is usually considered the person responsible for determining that an athlete should not be allowed to participate in a specific sport. As previously indicated, efforts should always be made to find some avenue for participation if a specific sport is not well suited for the athlete. According to published guidelines (Smith et al. 1997) only two medical conditions would prevent an individual from participation in any physical activity: carditis (inflammation of the heart) and fever (temporary disqualification only). The responsibility of deciding on total disqualification from a sport sometimes creates a difficulty for the team physician who does not want to restrict participation unnecessarily but is responsible for protecting the student-athlete's health.

If the athlete does not receive clearance for the sport, this denial is an indication that participation poses additional risks. In establishing whether a condition warrants restriction from participation, the physician typically addresses the following questions:

- Does the problem place the athlete at an increased risk of injury?
- Does the problem place another athlete's safety in jeopardy?
- Could the athlete safely participate with compensations such as medication, bracing, padding, or specific rehabilitation?
- Could limited participation be permitted during the time in which treatment is being completed?
- If clearance is denied, what activities can the athlete safely participate in?

Ideally, the decision regarding athletic participation should meet with agreement between the team physician and other medical specialists, team officials (athletic trainer, coach, and attorney), and the athlete or family or both.

CONSIDERATIONS FOR ATHLETES WITH IMPAIRMENTS

As published in the *Sports Medicine Handbook* (NCAA 2003-2004), collegiate athletes who are considered "impaired" may include, but should not be limited to, the following:

1. Individuals who use a wheelchair (see figure 3.7)
2. Those who are deaf, blind, or missing a limb (see figure 3.8)
3. Those who have only one of a set of paired organs
4. Those who may have behavioral, emotional, and psychological disorders that substantially limit a major life activity

An athlete who has only one of a set of paired organs and who wishes to participate may do so if the medical specialists agree and, again according to the NCAA, if the following factors are considered and found in favor of the athlete:

1. The quality and function of the remaining organ
2. The probability of injury to the remaining organ
3. The state of the art in protective equipment and the capability of such equipment to prevent injury to the remaining organ.

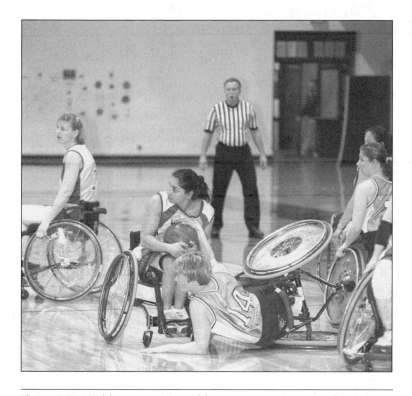

Figure 3.7 Highly competitive athletes compete in a wheelchair basketball game.

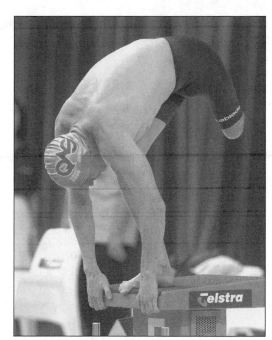

Figure 3.8 An impairment such as a disabled limb does not restrict a student-athlete from competition.

© Sport The Library

No firm rationale for disqualification can be stated for each sporting activity because each case is individual. It is reasonable to suggest, however, that all student-athletes should be provided the opportunity to participate if participation will not jeopardize their health or that of teammates.

ADMINISTRATION OF THE PREPARTICIPATION PHYSICAL EXAMINATION

There are as many different ways of doing the PPE as there are ranks of sport participation and fitness levels. However, all should establish the same thing: that there is no medical reason to prohibit the individual from participation. We consider two main methods of conducting a PPE: individual and group.

Individual Preparticipation Physical Exams

Teams with a limited budget frequently ask the athlete to be responsible for his or her own PPE, but the examination is usually outlined in a form provided to the participant. (An example is "Preparticipation Physical Evaluation" on pp. 108–110.) This procedure is quite common, especially at the high school and pre-high school levels (see figure 3.9). An advantage of having athletes see their own physicians for the PPE is that the family doctor is usually familiar with the athlete and the athlete's family. A physician who knows the medical history of the athlete and the family may question and report medical conditions that might otherwise go undetected. The physician familiar with the athlete may be able to discuss sensitive issues and may have a good understanding of the athlete's motivation for participation. Perhaps the best physical examination would be provided by the family physician who is knowledgeable about the physical demands of the sport and who is skilled in orthopedics as well as general medicine.

Preparticipation Physical Evaluation

History   Date _____

Name _____ Sex _____ Age _____ Date of birth _____

Grade _____ Sport _____ _____ _____

Personal physician _____ _____ _____

                                                                 Address   Physician's phone

Explain "Yes" answers below: .... **Yes   No**

  1. Have you ever been hospitalized? .... ❏ ❏

      Have you ever had surgery? .... ❏ ❏

  2. Are you presently taking any medications or pills? .... ❏ ❏

  3. Do you have any allergies (medicine, bees or other stinging insects)? .... ❏ ❏

  4. Have you ever passed out during or after exercise? .... ❏ ❏

      Have you ever been dizzy during or after exercise? .... ❏ ❏

      Have you ever had chest pain during or after exercise? .... ❏ ❏

      Do you tire more quickly than your friends during exercise? .... ❏ ❏

      Have you ever had high blood pressure? .... ❏ ❏

      Have you ever been told that you have a heart murmur? .... ❏ ❏

      Have you ever had racing of your heart or skipped heartbeats? .... ❏ ❏

      Has anyone in your family died of heart problems or a sudden death before age 50? .... ❏ ❏

  5. Do you have any skin problems (itching, rashes, acne)? .... ❏ ❏

  6. Have you ever had a head injury? .... ❏ ❏

      Have you ever been knocked out or unconscious? .... ❏ ❏

      Have you ever had a seizure? .... ❏ ❏

      Have you ever had a stinger, burner, or pinched nerve? .... ❏ ❏

  7. Have you ever had heat or muscle cramps? .... ❏ ❏

      Have you ever been dizzy or passed out in the heat? .... ❏ ❏

  8. Do you have trouble breathing or do you cough during or after activity? .... ❏ ❏

  9. Do you use any special equipment (pads, braces, neck rolls, mouth guard, eye guards, etc.)? .... ❏ ❏

10. Have you had any problems with your eyes or vision? .... ❏ ❏

      Do you wear glasses or contacts or protective eye wear? .... ❏ ❏

11. Have you ever sprained/strained, dislocated, fractured, broken, or had repeated swelling or
      other injuries of any bones or joints? .... ❏ ❏

        ❏ Head   ❏ Shoulder   ❏ Thigh   ❏ Neck   ❏ Elbow   ❏ Knee   ❏ Chest

        ❏ Forearm   ❏ Shin/calf   ❏ Back   ❏ Wrist   ❏ Ankle   ❏ Hip   ❏ Hand   ❏ Foot

12. Have you had any other medical problems (infectious mononucleosis, diabetes, etc.)? .... ❏ ❏

13. Have you had a medical problem or injury since your last evaluation? .... ❏ ❏

14. When was your last tetanus shot? _____

      When was your last measles immunization? _____

15. When was your first menstrual period? _____

      When was your last menstrual period? _____

      What was the longest time between your periods last year? _____

Explain "Yes" answers: _____

_____

_____

I hereby state that, to the best of my knowledge, my answers to the above questions are correct.

Date _____ Signature of athlete _____

Signature of parent/guardian _____

Physical Examination

Date _____

Name _____ Sex _____ Age _____ Date of birth _____

Height _____ Weight _____ BP _____ / _____ Pulse _____

Vision R 20 / _____ L 20 / _____ Corrected: Y N Pupils _____

<table>
<tr><td rowspan="20">COMPLETE</td><td rowspan="7">LIMITED</td><td></td><td>Normal</td><td colspan="4">Abnormal findings</td><td>Initials</td></tr>
<tr><td>Cardiopulmonary</td><td></td><td></td><td></td><td></td><td></td><td></td></tr>
<tr><td>Pulses</td><td></td><td></td><td></td><td></td><td></td><td></td></tr>
<tr><td>Heart</td><td></td><td></td><td></td><td></td><td></td><td></td></tr>
<tr><td>Lungs</td><td></td><td></td><td></td><td></td><td></td><td></td></tr>
<tr><td>Tanner stage</td><td>1</td><td>2</td><td>3</td><td>4</td><td>5</td><td></td></tr>
<tr><td>Skin</td><td></td><td></td><td></td><td></td><td></td><td></td></tr>
<tr><td>Abdominal</td><td></td><td></td><td></td><td></td><td></td><td></td></tr>
<tr><td>Genitalia</td><td></td><td></td><td></td><td></td><td></td><td></td></tr>
<tr><td>Musculoskeletal</td><td></td><td></td><td></td><td></td><td></td><td></td></tr>
<tr><td>Neck</td><td></td><td></td><td></td><td></td><td></td><td></td></tr>
<tr><td>Shoulder</td><td></td><td></td><td></td><td></td><td></td><td></td></tr>
<tr><td>Elbow</td><td></td><td></td><td></td><td></td><td></td><td></td></tr>
<tr><td>Wrist</td><td></td><td></td><td></td><td></td><td></td><td></td></tr>
<tr><td>Hand</td><td></td><td></td><td></td><td></td><td></td><td></td></tr>
<tr><td>Back</td><td></td><td></td><td></td><td></td><td></td><td></td></tr>
<tr><td>Knee</td><td></td><td></td><td></td><td></td><td></td><td></td></tr>
<tr><td>Ankle</td><td></td><td></td><td></td><td></td><td></td><td></td></tr>
<tr><td>Foot</td><td></td><td></td><td></td><td></td><td></td><td></td></tr>
<tr><td>Other</td><td></td><td></td><td></td><td></td><td></td><td></td></tr>
</table>

Clearance:

    A. Cleared

    B. Cleared after completing evaluation/rehabilitation for: _____

    C. Not cleared for: ❏ Collision

                 ❏ Contact

                 ❏ Noncontact _____ Strenuous _____ Moderately strenuous _____ Nonstrenuous

           Due to: _____

Recommendation: _____

_____

Name of physician _____ Date _____

Address _____ Phone _____

Signature of physician _____

(continued)

Preparticipation Physical Evaluation (continued)

Examination   Patient's name: _____

*1. BP _____ WT _____ HT _____ Vision (R) _____ (L) _____

*2. Cardiovascular Exam   ❏ Normal   ❏ Abnormal   Comments:

Murmur ❏ Yes ❏ No   Describe:

*3. Musculoskeletal Exam   Record laxity, weakness, instability, decreased ROM—if abnormal

Knee   ❏ Normal   ❏ Abnormal

Ankle   ❏ Normal   ❏ Abnormal

Shoulder   ❏ Normal   ❏ Abnormal

(Other orthopedic problems,
e.g., neck, feet, scoliosis)   ❏ Normal   ❏ Abnormal

4. Optional Exam—should be done if history is positive. Comments:

ENT   ❏ Normal   ❏ Abnormal

Chest   ❏ Normal   ❏ Abnormal

Abdomen   ❏ Normal   ❏ Abnormal

Genitalia   ❏ Normal   ❏ Abnormal

Skin   ❏ Normal   ❏ Abnormal

*Assessment: 5. A. ❏ No problems identified   B. ❏ Other

*Recommendations: 6. A. ❏ Unlimited   B. ❏ Limited to specific sports   C. ❏ Deferred until: (e.g., rehab.,
                                                                           recheck, consultation, lab, etc.)

*Reexamine: 7. A. ❏ Yearly and after any injury that limits participation for greater than one week.
              B. ❏ Other:

I certify that I have examined the above student and that such examination revealed (❏ conditions ❏ no conditions) that would prevent this student from participation in interscholastic sports.

Are you licensed to practice medicine in the United States?   ❏ Yes   ❏ No

Signature _____   Phone number _____

Address _____   Date _____

If student not qualified, list reasons for disqualification: _____

_____

(The following are considered disqualifying until medical and parental releases are obtained: acute infections, obvious growth retardation, diabetes, jaundice, severe visual or auditory impairment, pulmonary insufficiency, organic heart disease or hypertension, enlarged liver or spleen, hernia, musculoskeletal deformity associated with functional loss, history of convulsions or concussions, absence of one kidney, eye, testicle, or ovary, etc.)

*Required element.

From American Academy of Family Physicians and Preparticipation Physical Evaluation Task Force 1996. Reprinted with permission of McGraw-Hill Companies.

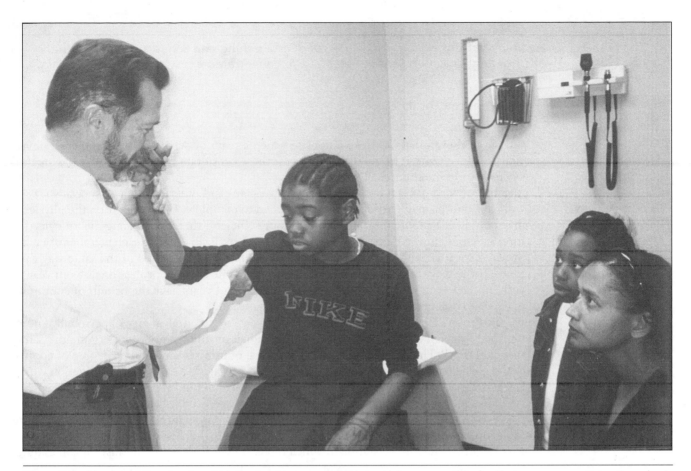

Figure 3.9 Many middle school and high school teams ask athletes to be responsible for their own preparticipation physical exam.

© Susan Kay Hillman

Medical costs have skyrocketed in part because of the rising costs of medical malpractice insurance. A typical orthopedic physician pays about $50,000 a year in medical malpractice insurance. Some medical specialists pay more, and others pay less, yet all medical providers must hold this type of insurance to protect them financially in the event of an error in medical care. The net result is increased costs to the consumer. Medical care has become so expensive, in fact, that many families subscribe to large health maintenance organizations (HMOs) rather than receiving health care from the family physician as in the past. All too commonly an individual visits the HMO physician only when in need of urgent care, and a different physician handles the visit each time. The family physician who knows the entire family and all associated medical histories may be the exception rather than the rule in today's medical system. This lack of familiarity, and perhaps a lack of frequent wellness exams, make the PPE even more important.

In addition to lacking personal knowledge of the athlete, and perhaps of the family's medical history, the HMO physician may not be equipped to handle some aspects of the physical exam such as the eye test, body composition measures, or some of the flexibility exams. The coach or another trained team representative can complete these somewhat nonmedical aspects of the evaluation.

The Group Preparticipation Physical Examination

When a large group of people must be screened at the same time, a group examination may be an efficient means of accomplishing the task. The group examination relies on a number of health care professionals who staff stations through which the athlete must pass to complete

The reader may obtain more information on the process of establishing and conducting the PPE in the book in this Athletic Training Education Series titled *Management Strategies in Athletic Training, Third Edition.*

the physical examination. In situations in which a team or school uses a number of physicians as consultants, it would be logical to use these consultants as physicians for the medical evaluations in the group PPE.

Since the group exam uses a number of physicians and other health care specialists, each will have only a small portion of the entire exam to complete. In this situation the physician may be able to be more thorough and also more efficient, thereby reducing the time needed for the examination. Additionally, having the same physician evaluate each member of a team provides great reliability (meaning that the same finding is reported in the same way each time). If the team is fortunate enough to have the same medical professionals from year to year, athletes remaining with the team over a period of years have the benefit of continuity of care and excellent consistency of medical practice.

The group PPE allows the team's athletic trainer the added advantage of personally knowing the physician and knowing that each individual on the team has undergone the same, thorough PPE. However, although there is peace of mind from having a degree of control of the participants' PPEs, problems often arise in conducting a physical examination with a large group. With proper advanced planning, one may minimize each problematic issue.

To use a school gymnasium as an example, stations may be set up to allow a smooth transition from one test to another in the group physical examination. Group physicals require preplanning of space, equipment, and personnel needs. Each station may create a unique concern; for example, the station in which blood pressure is measured must remain as quiet as possible in order to allow the examiners to hear. If this station is positioned where patients congregate, noise levels may rise and make the evaluation of blood pressure difficult. See the example of a gymnasium setup.

Group Physical in a School Gymnasium

Station 1: Check-In

Student-athletes obtain appropriate forms and progress to chair area to complete required documents. Computers may be used.

Station 2: Height and Weight

Student workers take measurements and record them on medical forms; worker from the sport information office or department records data for use in media relations.

Station 3: Vision and Eye Screening

A well-lighted area 20 ft (6.1 m) in length is needed for the vision screening. The physician supervises the vision screening and then performs individualized eye exams.

Station 4: Laboratory Testing (Urinalysis and Blood Test) and Immunizations

Student-athletes progress to the rest room area. Nurses perform any needed immunizations. Contracted laboratory **phlebotomists** do blood draws and obtain urine samples.

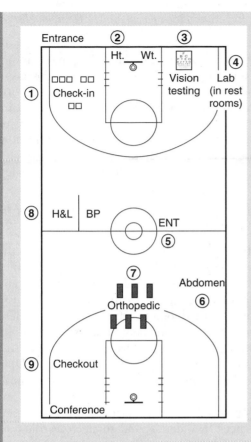

Station 5: Ear, Nose, and Throat

Physician perform ear, nose, and throat evaluation with the student-athlete in a seated position. A small table, such as a taping table, is usually satisfactory.

Station 6: Abdominal Exam

Physician checks abdomen and pelvis. This location within the examination area must be sectioned off to ensure privacy for the student-athlete being evaluated.

Station 7: Orthopedic Exam

Because of the length of time required to perform each orthopedic exam, athletic trainers may assist the orthopedic surgeon(s) in the evaluation of bones and joints. This location need not be enclosed, but having some partitions on the periphery of the area is beneficial.

Station 8: Blood Pressure and Heart/Lung Evaluation

These are actually two adjoining stations, both of which require a degree of silence. Several evaluators are needed to obtain blood pressure and pulse, while only one or two physicians are necessary to complete the heart and lung examination.

Station 9: Checkout

Typically the team physician responsible for the medical services performs the checkout duties. The physician must perform a thorough review of all data collected before signing off on the permission to participate.

SUMMARY

1. *Discuss the importance of a PPE for sport team members or for someone beginning a fitness program.*

   The PPE evaluates the medical status of the individual with reference to the requirements of the sport or activity to be undertaken. The PPE differs from an annual physical exam (wellness exam) in that the evaluation focuses on potential areas of increased risk of health hazard during vigorous activity rather on than the health of the sedentary individual.

2. *Discuss how knowledge of preexisting conditions may help in the medical care of the athlete or physically active individual.*

   When a preexisting condition is detected before it has caused harm, treatment or adaptations can be instituted to allow safe participation in physical activities. For example, an athlete who is diagnosed with a small **hernia** may be cleared to participate in activities but restricted from heavy weight training. Knowledge of the potential for further trouble can help keep the athlete and the medical staff alert if symptoms increase.

3. *Present the two main ways to conduct a physical examination for an athletic team, and list the advantages and disadvantages of each.*

Individual examinations cost less for the school or team, and the physician may know the patient or his or her medical history well. On the other hand, the physician may not know the individual, and the quality of the exam will not be uniform across all athletes tested. With a group examination, in which all participants are checked by the same physicians, the exam is concluded during one session (therefore it's fast). The problems associated with group exams are typical of managing a large group: The noise level is high; people may become distracted and confused; follow-through on suspicious findings is difficult; and there is less privacy and individual counseling.

4. *List the types of examinations to be included in the PPE, and identify the members of the medical team needed to conduct these exams in a group physical.*

Administrative forms and history will be handled by a department administrative assistant or other staff members. Local emergency medical technicians, paramedics, nurses or nursing students, and athletic trainers or trained student athletic trainers usually take an individual's blood pressure and pulse. Nurses or phlebotomists, or both, from a laboratory take samples for the blood test and urinalysis. Athletic trainers or trained students measure height, weight, and body composition. Optometrists or trained ancillary staff perform vision screening. Orthopedic surgeons and athletic trainers do an orthopedic evaluation. A general surgeon or other MD, or a doctor of osteopathy (DO), assesses the abdomen and pelvic areas. An ear, nose, and throat specialist or other MD or DO evaluates the individual's ears, nose, and throat. A cardiologist or other MD or DO does the evaluation of the heart and lungs. Optional tests include dental check by a dentist and an electrocardiogram by an exercise physiologist or other trained ancillary staff.

5. *Compare and contrast aspects of the group physical and the individualized examination.*

Both methods of PPE evaluate the participant to ascertain that there is no known risk to participation in the desired sport. The group physical utilizes the same examiner for each athlete and thus provides a degree of reliability, whereas a group of individual examinations yields data from a variety of examiners. The individual exam can provide more time for discussion and counseling for the individual athlete, while the group exam may become backlogged if one individual needs additional time. The individual examination is as quiet as the examining physician needs it to be, while the group physical can become noisy. The group physical is typically conducted by the team, at no cost to the individual participant, whereas the individual exam is at the patient's expense.

6. *Identify problematic areas in conducting a group physical and list ways in which those situations may be managed.*

Problematic areas include the following:

- Noise levels may make it difficult to hear: Arrange stations to limit congregation outside critical areas.

- Participants may become confused regarding where to go next: Provide "ushers" to direct traffic flow and assist patients in finding the next station.

- Minor findings may become lost in the numbers: Generate a list of any remarks made on the athlete's physical exam form. Assign an certified athletic trainer (ATC) for a sport team to ensure proper follow-through and follow-ups.

- Physical arrangement of stations may allow a waiting athlete to pressure the examiner: Arrange stations to provide as much privacy as possible, and have a staff member serve as monitor to control situations.
- Individual counseling may be reduced by the large number of athletes waiting for evaluation: Have physicians schedule postexam time to speak with patients.

CRITICAL THINKING QUESTIONS

1. As the athletic trainer for a high school, identify the advantages and disadvantages of a school-conducted PPE for the athletes.

2. You are the head athletic trainer at a local high school with five student trainers and 1,000 athletes. You have one team doctor, an orthopedic surgeon, who is willing to bring two of the nurses from his office, as well as his wife (a general practitioner), who has agreed to help. The school has budgeted $150 to cover any costs of the PPEs. You have unlimited use of the building facilities of the east wing of the school, which includes your training room, one average-size gymnasium, and two average-size classrooms. Your roommate has volunteered to help out on that day, as have the school nurse and three coaches. You have chosen to hire one additional ATC from the community to assist you. Please draw/map out the schematic of how you would run your PPE that day. Include stations for check-in, height and weight, vision and eye screening, abdominal exam, orthopedic exam, blood pressure, heart and lung, and checkout. Please also include the following:

   a. Identify who you will put at each station and why, as well as where each station will be set up and your reasoning for setting it up this way. Write a short description of the helpers' responsibilities at each station.

   b. Estimate the length of time you will allow for the PPE.

   c. Discuss work breaks, directions for the student-athlete on how to progress through the stations, and ways in which you will ensure that all athletes have completed all stations.

3. There are additional logistical questions to answer in planning a successful PPE, including those listed next. Please answer the following additional questions regarding the scenario presented in question 2.

   a. Will you be providing food/snacks for workers? What are the costs?

   b. Assuming that the doctors, nurses, and hired ATC will bring their own supplies, what additional supplies will you need? What are the costs of these supplies?

   c. Which employees will you be paying and how much? (Remember you have only $150 budgeted for PPEs.)

   d. Each worker at each station will have specific responsibilities. How will you convey this information to the workers?

   e. Will there be any pre-PPE meetings (either on the day of or during the weeks before)?

   f. Will you assign your athletes specific times to be there? How will you get this information to the athletes?

   g. Will you charge the athletes for the PPEs given at the school? How much? How can you justify charging them?

4. What are the advantages and disadvantageous of allowing student-athletes at any level to be responsible for their own PPEs (i.e., giving them forms and having them take the forms to their own physicians)?

5. Given the following setup (see "Interoffice Memo" below):
    a. List any areas you think may be problematic during the PPE.
    b. Explain why each may be a problem.
    c. What would you change about the presented setup and why?
6. List as many topics as you might want to cover in the health information questionnaire. Describe the importance of the various topics identified.
7. Along with the logistics of setting up the layout for a PPE are several considerations for forms that the student-athletes should have filled out and need to bring to the PPE. What forms would you include in this packet, and why?

Interoffice Memo

TO: All Staff and Student Trainers

FROM: John Doe, Head Athletic Trainer

RE: Preparticipation Physical Exam for National Youth Sports Program

The physical exam will be held in the physical education building. We will have three teams reporting at 7:30 a.m., so please be at your stations and be ready to go by then. Here are the locations of the various stations. Remember the floorplan of the PE building is with the three gymnasiums on the ground floor. The men's and women's locker rooms and restrooms are on the basement level and there are six open classrooms on the second floor (even numbers are on the left side of the hall, odd numbers on the right).

Station #	Exam / Function of Station	Location
1	Check-in	Gymnasium 1
2	Height and weight	Locker rooms
3	Vision screen	Gymnasium 2
4	Flexibility screen	Gymnasium 3
5	Urinalysis	Locker rooms
6	Ear, nose, and throat	Classroom 201
7	Heart and lung eval	Classroom 203
8	Orthopedic exams	Classroom 205
9	Blood pressure/Pulse	Classroom 206
10	Insurance paperwork	Classroom 204
11	Checkout	Classroom 202

CITED SOURCES

American Heart Association. 1996. Cardiovascular preparticipation screening of competitive athletes. *Circulation* 94: 850-856.

American Heart Association. 1998. Cardiovascular preparticipation screening of competitive athletes: Addendum. *Circulation* 97: 2294.

National Collegiate Athletic Association. 2003–2004. *NCAA sports medicine handbook 2003-04.* Indianapolis: National Collegiate Athletic Association. http://ncaa.org/library/sports_sciences/sports_med_handbook/2003-04/index.html (accessed June 15, 2004).

Smith, D.M., J.R. Kovan, B.S.E. Rich, and S. Tanner. 1997. *Preparticipation physical evaluation*, 2nd ed. Minneapolis: McGraw-Hill.

ADDITIONAL READINGS

American Academy of Pediatrics Committee on Sports Medicine and Committee on School Health. 1989. Policy statement: Organized athletics for preadolescent children (RE9165). *Pediatrics* 84(3).

Bratton, R.L. 1997. Preparticipation screening of children for sports. Current recommendations. *Spts Med* 24(5): 300-307.

Cook, L.G., M. Collins, W.W. Williams, D. Rodgers, and A.L. Baughman. 1993. Prematriculation immunization requirements of American colleges and universities. *J Am College Health* 42: 91-98.

Fields, K.B. 1994. Clearing athletes for participation in sports: The North Carolina Medical Society Sports Medicine Committee's recommended examination. *NC Med J* 55(4): 116-121.

Gardner, P., and W. Schaffner. 1993. Immunization of adults. *New Eng J Med* 328(17): 1252-1258.

Glover, D.W., and B.J. Maron. 1998. Profile of preparticipation cardiovascular screening for high school athletes. *JAMA* 279(22): 1817-1819.

Hepatitis B virus: A comprehensive strategy for eliminating transmission in the United States through universal childhood vaccinations: Recommendations of the Immunization Practices Advisory Committee. 1991. *Morbid Mortal Wkly Rpt* 40: W-131.

Kibler, W.B. 1990. *The sports preparticipation fitness examination.* Champaign, IL: Human Kinetics.

Maron, B.J., and J.H. Mitchell. 1994. 26th Bethesda Conference: Recommendations for determining eligibility for competition in athletes with cardiovascular abnormalities. *J Am Coll Cardiol* 24(4): 845-899.

Maron, B.J., J. Shirani, L.C. Poliac, et al. 1996. Sudden death in young competitive athletes: Clinical, demographic, and pathological profiles. *JAMA* 276(3): 199-204.

Maron, B.J., L.C. Poliac, J.A. Kaplan, and F.O. Mueller. 1995. Blunt impact to the chest leading to sudden death from cardiac arrest during sports activities. *N Eng J Med* 333(6): 337-342.

Maron, B.J., P.D. Thompson, J.C. Puffer, et al. 1996. Cardiovascular preparticipation screening of competitive athletes. *Am Heart Assoc* 94(4): 850-856.

McKeag, D.B. 1996. Ugh! Sports physicals [editorial]. *Phys Sptsmed* 24(8): 33.

Myers, A., and T. Sickles. 1998. Preparticipation sports examination. *Prim Care* 25(1): 225-236.

Peterson, B. 1991. Pre-season examinations: Organizing this most vital part of any athletic program. *The first aider.* Garner, KS: Cramer Corporation.

Sanders, B., and W.C. Nemeth. 1996. Preparticipation physical examinations. *J Orthop Spts Phys Ther* 23(2): 149-163.

Sarpinato, L. 1996. Clearing athletes for sports participation. *Hosp Pract* 31(4): 120-122.

Tanner, S.M. 1994. Preparticipation examination targeted for the female athlete. *Clin Spts Med* 13(2): 337-353.

26th Bethesda Conference. Recommendations for determining eligibility for competition in athletes with cardiovascular abnormalities. 1994. *Med Sci Spts Exerc* 26(10, Suppl.): S223-S283.

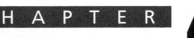

CHAPTER 4

Conditioning and Strength Training in Athletics

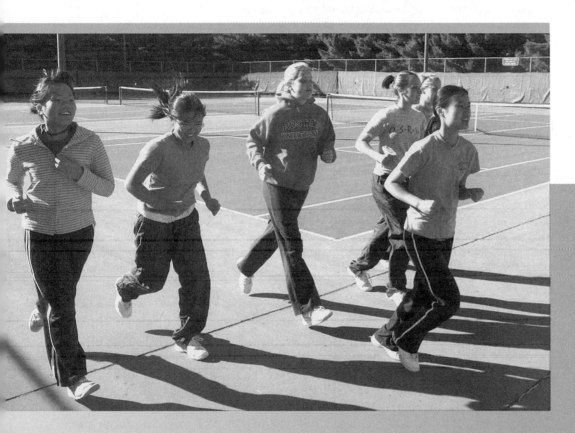

Objectives

After reading this chapter, the student should be able to do the following:

1. Identify ways in which information from fitness testing can help the athletic trainer.

2. Discuss the rationale for conducting fitness testing at various times before, during, or after the sport or training season.

3. Explain the method of establishing the 1-repetition maximum in weightlifting.

4. Define "aerobic" and "anaerobic" with reference to energy systems and relate each to various activities.

5. Define isotonic, isometric, and isokinetic exercise and give an example of each.

6. Compare and contrast the two types of muscle contraction: concentric and eccentric.

7. Discuss factors to consider in designing an exercise prescription.

8. Define the overload principle and explain how it applies to conditioning and strength techniques.

"**W**hitney, could you design a weightlifting program to help me improve my golf game?" asked a man who was working out in the gym.

"Hey, I'll join in on that if it would be okay!" shouted someone else working nearby.

This type of request was not unusual for an athletic trainer, but whom the request came from was unusual. After graduation, Whitney had started working in an exercise facility in an active adult community, and her athletes were a little older than one might expect . . . the youngest was 63!

Whitney was delighted to assist. She felt much more prepared to work with the adult athletes than either her fitness professional colleague or the staff physical therapist working in the club. Whitney felt that her experience of working with competitive athletes helped her to understand the psychological issues and the intense motivation these athletes showed.

Whitney had completed a rotation in the same gym during her graduate education and immediately sensed the appreciation and respect of the older adults. The transition from young athlete to older athlete was simple, especially since she paid attention in the class "Exercise Across the Life Span" during graduate school. It wasn't long before she realized that older adults were just as motivated as those in college athletics; in fact, they actually sometimes needed to be held back more!

Whitney applied the concepts of strengthening that she would use with any athlete and tailored the exercises to the fitness level, sport, and any physical limitations of each individual. Through a gradual program using sound principles of progression, Whitney had helped several individuals win age-related golf tournaments; helped an 85-year-old catcher spur his team into a second place finish in an "old-timers" baseball league; and was delighted when a 90-year-old lady she was helping returned to bowling after breaking her hip.

"The principles are the same," Whitney told her workmate when asked what she did to make the older athletes like her so much. "I just treat them as I would any athlete and give them the challenges I know their body can tolerate. They all want to participate in their sports just the same as anybody else. Sometimes the sport is about all these folks have in their lives, so I give them as much time and consideration as I can."

The area of strength and conditioning has grown considerably in recent years: Whereas in the past it was just one of a coach's responsibilities, today we have full-time strength and conditioning coaches. Strength and conditioning coaches have helped to reduce the sport coaches' responsibilities, giving increased attention to off-season conditioning as well as to strength and conditioning during the sport season.

Unfortunately, some schools and teams still rely on the sport coach to provide proper conditioning and strengthening programs for the athletes. Regardless of the job description, all individuals working with the athlete should be familiar with the various aspects of strengthening so that they can advise athletes in this area if necessary.

In addition, there may be times when you will work with people who are not as fit or active as high school athletes. With attention to proper warm-up, exercise moderation, and a good stretching program, even athletes in their eighth decade of life may be challenging one another in physical activities. Only a few of the injuries related to a walking/running program are unique to that age group. Because of decreases in **cardiorespiratory** function, these participants may encounter "dizziness" and "side stitch." Orthopedic conditions affecting the weight-bearing joints may be related to a loss of bone density or to various stages of **osteoarthritis** in the older athlete. All these types of conditions can be easily prevented by careful planning and exercise selection.

This chapter addresses methods of testing the individual to determine the starting point for specialized weight-training programs, as well as methods for evaluating the progress of an individual on a conditioning program. We consider strengthening programs, techniques and equipment used in strength training, and finally aspects of flexibility, an often neglected area of the total conditioning program.

FITNESS-TESTING PROCEDURES

Starting a conditioning program requires a knowledge of the "baseline" of fitness. If you ever have begun a strength or conditioning program you may have had no real idea where to start. You may have found yourself looking at a rack of weights and wondering how much you should start with. This sense of uncertainty reflects one of the reasons the fitness test is so important. A fitness test can allow you to identify the muscle groups or the basic energy sources that need to be trained. Fitness testing can take many forms but usually comprises tests of muscular function (strength, endurance, and power), cardiovascular function, speed, and agility, as well as body composition (see table 4.1).

Table 4.1
Various Methods to Test Fitness

Fitness test	Test purpose	Description	Pros and cons	Comments
Run tests for set time or distance	Cardiovascular endurance	Various tests using time (9, 10, 12 min) or distance (1 mile, 1.5 miles)	Pros: Easy, inexpensive to conduct; can test large groups. Cons: Affected by motivation.	Well suited to all age groups and fitness levels. Use longer time (10 min) for adults, shorter time or distance for children.
Harvard Step Test	Cardiovascular endurance	Subject steps up and down 20-in. height at 30 steps/minute for 5 min or until exhaustion. Exhaustion = inability to keep pace for 15 sec. Stop, sit, and count heart rate (for 30 sec) at 1, 2, and 3 min postexercise.	Pros: Simple test, easy to administer. Cons: Metronome or cadence tape required.	Scoring: (100 × test duration in seconds) divided by 2 × total number of heartbeats in recovery period. Excellent: >90 Good: 80-89 High average: 65-79 Low average: 55-64 Poor: <55
1-repetition maximum tests	Isotonic strength	Subject lifts one repetition of a selected weight. If weight can be lifted properly, heavier weight is selected. Repeat until maximum is identified.	Pros: Equipment is usually available. Cons: Applies only to that particular lift.	Excellent method of determining pre- and post-measurements of strength.
Vertical jump test	Muscle power	Subject stands next to wall and reaches up with the hand closest to the wall to highest point. That point is recorded. Subject then takes one step into jump to touch as high on the wall as possible. Three jumps are completed. Record the difference between highest jump and reach.	Pros: Simple and easy to administer. Cons: Subjects with low coordination may score poorly.	Raw score is only a distance measure. Calculations can be found to convert to "power."
Standing long jump	Muscle power	Subject stands with both feet comfortably placed behind marked line. Using arm swing and leg propulsion, subject launches forward as far as possible, landing on both feet.	Pros: Simple and quick to administer. Cons: May be somewhat traumatic for elderly or previously injured subjects.	Distance jumped is recorded.

(continued)

Table 4.1
(continued)

Fitness test	Test purpose	Description	Pros and cons	Comments
Push-up test	Muscle endurance	Subject performs (using tester-defined protocol) push-ups during specified time period (60 sec, 2 min).	Pros: No equipment is required. Cons: Subjects with low upper-body strength may be unable to perform test.	Number of correctly performed push-ups is recorded.
Abdominal endurance test	Muscle endurance	Subject performs sit-ups (using tester-defined protocol) during set time period (20-60 sec, 2 min).	Pros: No equipment is required. Cons: Subjects with low back pain may be unable to perform.	Tester must standardize sit-up test with the methods used to establish norms. Record total sit-ups performed.
Sprint test	Speed	Subjects run (sprint) designated distance for time, typically 10, 20, 30 m.	Pros: Quick and simple. Cons: Requires subjects to warm up. Performance may be influenced by motivation.	Use sprint distance that applies directly to sport or activities in which subject is involved. Norms can be established for individual groups.

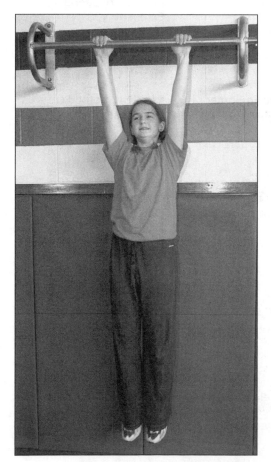

You probably remember fitness tests from your early years in physical education classes. The Presidential Physical Fitness Test may have been one of your earliest exposures to fitness testing (see figure 4.1). The President's Council on Physical Fitness and Sports works toward promoting physical activity, fitness, and sports that enhance and improve health. In an attempt to promote participation in sport and physical activities for people of all ages and abilities, the council coordinates several programs, including the President's Challenge, the Presidential Sports Awards, and National Physical Fitness and Sports Month (each May). In addition to the national focus on fitness and fitness testing, almost every fitness center, club, and school conducts fitness evaluations either for the patient's information or for preparticipation purposes. Additionally, fitness tests have almost always been used by coaches to determine the level of conditioning of athletes. Fitness tests may be done prior to accepting an athlete on a sport team, during the season, or at the end of the sport season to allow the setting of goals for the next season. Whenever the testing is performed, the goal is to measure the athlete's level of fitness. Before we discuss fitness testing, let's consider when the tests should be done.

The Preseason Participation Evaluation

Preseason participation evaluations are often used to assess the individual's level of conditioning in order to determine areas of weakness

Figure 4.1 Remember the Presidential Physical Fitness Test? It may have been your first exposure to fitness testing.

More information on circuit training, exercise techniques, flexibility, injury prevention, safety, special populations, and women's issues is available through the National Strength and Conditioning Association article index at www.nsca-lift.org. Here you can see a bibliography of all articles and columns that have been printed in the association's professional journal, *Strength and Conditioning Journal.*

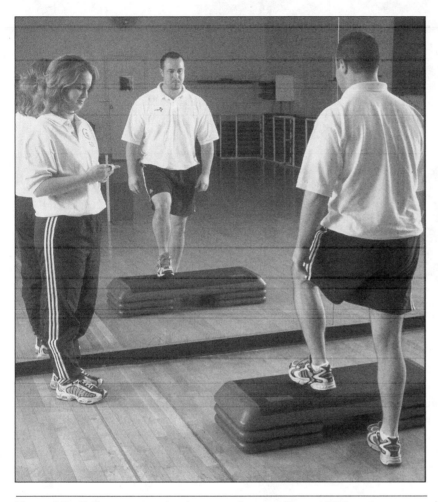

Figure 4.2   Early season evaluations are often used to establish an in-season conditioning or training program.

and to establish an in-season conditioning or training program (see figure 4.2). Discovering that an athlete's endurance level is less than that of other members on the team may allow special attention to endurance training to help the athlete develop better stamina in long bouts of activity or in long competitions. A recreational athlete, or anyone entering a fitness program, should consider participating in a fitness-testing program prior to the start of the activities. Just like the athlete on a sport team, the participant will benefit from knowing his or her level of fitness before beginning the exercise endeavor. In addition to showing the fitness baseline, performance in a fitness test can indicate the person's potential for success or difficulty in the upcoming activities. Knowledge gained from the fitness tests can be used to design the activity level of the participant in order to allow safe and beneficial participation.

Ongoing Evaluations

Evaluations during a sport season or during training are probably less common than pre- or postseason evaluations. An evaluation may be employed during the middle of the off-season strength and conditioning program to allow the coach to judge the effectiveness of that program (see figure 4.3). Testing in the middle of the competitive season can be used to demonstrate a particular weakness that has developed during the season because of misuse or disuse. This decrease in strength is often seen during a competitive season, especially in lifts that are not specific to the skills the athlete uses in the sport. It might be logical to think that an in-season weightlifting program would alleviate this problem, yet increases in conditioning during a long competitive season may place too much physical demand on the athlete and prove counterproductive. Many coaches require the athlete to continue to lift during the competitive season, but limit the exercises to those most applicable to the sport. Evaluation of these in-season programs could allow the coach to better individualize the lifting program of each athlete. People participating in less organized teams or groups, as well as those entering an exercise program alone, benefit from repeating the preparticipation fitness evaluation during the course of the program. This periodic evaluation serves to indicate the individual's progress toward the fitness goals and also to indicate when it would be advisable to consider changes in the current program.

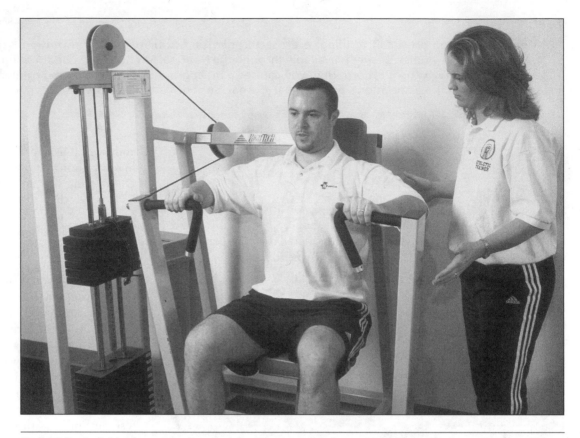

Figure 4.3   Individuals can monitor their training progress by periodic evaluations.

Remember John, the ultramarathoner (mentioned in chapter 3) who had to give up running? Think for a moment about how he could have known whether he would be in the proper condition to attempt his first 100-mile (161-km) run. Unless he participated in periodic fitness evaluations, he might not know whether his daily runs and the much longer runs on the weekends were actually building his body up or breaking it down. It is entirely possible to overtrain by exercising more than the body can withstand. Periodic evaluation of John's cardiovascular endurance would have told him what training programs could benefit him the most.

Postseason Fitness Evaluations

Postseason evaluations of fitness levels give the coach or athlete a baseline for measuring changes that occur during the off-season. These data are also used to better establish the specific areas to address during the off-season training program. Athletes participating in more than one sport in a school year may not be able to participate in the sport-specific off-season training program; in this case the postseason evaluation is very important. Athletes who have undergone an end-of-season evaluation of fitness will have a better understanding of the goals they are to reach during the off-season conditioning program.

FITNESS-TESTING PARAMETERS

Sport performance obviously requires unique physical abilities. Different sports necessitate different levels of physical performance; yet in general, fitness testing for any sport includes evaluation of muscular function (strength, endurance, and power) as well as cardiovascular function, agility, and speed. If we stop for a moment to examine these parameters, we may conclude that they are the same factors that contribute to injury prevention. Looking at fitness test results to determine areas of weakness could help the athletic trainer and strength and conditioning specialist work together to prepare the athlete—and thus take a step closer to preventing an injury. In addition to these strength and conditioning parameters, other measures such as flexibility, body composition, and height/weight can be included either in the preparticipation physical examination or in fitness tests. Let's look at why these parameters may be important to measure.

Muscle Function

Muscle strength is the ability of the muscle or group of muscles to overcome a resistance. To fully understand the muscles active in a particular motion, one must have a firm knowledge of anatomy. To assist you in this quest, we have provided a CD-ROM, *Essentials of Interactive Functional Anatomy*, with this book. In this CD-ROM, you will be able to locate a specific muscle and learn about its actions through text, animations, and human action videos.

Strength is considered to be the maximum force that a muscle or muscle group can generate in a specific movement pattern at a specified velocity of movement. Few would debate the need for muscle strength in sports like wrestling, football, or gymnastics, yet people often regard sports like swimming and track as speed events that involve little need for muscle strength. Coaches have become more aware of the need for strength in all events and sports and have found that muscle strength evaluation data are very useful.

Muscular endurance refers to the ability of a muscle or group of muscles to perform a repetitive action. Sports like cross country, some events in track, and most swimming events require a great amount of endurance, both muscular and cardiovascular. In tennis, as another example, muscle endurance allows the athlete to perform repetitive actions like the backhand swing and overhead serve. Individuals in activities such as cycling or rowing continually repeat the same movement patterns. Repeated movement can cause trauma in weak or unconditioned muscles.

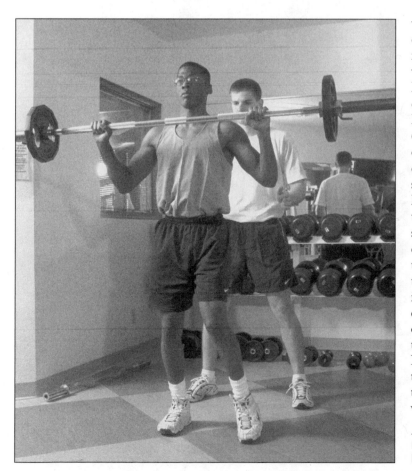

Muscle power is the rate of performing work. You might think of this as how fast you can perform a particular lift, yet the concept is not that simple. Power is a term from physics, where it is defined as work during a unit of time. Physicists further define work as force times distance. Thus, muscle power equals a weight lifted (force) through a range of movement (usually a vertical distance) divided by the unit of time required to perform the lift. One can develop power by lifting the same weight the same distance in a shorter period of time, or by lifting a greater amount of weight the same distance in the same period of time. Activities that strength and conditioning specialists evaluate to determine muscle power include exercises like the "clean and jerk" (see figure 4.4). In the clean, the weight is lifted from the floor to chest level in one smooth motion. This exercise involves carrying a weight bar (force) over a large range of movement (vertical distance from the floor to the chest) in a short period of time—thus power. If someone is lifting 100 lb, if the distance from the floor to the chest is 4 ft, and if it takes 1 sec to perform the lift, the power is 100 lb × 4 ft, which equals 400 ft-lb/sec.

Figure 4.4 Exercises like the clean and jerk can help evaluate muscular power.

Many sport activities require power. For example, jumping requires moving the body (equivalent to a weight) through a range of motion (preparation through takeoff), and the activity occurs very rapidly. Jumping activities benefit from conditioning programs that include exercises for power development.

Evaluating Muscle Strength

To evaluate muscular strength, a baseline measure is first taken. This measurement is typically performed using a technique called 1-repetition maximum (1RM). If a sport requires particular muscle activity, the fitness evaluation may include a 1RM test of a lift that uses those muscles or muscle groups. Traditionally the bench press is used to evaluate upper-body strength, and the leg press or squat is used for lower-body strength (see figure 4.5).

A repetition maximum is the maximum number of repetitions per set that a person can perform at a particular weight. Thus a 1RM is the heaviest weight that a person can lift for one complete repetition of an exercise. To determine the 1RM weight, the participant must use more than one lift. The first lift should be at 50% of the anticipated 1RM, and subsequent lifts should be at 75%, 90%, and 100% of the predicted weight. If the athlete can lift the full weight, additional weight should be added until he or she is unable to perform the lift. The final completed lift is the weight to be recorded as the 1RM. Unfortunately, the more trials one must complete prior to establishing the proper weight of 1RM, the more muscle fatigue possible. This simply means that the 1RM is, at minimum, the weight established. The athlete may be wise to attempt to lift the weight after a sufficient rest and make further adjustments at that time.

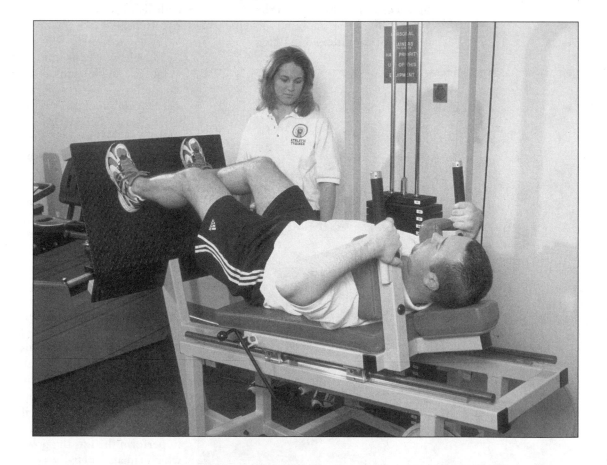

Figure 4.5   The leg press or squat is used to evaluate lower-body strength.

A number of other tests of muscle strength may combine various aspects of muscle fitness—for example, a test of how many times you could bench press 100 lb (45 kg). A test such as this, which evaluates fatigue of the muscle, is considered a test of muscle endurance. If we change the test a little to show how much weight you can bench press 12 times, it becomes more a measure of strength; but it may become a test of endurance if you started with too high or too low a weight and had to lift many more than 10 repetitions. How much weight can be lifted is a measure of strength; how many times it can be lifted is a measure of endurance.

Testing Muscle Endurance and Evaluating Muscle Power

Muscle endurance uses an energy source different from that needed for muscle strength and must be evaluated independently. One can measure endurance of a muscle group to allow sport-specific evaluation of that muscle group; or one can use a general test such as sit-ups or timed push-ups as a test of muscle endurance generally. As an example, if you wanted to evaluate the muscle endurance of a cross country runner's legs, you might use the squat because its combination of joint movements resembles to some extent the use of the legs in running. The athlete would do as many repetitions as possible of the squat exercise at a given weight (a relatively light weight, such as 25 to 45 lb [11.3-20.4 kg]). This test compares performance between athletes and also provides a baseline for further individual evaluation as the season or weight program progresses.

A more general test of muscle endurance is the sit-up test. The athlete does as many bent-knee sit-ups as possible in a set period of time (usually 60 sec). Exact performance issues, such as feet secured or free, are factors to be determined in relation to the abilities of the athlete being tested; test-to-test consistency is, of course, essential.

In terms of exercise, power is the ability to exert a maximal force in as short a period of time as possible, as in the vertical jump.

Cardiovascular Function

Aerobic power involves the ability to utilize oxygen in performing work. Aerobic power relates to most athletic events that require oxygen consumption during performance. Aerobic—"with oxygen"—simply refers to the athlete's use of an energy source that is dependent on oxygen.

Anaerobic—"without oxygen"—power comes into play in activities of very short duration. Activities such as sprints that occur very quickly are often anaerobic; they use a source of energy that does not require as much oxygen. Many sports that entail short spurts of activity involve both the anaerobic and the aerobic systems. The fast break in basketball is typically an anaerobic event, whereas the period of offense or defense in which the ball is moving around the half-court is an aerobic phase.

Evaluating Aerobic Power

We can measure aerobic power without using sophisticated equipment by timing the athlete during a run. One common test, the 1.5-mile (2.4-km) timed run, is an accepted standard for measuring aerobic power. Other tests that can measure aerobic power include the step test and the 2-mile (3.2-km) timed-run test.

Measuring Anaerobic Power

The anaerobic (without oxygen) system can be measured by having an athlete perform an explosive movement such as a vertical jump or a shuttle run (see figure 4.6). Both of these tests are very short in duration and are usually performed anaerobically. The shuttle run can be designed to replicate some of the anaerobic demands of the sport. The subject is asked to run back and forth between two lines (about 20 yd [18.3 m] apart) in the least amount of

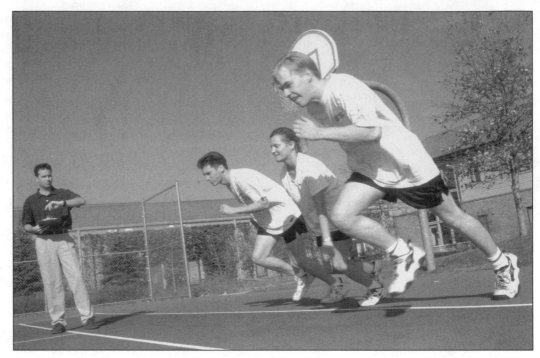

Figure 4.6 The shuttle run replicates some of the anaerobic demands of a sport and is used to test anaerobic power.

Aerobic Tests

Running Tests

Description and procedure: Although there are a variety of tests, each involves running for a set time (9, 10, 12 min) or a set distance (1 mile, 1.5 miles, 2 miles [1.6, 2.4, 3.2 km]), with the distance covered or time required being the result recorded. The time required for these tests normally ranges from 8 to 15 min, depending on the population being tested.

Modifications: In addition to the various times and distances employed for this test, different exercise modes such as swimming can be used.

Norms for males and females for the 1-mile [1.6-km] run and 9-min run are published in the *AAHPERD Manual* (1980). There are some equations that can be used to estimate $\dot{V}O_2$max from performance in these tests: For example, for the 12-min run, $\dot{V}O_2$max (in milligrams per kilogram per minute) = (35.97 3 miles) – 11.29.

Equipment required: Oval or running track, marking cones, recording sheets, stopwatch.

Validity: Cooper (1968) reported a correlation of 0.90 between $\dot{V}O_2$max and the distance covered in a 12-min walk/run. Other published studies generally show a correlation of 0.65 or better for runs greater than 9 min or 1 mile [1.6 km].

Harvard Step Test

Description and procedure: The athlete steps up and down on the platform at a rate of 30 steps per minute for 5 min or until exhaustion. Exhaustion is defined as the inability of the athlete to maintain the stepping rate for 15 sec. Upon completion of the test the athlete immediately sits down, and the heartbeats are counted from 1 to 1.5, from 2 to 2.5, and from 3 to 3.5 min.

Scoring: The score is determined by the following equation: score = (100 × test duration in seconds) divided by 2 × (total heartbeats in the recovery periods). Excellent: 90 or above; good: 80-89; high average: 65-79; low average: 55-64; poor: less than 55.

Equipment required: Step or platform 20 in. (50.8 cm) high, stopwatch, metronome or cadence tape.

Reprinted from Cooper 1968.

Three-Minute Step Test
(Also Known As Queen's College Step Test)

Description: The athlete steps up and down on the platform at a rate of 22 steps per minute for females and 24 steps per minute for males, for a total of 3 min. The athlete immediately stops on completion of the test, and the heartbeats are counted for 15 sec from 5 to 20 sec of recovery.

Equipment required: A 16.25-in. (41.3-cm) step, stopwatch, metronome or cadence tape, heart rate monitor (optional).

From McArdle et al. 1972.

time possible. The number of touches of the line can be chosen according to the demands of the sport. Because the performance frequently improves after the first repetition, the testing protocol often allows the participant to perform the run three times, and the best of the three times is recorded.

Agility and Speed

Agility is the ability to start, stop, and change direction, and evaluating agility is very useful in most sports. Sudden changes in direction of movement involve an element of agility. The shuttle run can be used as a test of agility because of the rapid change in direction inherent in the activity. Speed, on the other hand, does not depend on the subject's ability to change direction, but reflects only the length of time required to travel a set distance.

Testing Agility

Important factors that permit the performance of agility tests include the absence of injury and the use of proper footwear. Agility tests require rapid deceleration, change of direction, and sprinting to the next line; thus individuals with ankle or knee injuries will not perform as well as those who are free of injury. Because these tests are unique, the athlete often needs to learn the pattern to be timed before actually performing the test. Even though the agility test seems to require excellent coordination and speed, a participant at any level could complete it if given sufficient time. The most critical factor in administering an agility test is that you compare the individual's performance to the performance of others who are on a similar level.

Just as it would be foolish to compare the test results for a tennis team with those for a group of same-age football linemen, it would be unwise to compare test data for able-bodied participants with data for athletes who have disabilities.

Many other agility tests have been devised for sport-specific purposes. Many variations are possible, depending on the demands of the sport or the skill of the participant. Two quite different tests are the T-test and the Edgren Side Step test. In the T-test, four cones are set up in a "T" (see figure 4.7). The participant, starting at the bottom of the "T" (cone 1), runs 10 yd (9 m) straight ahead to cone 2, touches its base with the right hand, and then shuffles to the left (5 yd [4.6 m]) to touch cone 3. He or she then immediately shuffles toward the right (past cone 2) 10 yd (9 m) to cone 4, touches it with the right hand, shuffles back to the center to cone 2, touches it with the left hand, and backpedals to the starting point. The timer starts the watch as the subject leaves the starting point and stops the watch as soon as the subject reaches cone 1 on the return.

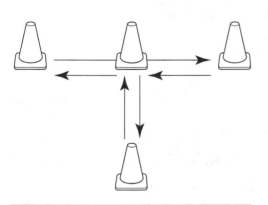

Figure 4.7 The T-test evaluates agility and is good for basketball, volleyball, and other sports that require quick shuffling moves.

The Edgren Side Step test uses an area 12 ft (about 3.6 m) wide, marked off in 3-ft (.9-m) sections (see figure 4.8). The subject sidesteps from the center line outward to the leftmost line (6 ft [1.8 m] away), immediately changes directions, and sidesteps back past the center line and all the way to the right boundary (12 ft [about 3.6 m] away). This side-to-side movement

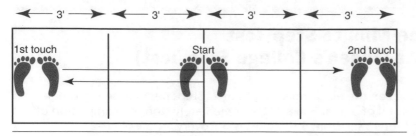

Figure 4.8   The Edgren Side Step test.

is continued for as many touches as possible during a 10-sec period. Each touch of the boundary line is recorded as a point, and any partial distance is recorded as 1/4 point per 3-ft (.9-m) section completed.

There is a good case for the learning effect in some agility tests, as you may even notice when you are the fifth or sixth person to go through a drill and have been able to watch the participants ahead of you. The test of agility will allow for the learning effect; it usually measures the time for completion three or more times and then uses the best of the scores. The examiner can vary these tests by asking the subject to perform a crossover step rather than the side step or by making other footwork changes relevant to the sport.

Measuring Speed

Speed tests involve running, and it is best for athletes to perform them in distances similar to those that occur in the sport. Often sports include short bursts of activity with the athlete sprinting to a position or location. For these sports, one may use a timed dash such as the 40-yd (36.3-m) or 100-yd (91-m) run. In shorter sprint tests, an area for deceleration should be provided so that the athlete is not required to stop suddenly.

Flexibility

Imagine a gymnast bending backward as if there were no limits to the motion, or a football player doing a hamstring stretch that enables him to place his head on his knees. We would consider these individuals flexible. Flexibility is the result of several anatomical factors: joint structure, muscle size, ligament and tendon composition, age, and sex. It is also a result of training. Let's look at each of these factors.

Joint Structure in Relation to Flexibility

The structure of the surfaces of a joint determines the range of motion that a person may achieve. A ball-and-socket joint such as the shoulder or hip is capable of a large range of motion. This movement may be in any of several directions: flexion/extension, abduction/adduction, internal/external rotation, or horizontal adduction/abduction (see figure 4.9). It may also be a movement, called **circumduction,** that combines many other directions of movement.

If the joint is not a ball and socket, it is not capable of circumduction, and it may not be able to move in more than one body plane. As an example, take a **ginglymus** joint, the elbow. Ginglymus is defined in *Stedman's Concise Medical Dictionary* (1994) as "hinge joint; a **uniaxial** joint in which a broad, transversely cylindrical convexity on one bone fits into a corresponding concavity on the other, allowing of motion in one plane only, as in the elbow." The elbow is capable of flexion and extension only. The rotation movement that you may think occurs at the elbow is actually produced by a joint in the forearm. The structure of the joint surface determines the motions available, and from there one can chart the range available in each motion.

Effect of Muscle Size on Flexibility

You have undoubtedly seen people with great muscle mass, so much that it may even appear that they can't put their arms to their sides (adduction of the shoulder joint). Muscle bulk can limit movement; for example, bend your elbow and make a muscle (biceps). Compare the range of motion in your dominant arm to that of your other arm. Is there any difference? Compare the angle of flexion in your elbow against that of someone different in size, strength, or gender. Are there differences?

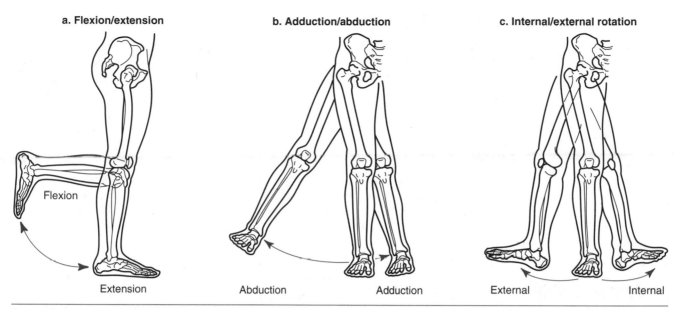

a. Flexion/extension

Flexion

Extension

b. Adduction/abduction

Abduction   Adduction

c. Internal/external rotation

External   Internal

Figure 4.9 Movement directions of knee and hip joints.

Muscles surrounding a joint may grow so large that range of motion is reduced. We have all seen people with so much muscle mass that they appear stiff and immobile. If the individual were actually stiff, the reason would be that the range of motion in the joints has become limited due to excessive bulk. There are two ways this loss of flexibility can be limited or avoided: stretching the same muscle that is strengthened and strengthening the opposite muscles (the **antagonists**). Let's look at those two ways. Stretching a muscle after strengthening will keep the muscle from becoming short and inflexible. A good stretching program should accompany every strengthening program. Strengthening the antagonist muscles along with the strengthening of **agonist** muscles (the muscles producing the action) will help balance the joint forces and reduce the potential for excessive tightness of one of the muscles. If you think about your biceps muscle, as you flex the elbow and contract the biceps (the agonist), then the opposite muscle group, the triceps (antagonist), must relax. If you were to work only the biceps and never work the triceps the result would be like doing a stretch of the triceps and strengthening of the biceps. The elbow may become stiff and unable to fully extend. A well-designed resistance training program incorporates exercise of both the agonistic and the antagonistic muscles to provide a better balance of strength. Thus, there are two ways to alleviate the fear that resistance training will reduce range of motion: (1) Always include a stretching program for all muscles exercised and (2) always exercise both the agonistic muscle group and the antagonistic muscle group in any exercise program.

Effect of Ligament and Tendon Composition on Flexibility

Although all connective tissues are made up of a combination of collagen and **elastin,** some people seem to have more elasticity in their ligaments and tendons than others (see figure 4.10). A quick and easy test for the elasticity of ligaments is to bend your wrist forward and try to passively pull your thumb down to your wrist. (Careful! Don't do this with much force. Just pull gently.) People who can easily put the entire thumb against the surface of the wrist have greater elasticity in their connective tissues (ligaments and tendons).

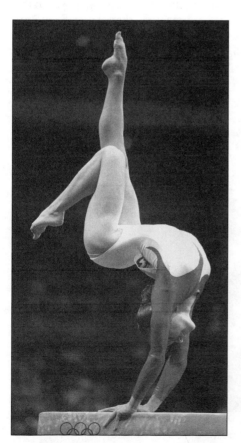

Figure 4.10 A gymnast with extremely elastic connective tissue.
© Sport The Library

Effects of Age and Sex on Flexibility

It is generally thought that females tend to be more flexible than males of the same age and body size, yet these differences are certainly not absolute. People who participate in the kinds of activities that encourage flexibility increase in their ability to stretch regardless of their sex. Likewise, as people age they tend to decrease in flexibility; yet with continued stretching these individuals can delay or actually reverse these effects of aging. Overall, active people have higher levels of flexibility than sedentary individuals.

Testing Flexibility

Evaluation of the individual's flexibility is an important part of the fitness-testing program. A decreased range of motion at a joint may play a role in causing an injury. Take, for instance, an inflexible hamstring muscle. As you run, the hamstring muscle must elongate or stretch to allow the foot to progress to take the next step. If the hamstring is too short or otherwise unable to elongate, the muscle may become injured during strenuous running. Hamstring flexibility is the most standard flexibility element included in fitness evaluations.

One test of hamstring flexibility, the sit-and-reach test, involves sitting on the floor with legs out straight ahead. The athletes' shoeless feet are placed flat against a box that has a yardstick or ruler attached to it. The athlete slowly leans forward as far as possible and holds the greatest stretch for 2 sec. The fingertips will reach a point on the ruler either above or below the level of the box. The ruler helps to quantify the distance. The score is recorded as the distance before (negative) or beyond (positive) the box (see table 4.2). This test is repeated twice, and the best score of the three trials is recorded.

One can devise other similar tests to evaluate flexibility at a particular joint. The key to designing such a test is to position the subject so that other joints are stabilized and there is a way to measure the relative flexibility. For example, for evaluation of the flexibility of the **pectoralis major** muscles, subjects take a supine position (i.e., lie on their back) on a table (see figure 4.11). They are asked to clasp their hands behind their head and then relax their shoulders to allow the elbows to move toward the

Table 4.2
Sit-and-Reach Measurements for Adults

Category	Men	Women
Excellent	+17 to +27	+21 to +30
Good	+6 to +16	+11 to +20
Average	0 to +5	+1 to +10
Fair	–8 to –1	–7 to 0
Poor	–19 to –9	–14 to –8
Very poor	<–20	<–15

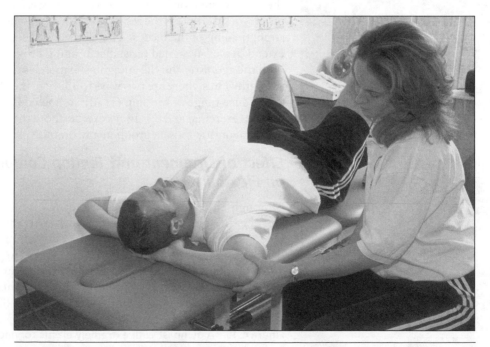

Figure 4.11   This test evaluates the flexibility of the pectoralis major muscles.

table. The test is considered normal if the subject's elbows can touch the table. If the elbows fail to reach the table, the test is positive for pectoralis major tightness. Measurement of the distance between the elbow and the table would further quantify the evaluation. For other tests of range of motion, see the book entitled *Examination of Musculoskeletal Injuries, Second Edition*, in this series.

Height, Weight, and Body Composition

Measurement of an individual's height or weight is sometimes referred to as **anthropometry,** which means measurement of body size. Physical data regarding the athlete's height and weight are commonly used by coaches to determine the position on the team the athlete might be best suited for. Obviously these measures are far from the kinds of measures included in fitness tests, yet some might say that the measure of weight could be directly related to the athlete's level of fitness. Think about a 300-lb (136-kg) football player who returns to school after the summer weighing 355 lb (161 kg). Most individuals, regardless of their physical activity level, would benefit from knowing their height and weight. Some people are able to maintain a suitable weight for their height with little difficulty. Yet athletes may be asked to add weight (football linemen) or reduce weight (gymnasts). Intentional gains and losses should be anticipated, while unexpected changes in weight can be a sign of a medical condition. Rapid changes in body weight should always be reported to a physician. Height and weight data should be collected either in the physical examination or during fitness tests.

Some change in weight is typical when muscle mass increases as a result of strength training. Therefore a test of body composition is more significant. Body composition has to do with the amount of fat in relation to lean tissue in the body. Levels of fat that are too high affect the ability to move the body optimally. Additionally, obesity has been found to be associated with heart disease, high blood pressure, diabetes, arthritis, and some forms of cancer.

Methods of measuring body composition include the use of skin calipers, body mass index, underwater (hydrostatic) weighing, and electric impedance. The most common method is the skinfold method (see figure 4.12). With use of this method, one person trained in taking these measurements should be responsible for all individuals being tested in order to maximize reliability. The specially designed skinfold calipers measure the thickness of folds of tissue. Formulas for analyzing skinfold measures provide an accurate means of calculating the percentage of fat using the data from specific body locations. Depending on the measurement device used, body composition can be an accurate way to determine the amount of lean body tissue in an individual. The average healthy male should have approximately 12% to 18% fat, and the average healthy female approximately 14% to 20% fat. Table 4.3 shows optimal body fat percentages on the basis of age and gender. These values are generally accepted in sport physiology and reflect the averages used by various medical agencies and research groups.

Hydrostatic weighing is a well-established method of estimating an individual's total body fat, but it may not be totally reliable for all ages, sexes, and ethnic backgrounds. In hydrostatic weighing the individual's lung volume is measured, and the person is then submerged in water and weighed. Lung volume and underwater weight are computed using a special equation that yields the body fat percentage.

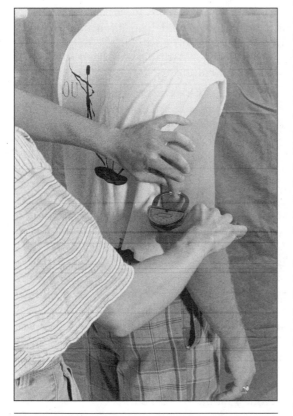

Figure 4.12 Skinfold measures determine an individual's body composition—a way to measure fat versus lean body tissue.

Table 4.3
Optimal Body Composition

Subject's age	Optimal % fat male	Optimal % fat female
<20	15	19
20–29	16	20
30–39	17	21
40–49	19	23
50–59	19	23
60+	20	24

Bioelectrical impedance utilizes **electrodes** attached to the wrists, ankles, or feet. Based on the fact that fat resists electricity, the test measures resistance to the current transmitted by the electrodes. This method of calculating the athlete's total body fat can be quite reliable (yielding reproducible data), but it is less likely than other techniques to be the method of choice because it has less validity (accuracy) and the equipment is less available. Bioelectrical impedance may soon become the preferred method of evaluating an athlete's body composition, however, because of the speed with which the data can be collected and because of the test's reproducibility.

EXERCISE PRESCRIPTION

You would probably not be surprised to hear that there is some debate about the best exercises to use to develop overall strength, aerobic function, and flexibility. Exercises can be highly specific, taxing only one joint in one motion pattern, or can involve several joints, maximizing the large muscle groups. One must consider several factors when establishing an exercise prescription: the results of needs analysis, the setting of goals (including short-term goals, long-term goals, and limitations to the plan), and the exercise plan itself.

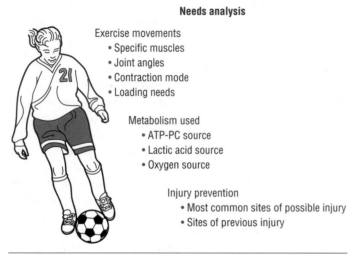

Needs analysis

Exercise movements
• Specific muscles
• Joint angles
• Contraction mode
• Loading needs

Metabolism used
• ATP-PC source
• Lactic acid source
• Oxygen source

Injury prevention
• Most common sites of possible injury
• Sites of previous injury

Figure 4.13   A careful look at what needs to be trained during a conditioning program is called needs analysis.

Adapted from Fleck and Kraemer 1997.

Needs Analysis

Before venturing into the development of an exercise or conditioning program, one should complete a needs analysis (see figure 4.13). Whether the individual is young or older, a beginner or a seasoned athlete, it is advisable to consider the objectives of the program. In forming the objectives, you should take into consideration the fitness demands of the activity as well as the current fitness level of the individual. In establishing the program objectives it may be helpful to answer the following questions as suggested by Fleck and Kraemer (1997):

• What muscle groups should be conditioned?
• What energy system (aerobic vs. anaerobic) should be trained?
• What type of muscle activity (**concentric, eccentric,** or isometric; see figure 4.14) should be used?
• What are the typical sites of injury for the sport? What are the individual's previous injuries?

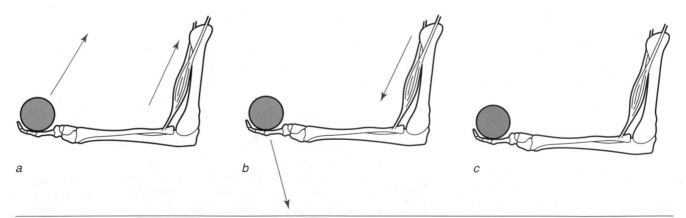

a   *b*   *c*

Figure 4.14   *(a)* During a concentric action, a muscle shortens; *(b)* during an eccentric action, the muscle lengthens in a controlled manner; and *(c)* during an isometric action, no movement of the joint occurs and no shortening or lengthening of the muscle takes place.

Muscle Groups

Two factors come into play when one determines which muscle groups should be exercised: the demands of the sport and the abilities of the individual. An understanding of the physiology and mechanics of the sport and the sport skills is essential in designing the exercise program. If you are very familiar with the sport and the skills it requires, this analysis may be relatively easy; but if not, there is always help. The sport coach is generally the most knowledgeable person regarding what is needed in the sport. Videotapes of practices can be helpful for an understanding of the muscle groups used in particular skills, as can textbooks on sport techniques. This **biomechanical** evaluation of the skills of the sport will direct you toward the muscles used in the sport. Often, in investigating the muscle groups needed, you will begin to answer your fourth question for the needs analysis. You will also begin to understand how the muscles work.

Energy Systems

The analysis of the energy systems used in the sport may not be as clear as you would like. Many sports use short bursts of activity during long periods of participation: For example, basketball players often have a burst of speed as they steal the ball and drive to the basket but then immediately afterward have to run (or jog) back to the other end of the court to play defense. This back-and-forth activity is clearly aerobic overall, yet the bursts of activity at various times during the play may actually be anaerobic. When you find such a combination of energy systems in a sport, you will be wise to include exercises to address both energy systems in the conditioning program.

Muscle Activity

What types of muscle activity should be trained? As already mentioned, you will understand the way the muscle works on the basis of the same information you used to select the muscle groups. The analysis of the skills of the sport allows you to understand the way the muscles are expected to work. A skill that demands a "ready" position will be using the quadriceps muscles in an eccentric capacity. The quadriceps may also be used in a concentric capacity if the athlete is required to jump, for instance. The exclusion of either eccentric or concentric muscle activity would be detrimental to most sport skill development.

Understanding isometric muscle activity is another aspect of understanding how the muscle needs to work—one that is easy to observe. The isometric muscle contraction is used in activities that require a position to be held motionless. For example, gymnasts may be awarded additional points if they are able to hold a position motionless for several seconds. This type of muscle activity—in which there is no joint movement—is isometric activity. Specific training of the involved muscles in an isometric exercise may be needed in a sport skill and should be addressed in the exercise prescription.

Injury Patterns

Understanding the team's injury history may indicate a weakness in the conditioning program. Check with the coach and the team's medical staff to learn the injury trends over past seasons. In addition to the general injury trends for the team, you should understand the injury history of the individual. If a participant in your conditioning program has a preexisting condition, it is necessary to obtain clearance from the person's physician prior to beginning the exercise program.

Goal Setting

Goal setting plays a critical role within the exercise prescription. A program without objectives and goals will usually not last very long. It is easier for people to develop dedication and motivation to continue in an exercise program if they can achieve success during the process. Since success comes from achieving goals, setting the goals is critical. You should make sure that all program participants have formed a set of long-term goals for their participation. Knowledge of these long-term goals will help you more clearly identify ways of progressing toward the goals, and in doing so you will establish the short-term goals.

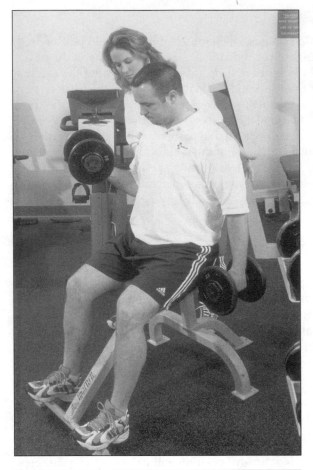

Figure 4.15 Short-term goals are the immediate day-to-day tasks of your participation in the program.

Short-Term Goals

After performing the needs analysis for each athlete, you can establish the short-term goals of the program (see figure 4.15). These goals should be the immediate (individual day) and short-range (month) goals of participation in the program. These short-term goals should contribute to the long-term goal of the program. As an analogy, if your long-range goal is to get a college degree, your daily goals (attending classes, completing assignments) and short-term goals (getting an A on each test and project, earning an A in each course this term) will contribute to your long-term goal of achieving your degree. If you lose sight of the short-term goals, it may still be possible to achieve the long-term goals, but it will be much more difficult.

Long-Term Goals

Each individual must establish his or her own goals for the exercise program. It would be unfair to ask you to dedicate yourself to someone else's goals if you had no interest in the outcome that person wanted. If you don't want your college degree but are trying to get it to satisfy your parents, it will be a long, hard struggle. When people take responsibility for establishing their own personal goals, motivation is more likely to remain high.

Most people would desire "success" as a long-term goal, but success must be more clearly defined in order to serve its purpose as a goal. Encourage all participants to identify specific long-term goals for their participation in the exercise program. Help participants identify exact outcomes they desire through participation. When team athletes set goals pertaining to their position on the team, you must remind them that the purpose of the exercise program is to prepare the body and that the execution of the skills of the sport has to come from the individual.

A solid conditioning program should provide the participant with the muscle strength and endurance to complete sport skill tasks, and it should build the cardiovascular system to allow stamina throughout practice sessions; but the conditioning program cannot be responsible for execution of the right play or for hitting the ball at the correct moment. Guide the participant in establishing performance goals that are measurable and that can be attributed to the conditioning program. Improving performance on a specific fitness test at the end of the season, being able to run 100 yd (91 m) in under x sec after every practice session, or being able increase the vertical jump by the end of the conditioning program would be measurable long-range goals. Depending on the time of the sport season, various exercise plans may be used to aid progress toward the long-term goals.

Limitations to the Plan

There will always be obstacles to a conditioning program: time constraints, availability of facilities or equipment, travel difficulties, and any number of others. Unfortunately, we cannot always avoid the difficulties associated with dedication to an exercise program. Insofar as possible, there should be alternative plans that will allow the participant to achieve the daily, weekly, and monthly goals even if difficulties arise.

A key to one common difficulty, "remote participation," is communication and encouragement. In the world of the Internet, daily progress notes can be exchanged, programs modified, and motivation provided typically without additional cost to the participant. If an individual does not have access to the Internet, it is important to achieve daily or at least weekly communication by some other method. Another potential barrier to dedication is boredom. Unless you provide a stimulating and rewarding program, you will hear more excuses about why someone had to miss a workout than you could have imagined. Just put yourself in the position of the other person, and you should soon see ways to make the program more appealing.

Finally, remember a saying used in management: "People support what they help create." Individuals should be involved throughout the development of the goals and the exercise prescription so that they are able to take ownership in the program's success. "Where there's a will there's a way" is often the motivated participant's motto. Your job will be to help develop that "will."

Exercise Plans

There are a number of strengthening methods, each having its unique benefits. After establishing the needs of the individual, the demands of the activity or sport, the goals of the program, and of course the availability and type of weightlifting equipment, one can develop the exercise plan or prescription. Next we take a look at two concepts associated with various techniques—namely, training volume and exercise order—and at two different types of designs for programs.

• Training volume. Training volume is simply the amount of work performed during a workout, during a week, or during a season. To estimate training volume, calculate the total number of repetitions performed or the total weight lifted. If the individual is seeking to increase muscle mass, frequently the training volume is increased as the program progresses.

• Exercise order. Two of the standard designs for strengthening programs focus on the order in which exercises are performed: the station approach and the circuit-training approach. In the station approach, the participant accomplishes all the sets for a given exercise before moving to the next exercise. This method of ordering exercise is sometimes called horizontal training, while circuit training is sometimes called the vertical training method.

• The station approach. The concept behind the station approach is to maximize the overload on one muscle group before moving on to another exercise. This approach appears to impose a more intense load on the given muscle group, yet the length of rest time between sets may offset the benefits of stacking the repetitions.

• Circuit training. The order of exercise performance in circuit training differs from that of the station approach in that the participant performs only one set of a particular exercise before moving on to the next exercise. This means, for example, that after the first set on the bench press you would move (quickly) to doing biceps curls for one set, then on to triceps extensions, and so on until you have completed one set of all the prescribed exercises. After the first time through the exercises, you begin the circuit again by returning to the first exercise and performing the second set. Participants usually follow the circuit—performing one set of each exercise prior to moving to the next exercise—until they have completed three sets of each exercise.

An aim of sport scientists who popularized the circuit-training approach was to maximize the body's ability to ward off fatigue. The concept behind circuit training is to work a muscle group to near fatigue and then hurry to the next exercise (maintaining the elevated heart rate from the exercise) to work another muscle group. The muscles in the first group are rested somewhat during the subsequent exercise, but the taxing of the cardiovascular system continues.

DEVELOPING THE STRENGTH-TRAINING PROGRAM

When developing the exercise prescription it is necessary to incorporate two essentials into every program: resistance and overload. Even minimal exercise equipment can provide resistance to muscle actions. Handheld weights, machine weights, or elastic bands can offer adequate resistance. Thus resistance may take many forms. On the other hand, overload means only one thing: that the stress or load on the muscle is greater than what the muscle is accustomed to moving.

Now program design can begin. The principal factors to consider are exercise intensity, periodization, progressive overload, and rest periods and training frequency. These will be the components that are manipulated during a training program and as the individual adapts to the training.

Exercise Intensity

The intensity of the exercise being performed is measured using the 1RM performance of the technique. As described earlier in this chapter, the 1RM can be calculated quite easily. This 1RM is then used to determine the amount of weight prescribed in the training program.

Intensity refers to the percentage of the 1RM. Generally the minimal intensity used in a set is 60% to 65% of the 1RM; so if an individual's 1RM for a leg press is 55 lb (25 kg), the minimum intensity used in training would be 30 lb (13.6 kg). If this person were to perform an average number of repetitions of the leg press (10-15) with a low-intensity weight (say 25 lb [11.3 kg]), he or she would undoubtedly show no strength gains. There must be an overload. One must keep intensity of a set in mind when designing progressive overloads.

Two general categories of methods of assigning the exercise intensity are the hypertrophy method (bodybuilding method) and the high-intensity training (HIT) or neurological method. Each has its specific physiological benefits, and selection of one or the other depends on the activity or sport skill as well as the athlete's body structure.

Hypertrophy Method

The objective of hypertrophic training is to increase a muscle's mass (achieve hypertrophy). Muscular hypertrophy is a general increase in bulk of the muscle through increase in the size of individual muscle fibers (but not the number of cells). The program uses between 5 and 12 repetitions, and the amount of weight is 70% to 85% of the 1RM.

The High-Intensity Training Method

In HIT, the intensity reaches up to 100% of the 1RM. The purpose of the HIT method is to improve the recruitment of existing muscle fibers rather than to increase the size of the fibers. Every muscle is made up of muscle fibers. These fibers contribute to the performance of an action depending on the size of the load. The greater the load, the more fibers will be used to perform the task. In HIT, the weight used is from 85% to 100% of the 1RM, and the number of repetitions is between one and four.

In both methods, the intensity or load may be adjusted as the athlete improves. Generally, when the athlete is able to perform the maximum number of repetitions, the weight should be increased. With use of the HIT method, the amount of weight being lifted should be increased if the athlete is able to lift the prescribed weight more than four times. The same concept applies to use of the hypertrophy method; if the athlete can perform more than 12 repetitions, the load must be increased.

Periodization

Just as you would use a different strengthening program in the off-season than during the season, you might find it beneficial to use a different training volume or intensity during one part of the week or month than another. This cycling is known as **periodization.** Periodization is a gradual change in the type, intensity, and amount of training to allow the athlete to achieve optimal gains in strength and power. Slight but safe variations in the position of the hand or foot can produce strength gains, as can the use of several different exercises that work the same muscle group. Periodization incorporates various types of exercises in a logical progression from general to specific throughout the cycles of the competitive season.

Table 4.4
Differences Between Strengthening Methods

Component	Sets	Repetitions	Weight (% max)
Hypertrophy	3-6	8-20	65-80
Strength	3-6	1-6	85-120
Endurance	1-3	10-30+	15-60
Recovery	3-6	8-20	15-60

There are many varieties of periodization programs, but all types have the components of hypertrophy training, strength training, development of power, muscle endurance, and muscle recovery built in (see table 4.4).

Generally the hypertrophy component is trained using three to six sets of 8 to 20 repetitions at about 65% to 80% of the athlete's maximum. Strength training in periodization techniques uses three to six sets of 1 to 6 repetitions at the 85% to 120% level. Endurance training uses from one to three sets of a higher number of repetitions and somewhere from 10 to upward of 30 reps done at the 15% to 60% level. The recovery component of periodization training techniques incorporates three to six sets of 8 to 20 repetitions at a load of about 15% to 60% of the athlete's maximum.

Although varied, all periodization programs also incorporate the timing of implementation of different components in the competitive season and off-season programs. For example, periodization programs utilize the off-season periods for hypertrophy and heavy strength training and avoid heavy loading during the competitive season.

Progressive Overload

Progressive overload refers to a gradual increase in the stress placed on a muscle as it gains strength or endurance. For instance, once you can easily lift 25 lb (11.3 kg) for 10 repetitions on the biceps curl machine, you should add more resistance so that further changes may occur. Therefore your overload would consist of more repetitions or more resistance. This means you would lift 30 lb (13.6 kg) for the same number of repetitions or lift the 25 lb (11.3 kg) 10 more times.

Rest Periods and Training Frequency

Resting between training sessions as well as between exercises or sets is an important component of training. In this discussion the rest period refers to the amount of time between consecutive sets, while the term training frequency refers to the length of time between exercise sessions.

Rest Periods

The rest period between sets depends on the training volume and exercise order and should also reflect the needs and goals of the participant. Individuals training with a high volume (1RM loads) for strength require a longer rest period between sets than if they were training for muscle hypertrophy. Rest periods of 3 to 5 min are not uncommon for the athlete working on absolute strength by lifting the 1RM weight, while a 30- to 60-sec rest is more typical for the athlete working on muscle hypertrophy and doing 8 to 12 repetitions of the exercise with a submaximal weight.

When the exercise order utilizes a longitudinal design as in circuit training, the rest periods should be approximately as long as the period of time spent on the exercise. This 1:1 ratio can help to produce gains in both strength and aerobic endurance but can create a feeling of nausea in some participants. If you are working with someone who is elderly or is deconditioned as a result of illness or other difficulty, it might be wise to begin the circuit-training program using a rest period that is longer than the time required to complete the set. As the individual's fitness level increases, the recovery rate will improve, and you may begin to gradually decrease the length of rest time until the ratio gets down to 1:1. The better the athlete's condition, the less time the person will require between consecutive sets.

Training Frequency

Training frequency, a highly individualized aspect of the total strengthening prescription, should be planned according to several principles.

- Traditionally, participants have done weight training on alternating days (one day of rest between exercise sessions). The intent is to allow sufficient recovery from the exercise session prior to the next session.

- Early in the exercise program, people often experience increased muscle soreness, perhaps because of eccentric contraction (negative phase) of the muscles used. This soreness usually abates after about the second week of the program; but until that time, less frequent lifting sessions may be necessary. If the exercise consists of only concentric muscle activity (**isokinetic** machines), postexercise soreness is usually not a factor, and the exercise frequency can be increased.

- Sessions of multiple-joint exercises require longer recovery periods than sessions utilizing only single-joint exercises.

- With use of maximum (1RM) or near-maximum loads in multiple-joint exercises, the individual requires more recovery time prior to the next heavy lifting day.

- More frequent lifting sessions can be performed with use of a lower training volume on the days between high-volume exercise sessions.

- Persons who have been weightlifting on a regular basis for a long time (years) may benefit from more frequent exercise sessions than those who do not have a long history of strength training.

Taking the individual's strength-training background and short-term goals into consideration, you should be able to devise a suitable training frequency with adequate rest periods in each session.

Power Lifting Versus Weightlifting

Power lifting and weightlifting are actually classified as sports; power lifting is seeking recognition as an Olympic event, petitioning the Olympic Committee the summer of 2004 in Athens, and weightlifting has been an Olympic event consistently since 1920. Power lifting consists of three lifts: the squat (figure 4.16), bench press (figure 4.17), and deadlift. Weightlifting currently consists of two lifts: the clean and jerk (figure 4.18) and the snatch (figure 4.19).

The sports of power lifting and weightlifting have led to an increase in the use of those lifts in the strengthening programs used in other sports. The term "power" may be a point of confusion if interpreted according to its actual, scientific meaning. As you will see, all types of strengthening techniques involve power. In physics, power is a function of time and work. Refer to table 4.5 to review the definitions of work and power from physics.

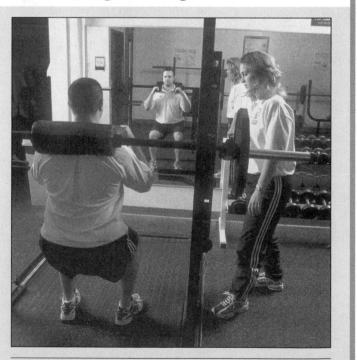

Figure 4.16 The squat.

In terms of strength training, all weightlifting that involves a force, distance, and a velocity can be defined as power training. This points out the major discrepancy between scientific and common definitions of power, which has led to some level of confusion when people discuss power lifting as compared to other forms of resistance training. The major differences are in the exercises performed.

The events of the sport of weightlifting require a large range of joint motion with a component of speed and thus are considered an exercise to build power (although the name implies differently). The clean and jerk exercise and the snatch exercise

Table 4.5
Deriving Power Using Terms From Physics

Term	Definition
Power =	work / time
Work =	force × distance
Power =	force × distance / time
Velocity =	distance / time
Power =	force × velocity

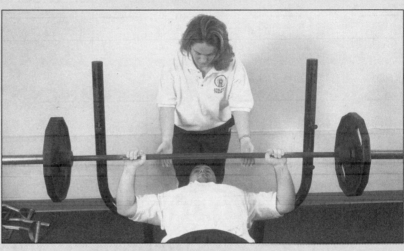

Figure 4.17 Bench press using free weights.

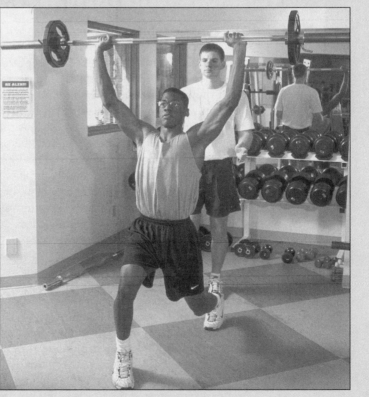

Figure 4.18 A phase of the clean and jerk exercise.

(continued)

are the two events of the sport of weightlifting. Because of the great pressures on the spine and lower extremity, medical professionals are continually discussing health concerns with these lifts. Strength coaches feel that the physician's fears can be diminished if proper lifting technique is observed. The greatest concern is with the athlete who attempts a weight too great for his level of strength, making proper technique difficult to maintain and often resulting in injury to the knees, the spine, or both.

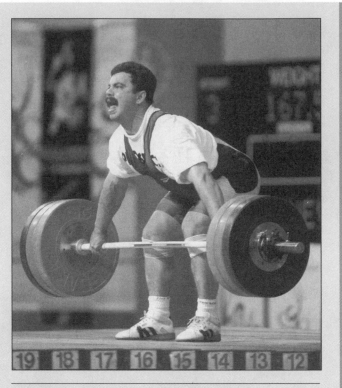

Figure 4.19   The snatch competition.
© Sport The Library

TYPES OF STRENGTH TRAINING

Various types of strength training are used for conditioning as well as in the rehabilitation of an injured athlete. Strength training is only a portion of an individual's overall conditioning program. As one considers the needs of the person and the demands of the sport or activity, specific strength-training types become apparent. Some high-level athletes have suggested that they have attained their level of performance without formal strength training. This is certainly possible for some gifted athletes, but it is not the rule for most people. Some athletes with specialized skills also suggest that they cannot strength train without adverse effects on their skill performance. This may be partially true, especially if the athlete makes gains in strength without simultaneous development of skill patterns; but with attention to skill development, this adverse effect can be controlled. Overall, strength training is an integral part of every athlete's training regimen. Discussed in this section are the common strength-training methods: isometrics, isotonic training, variable resistance, isokinetics, concentric and eccentric training, and plyometrics.

Isometrics

Isometric contraction occurs when the muscle generates a force but there is no joint movement. This means that the resistance is far greater than the athlete is able to move, and thus no movement occurs. There are stories of prisoners who have been able to maintain high levels of strength by performing isometric muscle contractions. Hettinger (1961) published one of the earliest reports of the positive effects of isometric muscle activity, saying that for the best results one should perform multiple sets of maximal or near-maximal muscle contraction held for 3 to 10 sec each. One limitation regarding isometric training is that the strength gains are greatest at the precise joint position at which the contraction was performed; there is only slight overflow of strengthening to the adjacent joint positions.

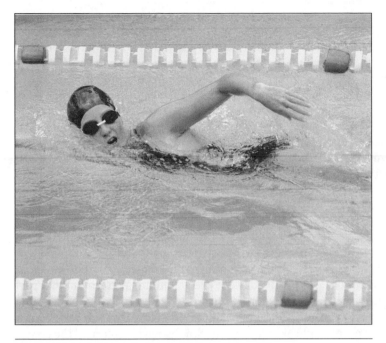

Figure 4.20 Swimmers exercise abdominal muscles strongly, yet large movements of the trunk may not be observed.

Isometric muscle activity is not often applicable to sport performance, yet when you analyze the performance of wrestlers and gymnasts, you may see application of isometric muscle strengthening. In addition to the holding of a position as in wrestling and gymnastics, in other sports some muscles act in a very limited range that appears nearly isometric. For example, in swimming, the abdominal muscles are exercised very strongly, yet there may not be large movements of the trunk (see figure 4.20). Running also taxes the abdominal and back muscles without significant excursions in the range of motion of the trunk.

Although isometric muscle activity can be done in virtually any setting and with virtually no equipment, it may not be a wise choice for a strengthening program, mainly because of the difficulty in measuring the overload. Without some feedback on muscle performance, the athlete's motivation may decline and thus directly affect the overload applied. If the athlete fails to produce a maximal contraction, an increase in the time the contraction is held may still not sufficiently overload the muscle; thus there will be little or no change in muscle performance.

Isotonic Training

Isotonic muscle activity involves moving the joint through a range of motion with a set amount of resistance applied. Isotonic muscle activity occurs in lifting free weights, as well as in the performance of most activities of daily living. For example, as you stand up from your chair you may need to reach down and pick up your backpack. As you reach for the pack, you will extend your elbow to its maximum position. As you raise the pack toward your shoulder, your elbow will begin to bend. This activity is an isotonic exercise because the weight does not change while your limb moves through a range of motion.

If you have ever had to move heavy objects from one place to another, you may have found that the loads you can carry are much heavier than the loads you can pick up. You may be able to take a 100-lb (45-kg) box off a waist-high counter and carry it to another counter, but if that 100-lb box is in the trunk of your car you may not be able to lift it up. This illustrates one of the primary difficulties in isotonic strengthening.

There are points in the range of every joint where the muscle is at its weakest. At other points (usually in the middle of the joint action), the muscle is at its strongest position. These points make up what is called a strength curve, which illustrates why you can carry the box from counter to counter but cannot lift it out of the trunk of the car.

Variable Resistance

Variable resistance was first introduced in the 1970s by the Nautilus Corporation. Nautilus used an offset cam to deliver a variation in the resistance to the movement. The cam was designed to maximize the strength at various points in the range of motion as suggested in the strength curve. The variable-resistance machines using the cam system tended to be quite expensive, so some manufacturers developed the sliding lever bar systems and others brought out various forms of elastics or large rubber bands.

The rubber band or elastic tubing provides increased resistance as the band is elongated. These very portable and inexpensive devices gained favor for patients in rehabilitation as well as for persons with a limited budget or limited space.

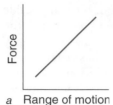

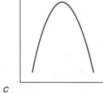

a Range of motion

b

c

Figure 4.21 The three major strength curves are *(a)* ascending, *(b)* descending, and *(c)* bell shaped. The resistance varies throughout the exercise.

Reprinted from Fleck and Kraemer 2004.

Isokinetics

Isokinetics refers to a muscular action performed at a constant velocity. In other words, an isokinetics (or accommodating resistance) machine uses shock absorbers, hydraulics, or a braking system to provide a maximum resistance through the entire range of joint movement. Isokinetic ("iso" means "same"; "kinetic" means "speed") machines are typically very expensive and are used most often in rehabilitation. Some isokinetic machines are capable of extremely high angular velocity (up to 1,000°/sec). The theory behind isokinetics is that the muscle has a varied capacity (strength curve) as well as being capable of very high speeds of joint movement (see figure 4.21). Some models of isokinetics even provide ways to adjust the type of muscle contraction being produced.

Concentric and Eccentric Training

If you were to analyze a sport activity, you would probably find that it involves both a concentric phase and an eccentric phase. Are there any sports or sport skills you can name that involve only concentric muscle activity? Consider wrestling, swimming, gymnastics, and golf. Does each involve eccentric muscle activity? If so, what specific motor pattern or what part of the motor pattern produces the eccentric contraction?

The type of muscle contraction performed is important in the selection of exercise equipment. Muscles can contract concentrically or eccentrically. Studies have implicated the eccentric phase of muscle activity as the cause of postexercise muscle soreness, yet eccentrics are also said to have a greater effect on strength development.

Concentric Muscle Activity

Concentric muscle activity occurs when the limb moves through a range of motion with a resistance applied. This concentric phase of the lifting movement involves a shortening of the muscle during the movement. This muscle action is the force-production part of almost every human movement. The only exercises that do not include concentric muscle activity are those exercises designed specifically to tax the muscle in an exclusively eccentric manner—and in those cases the "positive" or concentric movement is accomplished by an external force (another person or, in rehabilitation cases, the uninvolved extremity).

Eccentric Muscle Activity

The lowering of the weight produces a lengthening of the muscle while it is contracting. This lengthening contraction is called an eccentric muscle contraction. Some people describe eccentrics in terms of gravity, suggesting that most weights that are lifted are lifted away from the pull of gravity. This lifting away from the gravitational pull is the concentric phase, while the lowering back to the starting position involves contraction by the same muscle as it elongates. The muscle must generate force, even though it is working with the gravitational pull, to achieve a slow and controlled descent.

Eccentric muscle contraction does not occur in all forms of isokinetic exercise (some isokinetic machines do allow eccentric contractions), nor will proprioceptive neuromuscular facilitation exercises and manual resistance exercises provide eccentric contraction without some specific adaptations. Most other weightlifting machines utilize an eccentric phase, as do all forms of body weight conditioning (push-ups, pull-ups, sit-ups, etc.).

Plyometrics

Plyometrics, which is becoming known as "stretch–shortening cycle exercise," replicates many aspects of physical activity (see figure 4.22). The stretch phase is an eccentric loading phase of the exercise, while the shortening phase is the force-producing or concentric phase. Most physical activity relies heavily on this type of muscle activity. Imagine for a moment a very slow-motion film of a tennis player hitting a backhand shot. As the ball contacts the racket, the player absorbs the force of the ball (eccentric phase). Then for a split second the

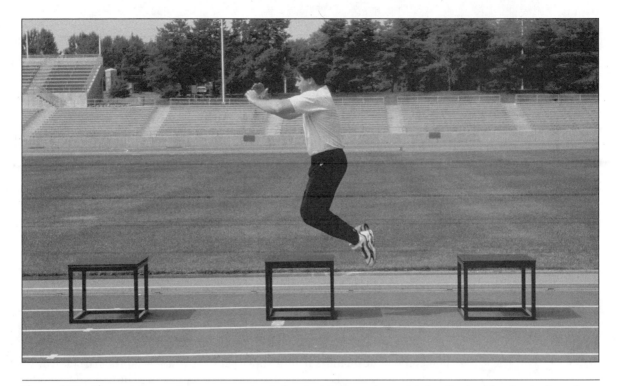

Figure 4.22 Plyometric exercises are composed of a stretch phase (eccentric loading) and a shortening phase (concentric or force producing).

movement stops (isometric); this is followed immediately by a production of force imparted to the ball (concentric), sending it on its way toward the opponent. Every physical activity incorporates the stretch–shortening cycle, making a strong case for the use of plyometrics in the training program.

Stretch–shortening cycle exercise can take many forms. It can be used as part of a rehabilitation program or can be part of an exercise program to prepare for specialized skill performance. The critical feature of this type of exercise is that there is a concentric force production following every eccentric load absorption. For example, in-depth jump training is a form of plyometrics that has been used to increase leg power. The technique utilizes two boxes; the participant stands on one box and steps off it, lands on the ground between the two boxes, and springs back upward to land on the top of the other box. This early form of plyometric training continues to be a cornerstone in many training programs but is not suitable for individuals weighing over 220 lb (100 kg).

The principles underlying the stretch–shortening concept were introduced by two physical therapists named Knott and Voss. They found that when a muscle was stretched prior to the onset of a contraction, the contraction was greater than it would have been otherwise. They used this technique to help weakened patients perform motor activity. The preliminary stretch of a contractile unit (muscle and tendon) stimulates a muscle contraction greater than would be produced by a contractile unit at the normal resting length.

There are many variations of stretch–shortening cycle exercise, making success possible for participants of every fitness level. Low-load plyometrics can be used with athletes who are disabled, allowing them increased power and in some cases increased dynamic stability. A simple exercise on a slide-board can be used as a low-load plyometric. If the participant can manage to slide to one end of the board and then slide back, the momentum of the slide will serve as the stretch phase as the exerciser makes contact with the end of the board. After the shock absorption, the kinetic energy is released as the shortening phase produces movement in the opposite direction. Progressively advanced exercises can be found in many texts on plyometrics.

EQUIPMENT SELECTION

There are as many ways to develop strength as there are muscles to strengthen. The saying "Necessity is the mother of invention" applies to the development of strength no less than to life in general. Individuals must gain an understanding of the biomechanics of the sport or activity of interest and then attempt to find specific exercises in order to challenge the relevant muscles to adapt. As the strength coach of the Pittsburgh Steelers, Chet Furman, stated (personal communication), "No matter what [technique] you use, the athlete will adapt to that particular lifting technique." That is, if you challenge your athletes to bench press with dumbbells, they will improve in the dumbbell bench. If you challenge them to bench press with a barbell, they will improve in the barbell bench. It would be ideal to be able to pick and choose the apparatus to use to exercise the muscle group or perform the activity of interest, but the reality is that selection probably depends more on the equipment available. Local health clubs might offer the greatest variety of machine and free-weight equipment, while a high school may have only a few multistation machines. From among a great number of types of equipment, we will look at a few of the more common machines and types of strengthening apparatus.

Free Weights

As you should be able to predict, the simplest strength-training equipment is free weights. The equipment includes handheld barbells, weight plates, the barbell bar, weight collars to secure the weight plate to the bar, and a variety of benches and racks. The lifting facility should have a rubberized floor that can resist repeated impacts of dropped weights; it should be equipped with mirrors so that athletes can observe their technique, and there should be chalk for athletes to use to decrease friction in their hands. Facilities with limited budgets may be able to purchase a range of dumbbells, weight plates, and bars to allow the athletes at least some variety.

Conditioning Program for Running

Almost every land sport requires some component of running. Sports such as soccer and track events require much more running than sports like volleyball or golf. No matter how much running the sport involves, running remains one of the best forms of cardiovascular conditioning for athletes.

In this conditioning program, "running" refers to the track event and not merely to the running component of many sports. Many of the suggestions within this program can also be applied to the development of running stamina for other sports.

Aerobic Conditioning for Running

Running is an aerobic sport and needs to be performed daily if one competes as a runner. However, a certain amount of cross-training (such as on a bike or stair climber) would be a good idea two or three days per week to encourage balance in muscle development. In addition, sprints and form running drills should be performed to enhance speed and technique. Running workouts are classified according to competition distance. The ultralong-distance day is distance 50% longer than the typical running distance of competition; the long day is distance 25% longer; the medium day is distance 25% less than the competition distance; and the short day is distance 50% less.

When an athlete is training for cardiovascular fitness for a specific sport, it may be advantageous to use the maximum distance of any given "sprint" involved in the sport and multiply that distance times the typical number of "sprints" that may be run during a "session." This becomes the training or target distance. For example, if the person is training for soccer, his or her position may call for 75-m sprints, and an approximate total of six sprints may occur before a situation occurs when the athlete may rest. The training program would be based on 6 × 50 m. In establishing the "ultralong" distance, one would add 50% more to the normal workout for a total of nine sets of 50-m sprints. Other adjustments should be made accordingly by changing the number of repetitions of the distance rather than the sprint distance itself.

Beginning Strength Training

The beginning program is typically four to six weeks long. The athlete would be asked to perform three sets of 12 to 15 repetitions (perhaps with adjustment depending on the strength-training philosophy). Strength training would follow either the sport schedule or would take place at least two days per week. Table 4.6 lists suggested exercises to choose from. Alternating the focus of the program each lifting day will prevent excessive use of any one muscle group. Each lifting day should include three exercises for the lower body, two for the upper body, and one each for the back and abdomen.

Table 4.6
Strengthening Exercises for Runners

Lower body	Abdominal muscles	Lower back	Upper body
Back squats	Sit-ups	Hyperextensions	Bench press
Leg press	Crunches	Shoulder shrugs	Standing military press
Standing calf raises	Cross-knee crunches		Bent-over rows
Seated calf raises	Knee-ups		
	Hanging leg raises		

Advanced Strength Training

After four to six weeks on the beginning strength-training program, athletes can usually progress to a more advanced set of exercises. A strength workout two to three times per week is generally sufficient unless the sport conditioning program requires more. Table 4.7 lists suggested exercise choices.

Table 4.7
Advanced Strengthening Exercises for Runners

Lower body	Abdominal muscles	Lower back	Upper body
Back squats	Sit-ups	Hyperextensions	Bench press
Lunges	Crunches	Good mornings, standing	Bench press with dumbbells
Leg press	Cross-knee crunches	Stiff-legged deadlifts	Standing military press*
Seated calf raises	Knee-ups	Bent-over rows	Shoulder press with dumbbells*
Standing calf raises	Hanging leg raises	Shoulder shrugs with dumbbells	Rear lateral raises
Leg press calf raises			

*Avoid if impingement symptoms arise.

(continued)

Flexibility

Flexibility is especially critical when one is lifting and running, both of which are quite important in this program. Stretching exercises should be performed once the muscles are warm and prior to activity, and also at least once again at the conclusion of the running or strength-training workout. Suggested muscle groups to be stretched and suggested stretching exercises are listed in table 4.8.

Table 4.8
Suggested Flexibility Exercises for Runners

Abdomen and back muscles	Press-ups (abdominal muscles)	Back stretch (spine)
Hamstrings	Seated hamstring stretch	Standing hamstring stretch
Quadriceps and hip flexors	Hurdler stretch	Standing quad stretch
Groin muscles (adductors)	V-stretch	Butterfly stretch
Back of leg (gastrocnemius/soleus)	Calf stretch, standing	Bent-knee calf stretch

Strength-Training Machines

The machine approach to strength training can be less expensive than having a variety of free weights if the choice is a multistation unit (see figure 4.23). Many manufacturers offer equipment that allows people to do a wide variety of exercises with minimal setup. These multistation gyms are often safer for young athletes because there is no chance of dropping a weight on their foot or chest. Multistation gyms may not provide an adequate range of exercises for all sizes of athletes (from the smallest gymnast to the largest football player) or for all strength levels.

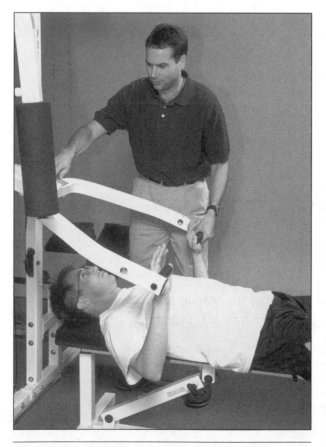

Young athletes who lack body control would be wise to begin the strengthening routine using machine weights. Caution is in order when the skeletally immature athlete embarks on any weight-training program. The immature athlete has open growth plates, and heavy weightlifting could adversely affect bone growth. For the skeletally mature athlete, machine weight training may be preferable to the use of free weights because it can be more highly individualized. When lifting with barbells, a partner needs to be spotting to ensure the lifter's safety.

Individual Machines

Many companies offer individual machines for performing specific joint actions or strengthening particular muscle groups. Depending on their design, these machines may provide isotonic exercise, variable resistance, accommodating resistance, or isokinetic resistance. It can be cost-effective to have a machine that allows more than one joint action. In general, a number of specialized weight-training machines take up more space and cost more than free weights. The major benefit of the individual machines is the ability to exercise an individual joint action or muscle group.

Figure 4.23 Multistation gyms are often safer for young athletes but may not provide an adequate range of exercises for all sizes of athletes.

Other Equipment

Depending on the level of creativity of the strength coach or exerciser, the potential for strengthening particular muscles can be limitless. Performing the bench press may be quite easy for a particular athlete, but when you ask him or her to balance on a Swiss ball in a push-up position, the pectoralis major muscle meets more of a challenge (see figure 4.24). Functional activities have long been used in the rehabilitation of athletes and certainly have a place in the conditioning of the noninjured athlete as well. These functional activities include many sportlike skills performed under heavier demands than normal. For example, to strengthen the rotator cuff muscles one could use a weighted ball (plyo ball): The athlete sits with elbow resting on a table, catches the ball, and immediately tosses it back using just the shoulder rotators. The plyo ball is useful for the development of upper-body strength, coordination, **proprioception,** and explosive power. Elastics such as tubing can be used, as a system or as an individual band, for resistance training. People often use elastics for strengthening during rehabilitation because of the resistance the elastic provides to both concentric and eccentric muscle activity.

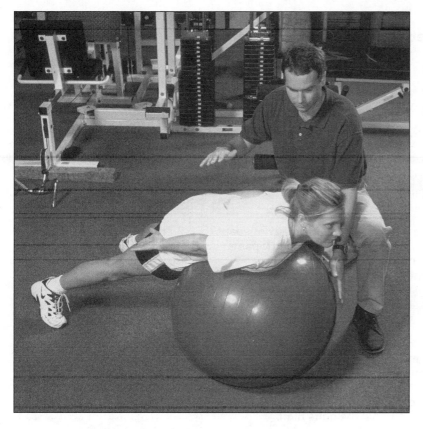

Figure 4.24 Swiss balls are useful for developing upper-body strength, coordination, proprioception, and explosive power.

Swimming or pool work is also excellent for strengthening when the resistance of the extremity is increased by the use of paddles or other devices. Milk jugs filled with sand or water work as free weights. Again, the number of ways the creative coach can find to exercise specific muscles is limitless. Keeping an open mind and an observant eye will help you design exercises to challenge athletes. First try the exercise yourself to ensure that the proper muscle is being worked and that the exercise is safe, and then teach it to the athlete. Variety can be the key in maintaining a young person's interest and motivation.

A Comparison of Equipment Types

You know that the development of strength depends on the application of some form of resistance in sufficient quantity to overload the muscle, and you know the methods of strengthening as well as the types of muscle contraction that are possible. How do use of free weights and use of machines compare as strengthening methods?

Most believe that strength training using free weights has advantages over the use of machines in that lifting with free weights requires a degree of balance, proprioception, and coordination. You have to have good balance to maintain an erect posture when you lift a loaded bar overhead. In addition, you need to have good proprioception in order to know the position of your arms overhead, allowing the best mechanical advantage for the lift. Finally, you must move the bar in a smooth and coordinated manner to avoid injury and to achieve success.

When doing an overhead press on a machine, you do not need the same degree of balance and coordination. You need to position the seat properly to provide the best mechanics for the lift—and then sit down and start working! The machines do offer a great advantage when range of motion is limited, as in a rehabilitation program, or for athletes who have disabilities. The pin used to select the number of plates to be lifted can be placed so that the machine will not go through its entire excursion, sparing the limb from the full range

Table 4.9
A Comparison of Strengthening Methods and Equipment Types

Strengthening mode	Advantages	Disadvantages	Comments
Free weights	Allows great flexibility in program design. Use may contribute to balance and coordination development. Well-planned purchase can provide sufficient equipment for small team.	Can be costly to provide sufficient equipment and supplies for multiple teams or large facility.	Supervision is essential. Not safe for individuals with poor body control unless one-on-one supervision is possible.
Machine weight stations	Safe for individuals lacking body control. Can isolate muscle groups. Supervision not essential to program.	Machines may not adapt to all sizes of participants. Does not develop coordination and balance.	Very safe. Excellent for facility where supervision is not always present. Good choice for general use and for those unfamiliar with weightlifting.
Individual weight machines	Some machines can isolate specific muscles and muscle actions (eccentric, concentric, isometric). All individual machines allow joint-specific exercise.	Large space required for the number of machines needed for a total-body program. Cost of individual units can be quite high.	Can be excellent supplement to other equipment due to the specificity of action for each machine.
Sportlike functional skills	Builds sport-specific strength. Promotes development of balance and coordination. Less stress on growth plates when body weight is used rather than external weight.	Does not develop antagonistic muscles. Difficult to learn the techniques and to master the exercises.	Allows functional strengthening without the need for expensive equipment. Can be used for athletes with disabilities to promote body control and balance.

of movement. For a summary of the various types of strengthening methods and equipment types, see table 4.9.

INTEGRATING OTHER FITNESS COMPONENTS

Suppose that you are lifting in the weight room and that friends come by to coax you into playing some basketball. You can probably imagine how your regular jump shot would feel if you had just finished three intense sets on the bench press. The basketball would feel light as a feather, and you would have a tendency to overshoot the basket. This same concept applies to weight training during the season and illustrates the importance of a good balance between lifting and skill performance.

Aerobic Endurance Training

The cardiovascular system is a cornerstone to physical activity. Nearly every recreational or sport activity requires some degree of cardiovascular, or aerobic, endurance. For decades the positive benefits of exercise have been well understood and accepted by those in the fitness and exercise physiology fields. Efforts to employ those concepts and promote physical activity in the American public has been a challenge undertaken nationally by the Surgeon General as well as the President's Council on Physical Fitness and Sports. As a health care provider, you should make it your goal to help promote physical fitness. The challenge then is to develop a rational program that must start with an understanding of the participant's current fitness level.

When the participant's fitness status is in any way questionable, or, at the other end of the spectrum, when the individual is in top physical condition, the best method for establishing fitness level is to use a cardiovascular stress test. One can design an aerobic conditioning program for young, healthy individuals by using data from fitness tests such as the 1.5-mile (2.4-km) or 2-mile (3.2-km) run test referred to earlier. Whichever method you use, you can determine the subject's maximal heart rate and general level of fitness. If the heart rate data are not available, you can estimate maximal heart rate by subtracting the individual's age from 220.

The recommendation in the ACSM position statement is an exercise intensity for aerobic conditioning between 60% and 90% of the maximal heart rate (or 50-80% of the $\dot{V}O_2$max obtained in a stress test). The training should be performed at a minimum frequency of three days per week and should last for 20 to 60 min each session.

The body's response to cardiovascular (endurance) training is an increased stroke volume (at rest as well as during exercise) and increased blood volume. The stroke volume is basically the volume of blood pumped out of the heart per stroke. This increase may be due to a slower heart rate that gives the heart more time for filling, or it may be due to an increase in the strength of the heart muscle (myocardium). The increased blood volume that occurs with training is a factor in the increase in stroke volume in that with an increase in the capacity of the heart the increased blood volume allows more blood to be pumped out per beat with fewer beats required to provide ample blood to the tissues. Thus, the changes that occur with training are all interdependent. These adaptations occur quite quickly during endurance training; however, they are also quite short-lived should the endurance training be discontinued.

Common sense dictates that if you are working with people who have a very low level of fitness and who are beginning an aerobic conditioning program, you should start them with an activity that allows them to reach and maintain at least 60% of their maximal heart rate and to sustain that pace (and heart rate) for at least 20 min. People who start the program with a higher level of fitness need more intense exercise in order to reach the desired heart rate; for these individuals, you may want to set a training heart rate goal of 70% of the maximal, or have them sustain this rate for longer than 20 min, or both.

Design of an aerobic conditioning program follows the same principles as for a program for muscle training: An overload is required. Your cardiovascular endurance program should encompass a short-term goal (the goal for the day, the week, or the month), as well as a long-term goal (goal of the program), and should move from one goal to the next in a logical and steady progression (see figure 4.25). A key to helping new exercisers stay with a program is to have them start at a low enough level to be training the aerobic system without overexertion; this will help keep them from giving up. Another good way to keep people motivated for cardiovascular exercise is to vary the program. Varying the use of the treadmill, stepper

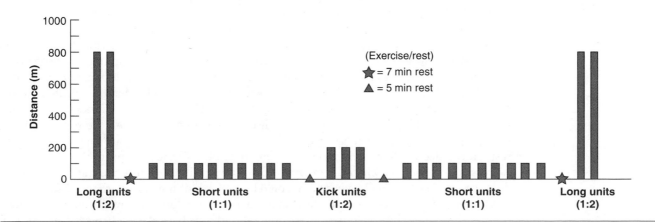

Figure 4.25 A sample power-unit workout for the development of aerobic and anaerobic capabilities. The units are performed on a grass field, four times a week, with a ratio of work time to rest time of 1:2 (i.e., if it takes the athlete 20 sec to sprint the distance, the rest period would be 40 sec).

Reprinted from Fleck and Kraemer 2004.

machine, elliptical apparatus, pool, or bike in achieving and maintaining the heart rate to achieve cardiovascular conditioning can do this. Some people can work at a seemingly high effort level for long periods of time and never reach the target heart rate while doing particular exercises. But it is essential to pay attention to the heart rate responses to exercise, no matter what activity is chosen.

Anaerobic Training

Anaerobic training is not as universally required as aerobic training, yet it plays a critical role in most activities and especially in sport participation. Sport skills often involve both anaerobic muscle activity and anaerobic cardiovascular work. Here we consider anaerobic cardiovascular training only.

Events that take between 1 and 5 min to complete require use of a combination of the aerobic and anaerobic systems. On the 1-min side of the spectrum, energy is produced by both systems in a 50-50 aerobic-anaerobic mix; as you move closer to the 5-min duration for the event, the aerobic system plays a greater role and the anaerobic system a lesser role in energy production. This means that most physical activity requires some amount of anaerobic metabolism (energy production) as well as some aerobic metabolism. Thus it is important to train both metabolic systems.

Anaerobic cardiovascular work means energy production by the body in the absence of oxygen. Training to improve the anaerobic system requires short, intense bursts of activity, and that activity should be sport specific. For example, if you are a water polo player, you will want to do sprint training to increase your anaerobic endurance. But running sprints will not be as beneficial to your sport performance as swimming sprints.

Anaerobic training can be accomplished by running short, intense sprints or by performing short, intense bouts on the slide-board, bicycle, step-up equipment, and so on. High-intensity, near-maximal exercise is impossible to sustain for long periods of time because it leads to exhaustion; therefore some period of rest is needed to allow the body to recover. Interval training does just that. Rather than using total rest between sets, participants can combine aerobic and anaerobic conditioning by alternating easy, submaximal exertion with hard, near-maximal output. Whichever way one chooses to use to train the anaerobic system, a key principle is that high-intensity, short-duration activity builds the anaerobic system but leads to exhaustion and cannot be sustained for long periods of time.

While everyone needs regular, moderately vigorous exercise, high-intensity exercise is primarily for people with a moderate level of fitness who want to improve this aspect of their conditioning. It is not appropriate for older individuals or others who have low fitness levels, or for anyone who might risk injury doing exercise at high intensity. Since high-intensity exercise means very high heart rates, persons at risk for cardiovascular disease should be carefully screened by their health care provider before entering into an interval or sprint training program. Many people who have their physician's endorsement for low- to moderate-intensity exercise may not be approved for high-intensity exercise.

People who are well prepared for an interval program must start out at a safe level and then progress, just as with every other part of the fitness program. At the beginning of an anaerobic or interval training program, the participant might run a set distance at maximum capacity (speed) and then jog back to the start. This sprint/jog cycle would then be repeated, say 10 times, before fatigue causes the person to stop. To make the program progressive, you change one of two variables: You can increase the distance sprinted or decrease the rest (jog) time. Interval programs are much easier to do on a track or other continuous path so that as the rest interval decreases the next sprint can begin regardless of the distance to the starting line. A cross country runner who does intervals could use a trail. Obviously the trail will not have distances marked off, so the work bout would be a length of time rather than a distance.

Often it is advantageous to vary the distance of the sprint during the workout. For example, assume that your physical fitness is fairly good and you have decided to start an interval program. The first day you might run a total of 2,500 m (2,734 yd; half of your average daily run) because you realize that if you are adding interval training to your exercise program, you will be exercising for shorter durations. After warming up and stretching, you may decide to start with 200-m (219-yd) runs at about 80% of your top speed. You run the 200 (30 sec) and then jog for about 30 sec; you then repeat this pattern seven times (total run is now 1,600 m [1,750 yd]). Next you do 10 intervals of 100 m (109 yd) with a 10-sec jog between repeats. That adds another 1,000 m (1,093 yd) to the total—and that is about what your workout was supposed to be. As your conditioning improves, you will increase your speed in the sprints (if possible) or decrease the jog cycle. You can accomplish both in that the faster you run, the less time it takes to achieve the distance and therefore the recovery time does not have to be quite as long. Keeping an accurate record of the number and distance (or time) of the reps will aid you in developing your progression.

In designing a progression in interval training, always increase the training volume gradually in order to avoid injury. A rule of thumb is to increase your training volume (mileage or time spent) by no more than 10% per week. Do not increase at all if injury or signs of overtraining are present. Signs of overtraining include fatigue, depression, irritability, insomnia, increase in resting heart rate, muscle pain, joint pain, overuse injuries, decline in athletic performance, and unexplained weight loss.

Because HIT is physically and psychologically demanding, many athletes alternate interval training days with days of rest or with days of more moderately paced exercise.

Flexibility/Stretching Programs

You may have heard a coach or a friend say that good muscle flexibility will decrease the chance of an injury. This concept is not strongly supported by research, yet many people insist that the only reason they have avoided serious injury is that they have an appropriate level of flexibility. When you consider that many injuries occur because a joint is forced beyond the range of motion it is capable of, you might suspect that flexibility could have a role in injury prevention.

In rehabilitation, stretching techniques are often central to achieving the therapeutic objectives. Therapeutic modalities—machines using electrical currents to aid tissue healing—are employed to increase the elastic properties of soft tissues. This concept and other methods of affecting the tissues are presented in the third text in this series, *Therapeutic Modalities for Musculoskeletal Injuries, Second Edition*. The use of stretching as a treatment technique following injury is addressed in the fourth text, *Therapeutic Exercise for Musculoskeletal Injuries, Second Edition*. In addition to the use of stretching for injury management, there are a variety of techniques that coaches and athletes employ to increase flexibility to enhance sport performance and prevent injury (see figure 4.26). Some of the most commonly used stretching methods are passive stretching, active stretching, and contract or relax stretching.

Passive Stretching

As the name implies, passive stretching entails no work on the part of the individual. The athlete relaxes while someone else carries the limb through a particular range of motion. Athletic trainers and physical therapists often utilize passive stretching to assist in the athlete's recovery after injury. The passive stretching technique requires that the assistant understand the meaning of muscle tension. An unskilled person may think that the stretch should be taken further into the range of motion than is safe, and this can actually damage muscle tissue. Passive stretching should be performed by people who have had training and experience in placing the athlete in a stretching position.

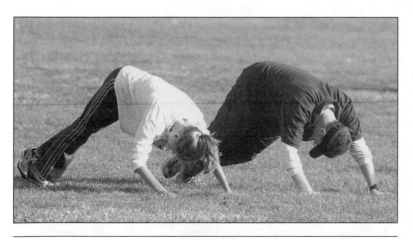

Figure 4.26   Stretching can take many forms.

Active Stretching

Again, the term "active stretching" is self-explanatory: The athlete takes an active role in the stretching. Most athletes develop a ritual of stretches they like to do to prepare for activity. Usually they warm up prior to beginning the stretching program and then take anywhere from 10 to 30 min to loosen up sufficiently.

In active stretching, the athlete uses his or her own body to produce the stretch of the particular area. For example, calf stretching can be done standing up, and the athlete's body weight and strength produce the range of motion. This muscle group is stretched more easily with the active technique than with the passive method. All forms of stretching have a place in the total development of the athlete.

Contract/Relax Stretching

In contract/relax stretching, the athlete works with a partner or therapist who both provides the resistance to the contraction and stretches the muscle group. Contract/relax stretching can be done in any movement plane. For example, contract/relax stretching of the hamstrings is much like the passive stretching except that during the contract phase, the athlete activates the hamstrings and **gluteals,** trying to extend (push down) at the hip joint. People who use contract/relax stretching feel that the contraction of the muscle prior to stretching allows the muscle to more fully relax during the stretching cycle.

Contract/relax stretching is very useful for athletes who have a difficult time relaxing during a passive stretch. The preliminary contraction helps to decrease anxiety and the discomfort of the stretch.

Proprioceptive Neuromuscular Facilitation

Proprioceptive neuromuscular facilitation (PNF) is a specialized technique of therapy that incorporates some stretching. In the strict sense, PNF requires that three movements occur in the extremity: flexion/extension, abduction/adduction, and rotation. The PNF "contract/relax" stretching is performed in a diagonal pattern so that all three components of the motion can be performed. This technique requires a good understanding of the diagonal patterns, the points of resistance, and the manual contacts during the stretching. It's important to realize that contract/relax stretching utilizes a single, straight plane of motion while PNF employs diagonal patterns of movement traversing three planes of movement.

Stretching Methods

In addition to active, passive, and contract/relax stretching, the ways in which a muscle or other connective tissue is stretched are classified into static, dynamic, and ballistic. Static stretching is a technique whereby the joint is moved to the point at which tightness is felt and that position is held. This static position of stretch is beneficial if the stretch can be held for up to about 30 sec. If it is possible to hold the stretch for a longer period of time, the deformation of the tissue is greater and the tissue is less apt to return to the previous shortened state. This low-load, prolonged stretch is a mild stretch that is held for a period of minutes or hours (if possible); it is often used in physical therapy to reduce muscle **contractures.** The shorter time period of the hold phase in static stretching increases the elongation of the muscles and provides a feeling of increased "looseness." Static stretching is used extensively by coaches, athletes, and athletic therapists to decrease muscle tension.

Performance of the **ballistic** stretch involves a bouncing movement. This stretch is much more difficult to perform safely because the bouncing movement fires the **Golgi tendon organs (GTO)** and causes the muscle to reflexively contract. Stretching a contracting muscle can cause muscle damage and should be avoided. Ballistic stretching is not entirely safe, so when athletes bounce during stretching, the athletic trainer or coach should advise them to stop bouncing and to hold the stretch position.

Dynamic stretching involves movements that are sport specific and can be thought of as part of the sport warm-up. The best example of the dynamic stretch might be the technique of "high knees" that sprinters use. The athlete raises the knees above waist level while run-

Table 4.10
Suggested Muscle Groups for Sport Flexibility Programs

Muscle to stretch	Major sport(s)	Special instructions
Pectoralis major	Striking and throwing sports	Use after lifting and sport practice or play.
Neck	Football	Use after practice, not before.
Upper and middle back	All sports	Stretch rhomboids and trapezius.
Lower back	All sports	Use rotational movements only by direction.
Hip flexors	All sports	Standing stretch is good in warm-up.
Quadriceps	All sports	Combine with hip flexor stretch.
Hamstrings	All sports	Include pre- and post-activities, especially running.
Groin	All sports	Use "butterfly" stretch.
Calf	All sports	Best method is active stretching, standing position.

ning (or jogging) 5 to 10 yd (4.6 to 9 m). The objective of the "high knees" is vertical rather than horizontal movement. This technique provides a dynamic stretch to the hamstrings and hip extensors in a sportlike drill.

Stretching Routines

Many athletes look for two or three different stretches for one muscle group. Actually, only one stretch is needed for any one muscle if it incorporates movement patterns for which the muscle is responsible. Table 4.10 lists the major muscles or muscle groups that most individuals should include in the stretching program.

PREVENTING INJURY THROUGH STRENGTH AND CONDITIONING

Many injuries occur at the start of a competitive season. Often these injuries result from a lengthy off-season in which the athlete devoted insufficient effort to keeping the body in good cardiovascular condition and keeping the muscles healthy. Strength and conditioning specialists can provide individual athletes with off-season programs to fit both their physical and sport requirements and their access to strength-training equipment. Several different techniques are employed to reduce the intensity of training during the athlete's off-season while keeping the level of conditioning and muscle strength from diminishing significantly.

Coaching Methods

The governing bodies of particular sports have addressed specific coaching techniques that are correlated with athletic injury. An example of a coaching technique highly correlated with athletic injury is "spearing" in the football tackle. Many coaches used to teach this technique of hitting as a tackling technique. As athletes began injuring the cervical spine in headfirst spearing tackles, coaching techniques were forced to change. Today, football coaches stress the importance of "keeping the head up" when making a tackle (see figure 4.27). Posters and other forms of media illustrate the importance of proper head and neck position in football, and rules outlaw the spearing technique.

Certainly coaching methods vary from individual to individual and from sport to sport. A group representing the National Association for Sport and Physical Education, the American Alliance for Health, Physical Education, Recreation and Dance, and various other sport

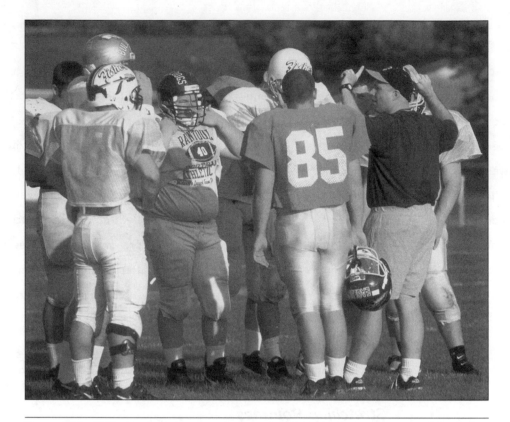

Figure 4.27 Skilled and competent coaches can help keep their athletes healthy and injury free by practicing safe coaching methods and using positive training techniques.

organizations, school boards, medical organizations, and legal consultants has produced the National Standards for Athletic Coaches (AAHPERD 1995). These national standards were published in an attempt to provide administrators, coaches, athletes, and the public with information regarding the skills and knowledge that coaches should possess.

The national standards for athletic coaches include 37 standards grouped into eight content areas of knowledge. Each standard is further supported by competencies that are divided into five levels, with each content area represented at each level. Content areas included in the standards are identified in table 4.11.

Through observance of the standards, coaches become more competent individuals who are skilled in the various aspects of coaching American youth. Programs like this enable parents to become more confident in this person who is so influential with their children.

Reducing Injury by Matching Athletes on Motor Skill Performance

It has often been noticed that when moderately skilled players compete on the same basketball team as players with low skills, someone gets hurt. The reason is often that the more highly skilled players have more body control and thus are able to maintain balance and avoid col-

For more information regarding standards for athletic coaches, visit www.aahperd.org/naspe/template.cfm?template=standards.html.

Table 4.11
Eight Content Areas of Knowledge for Athletic Coaches

Area of study	Suggested college course(s)
Injuries: prevention, care, and management	One or two courses in athletic training
Training, conditioning, and nutrition	Physical education/Conditioning
Social/Psychological aspects of coaching	Nutrition course
Skills, tactics, and strategies	Sport psychology
Teaching and administration	Specific sport coaching courses
Growth, development, and learning	Physical education/Administration
Risk management	Child psychology/Human development
Professional preparation and development	Physical education/Management

lision and injury. Players just learning a team sport may be so consumed by the rules and the various plays that they are out of position, and this can create the need for another player to maneuver at the last instant to avoid fouling. Even though the more highly skilled player has better body control, the out-of-position teammate can challenge the athlete's abilities, resulting in injury. It is good risk management to place like-skilled players together on teams such as basketball teams to avoid body-control injury.

In addition to team sports in which several teammates are trying to anticipate one another's movements, other sports can illustrate problems due to low levels of motor skill performance. Many of the problems that occur with younger players who have low skill levels involve contusions and sprains or strains that occur when the athlete fails to position the body correctly to absorb force or to perform the skill. It is fortunate, though, that the bodies of young athletes with low skill levels are still quite malleable and thus injuries are fewer than might otherwise be the case. Think of how often you have grimaced as you observed youngsters falling, only to see them bounce back to their feet and continue with the task.

Reducing Injury Through Control of Biomechanical Stress

Overuse is one of the most common causes of injury in sports like swimming and the running events in track. This stress is compounded when there is some dysfunction of an injured joint. Foot function is one of the more common areas in which poor biomechanics imposes biological stress on tissues unable to withstand such trauma. An athlete with an injury in the foot may return to sport using unusual gait patterns, and soon the repetitive trauma of participation causes breakdown somewhere along the biomechanical chain (e.g., right-sided knee soreness upon return from a left ankle sprain).

Effect of Extrinsic Forces on Injury Frequency

One factor that produces injury is extremely difficult to control: extrinsic force. A volleyball hitter may land off balance and still manage to avoid injury; however, if that same hitter lands on another player's foot, an injury may be unavoidable.

Studies have been done to evaluate the effectiveness of ankle and knee braces in preventing injury. Unfortunately, short of immobilization of the joint, there is no means of totally preventing injury to the knee and ankle joints. Some injuries are unavoidable, and the best we might do to prevent those injuries is to pay attention to all the other factors that can be controlled.

Modifying the Physical Demands Placed on the Athlete

An easily controllable risk factor is the actual physical demands placed on the athlete. Athletes who are experiencing an illness and whose endurance is thereby limited should not be required to perform. Many athletes will push themselves, and sometimes coaches will push; but the fact remains that the athlete does not have to continue participating in these circumstances. Additionally, a coach or athletic trainer observing practice must be aware of the signs of fatigue. Sometimes it is beneficial to work through fatigue to build stamina; but if the athlete is experiencing illness or recovering from physical or emotional stress, pushing through fatigue may be quite detrimental to good health.

SUMMARY

1. *Identify ways in which information from fitness testing can help the athletic trainer.*

   An athlete's fitness level can be a strong indication of his or her performance abilities in exercise sessions. Knowledge of a low level of fitness can help prevent an injury during an exercise session. Additionally, information about an aspect of a person's fitness level assists the athletic trainer in designing an exercise prescription to help get the individual into better shape.

2. *Discuss the rationale for conducting fitness testing at various times before, during, or after the sport or training season.*

   Preparticipation fitness testing should be a standard part of every exercise program. The information helps in establishing the baseline of fitness prior to an exercise program and in determining specific needs of the athlete to allow safe participation. Evaluation after the training season aids in the establishment of off-season objectives and gives the individual a better understanding of the progress made as a result of the training program.

3. *Explain the method of establishing the 1RM in weightlifting.*

   To establish a 1RM in a particular weightlifting exercise, you would select a weight that is your best guess at the appropriate weight for the individual. If the person cannot lift that weight, the weight is reduced until the person can accomplish one full lift. If the original weight is lifted easily, additional weight is added until the person cannot perform a full lift, and the recorded weight is the last successful lift or weight.

4. *Define "aerobic" and "anaerobic" with reference to energy systems and relate each to various activities.*

   The aerobic energy system depends on the availability of oxygen, whereas the anaerobic energy system can function without oxygen. All activities have some combination of anaerobic and aerobic function. Activities shorter than 1 min are as close to anaerobic as possible; the event lasting 1 min utilizes energy from both sources equally, and that ratio gradually changes toward aerobic energy supply as the event duration increases. Most sprints use the anaerobic system, while sustained activities can utilize energy from the aerobic system. Sports often involve a combination of the two—sprints or spurts of high-intensity work followed by periods of lower-intensity work. High-intensity, short-duration exercise uses the anaerobic system and cannot be sustained for long periods of time.

5. *Define isotonic, isometric, and isokinetic exercise and give an example of each.*

   Isotonic exercises are those in which a muscle contraction causes movement of a joint in response to a nonchanging load or weight. This type of exercise is like picking up a bowling ball or any other object. Isotonic exercises involve a joint action, muscle contraction, and accommodating resistance (weight); this type of action is like stretching a very heavy rubber band—the further you stretch it, the harder it is to stretch. Isometric exercises are those in which the muscle force is generated but no movement occurs. This type of exercise is similar to what a football lineman does when he holds his opponent away and similar to the execution of a hold by a wrestler. Special machines are needed to supply the accommodating resistance in isokinetic exercises.

6. *Compare and contrast the two types of muscle contraction: concentric and eccentric.*

   Concentric muscle contraction involves a shortening of the muscle whereas the eccentric contraction involves a lengthening of the muscle during the contraction. Most activities involve both types of contraction, generally with the eccentric activity acting to slow down or decelerate a movement or to act against the pull of gravity.

7. *Discuss factors to consider in designing an exercise prescription.*

   Several factors are essential when establishing an exercise prescription: the results of needs analysis, the setting of goals (including short-term goals, long-term goals, and limitations to the plan), and the exercise plan itself. The requirements of the activity or sport and the abilities and needs of the participant will help in designing the objectives for the prescription. The participant and athletic trainer should work together in establishing the goals for the day, the week, and even the month. Based on the objectives and on input from the participant, the long-range goals can be developed. Limitations to the plan can be numerous or few. Each individual must play an active part in developing the exercise prescription to keep small obstacles from becoming large roadblocks.

8. *Define the overload principle and explain how it applies to strength and conditioning techniques.*

   Strength and endurance gains occur only when the system is challenged. Overload, or asking more of a muscle or system than it is used to performing, stimulates growth and development. Overload in strength training can come from an increase in the amount of weight being lifted, the number of times the weight is lifted, or the number of exercises used. Adaptations will always occur; with adaptation, growth may be hampered. Progressions in the weight program are essential to improvement. In cardiovascular training, the same principles apply: The system must be overloaded. The sprint must be accomplished in less time or with less rest between repeats; the distance needs to be increased, or the pace increased on the same distance. Any additional challenge will provide an overload. A key to providing the overload is to do it in a measurable fashion. Subjective changes in performance are not only difficult to quantify; they are difficult to reproduce and thus difficult to use as a basis for overload.

CRITICAL THINKING QUESTIONS

1. Muscle function is divided into three subcategories: muscle strength, endurance, and power. What are the advantages of testing athletes for each? Develop and describe a testing procedure for each subcategory that you might perform in an athlete preseason, during the season, and postseason.

2. Flexibility is a combination of several anatomical structures (joint structure, muscle size, ligament and tendon composition). Describe how each of these would play a role in the flexibility differences between a 300-lb (136-kg) lineman on a college football team and a gymnast who has been performing since she was five years old. Include any significance their sport histories may play in your answer.

3. Discuss each of the types of body composition measuring. Be sure to include the advantages and disadvantages of each.

4. During your time as the athletic trainer at a local high school, the administration hires a new head football coach. The coach has a very impressive Division I football career history as well as some professional experience. During lunch one afternoon he presents to you his practice plan for the high school team and asks for your professional opinion. Please critique each of the three sections of his plan as seen in the following outline. What are some of the things you would keep, as well as some of the things you might change for each section? Be sure to include reasons for each of your decisions. Keep in mind the age level and physical maturity of the athletes he is now working with. (For example, will the athletes or parents mind the team requirements? Are there any risks associated with this number of practices per week?) Has the coach left anything out that you might want to see added to any or all of the sections?

   - Practice times: 6-8 a.m. M-Fri; 3-6 p.m. M-Thurs; games Friday night; 10 a.m.-1 p.m. Saturday for films and one hour of weight room

   - General guidelines for morning practices: Warm-up followed by track workouts for running/sprinting positions every morning (6-7 a.m.); mild-moderate cardio 3x a week for non-running positions (6-7 a.m.); weight room for all positions during second hour

   - General guidelines for afternoon practices: Warm-up 3-3:30 p.m.; stretching 3:30-3:45 p.m.; drills/conditioning 3:45-5:45 p.m.; team meeting 5:45-6 p.m.

5. The gymnastics, basketball, and football coaches of your school want to change their weight room programs for their high school athletes. They come to you inquiring about the differences between isometrics, isotonics, and isokinetics. They also want to know the advantages and disadvantages for each, as well as which type would most benefit their individual athletes. What is your answer? Would you choose different types for different positions or different teams? Would you recommend a combination of all three types? Please provide the definitions for each type as well as your rationale for your recommendations.

6. After completing a plyometrics workshop for CEUs, the track and field coach comes to you for collaboration on implementing plyometric workouts for his hurdlers and jumping athletes. He asks you for your definition of plyometrics and about the benefits of this type of conditioning. Please write out your answer to him and include an example of an exercise other than the box exercise presented in your book.

7. As you tour the facilities of a prospective new employment opportunity, you notice that the weight room includes only the following equipment:

   - Free weights ranging from 25 lb to 200 lb (11-91 kg)

   - One of the newer brands of treadmills

   - One of the newer brands of stationary bikes

   - One Universal machine predominantly for lower-extremity exercises (leg extensions, hamstring curls, leg press)

   - Additional space not currently being used (the approximate size of four average free-weight bench presses)

As one of your interview questions, the ATC leaving the position asks you for your opinion on the current weight room as well as any changes you would make to the equipment, given the opportunity to buy five new pieces of equipment. Please list what you like and dislike about the current room's equipment. Include machines you would add, as well as those you might donate away. Consider all areas of a workout regimen in your answer, including types of strength training and plyometrics, aerobic conditioning, and flexibility training. Please provide rationale for your equipment decisions as they pertain to your knowledge of strength and conditioning from chapter 4. Remember that all sports will be using this weight room as well as both male and female athletes.

8. Your lacrosse coach notices a trend in his freshman recruits. None of them seem to have any agility or grace during their drills, and in fact seem to be tripping over their own feet. He asks you for your opinion about improving both their reaction time and agility. What do you recommend and why? Please provide three examples of drills you will create for his athletes.

CITED SOURCES

American Alliance for Health, Physical Education, Recreation and Dance. 1995. *AAHPERD national standards for athletic coaches.* Reston, VA: American Alliance for Health, Physical Education, Recreation and Dance.

AAHPERD. 1980. *Health Related Fitness Test and Test Manual.* Reston, VA: American Alliance for Health, Physical Education, Recreation and Dance.

American College of Sports Medicine. 1990. ACSM position statement: The recommended quantity and quality of exercise for developing and maintaining cardiorespiratory and muscular fitness in healthy adults. *Med Sci Spts Exerc* 22: 265-274.

Cooper, K.H. 1968. A means of assessing maximal oxygen uptake. *JAMA* 203: 201-204.

Fleck, S.J., and W.J. Kraemer. 1997. *Designing resistance training programs.* Champaign, IL: Human Kinetics.

Hettinger, R. 1961. *Physiology of strength training.* Springfield, IL: Charles C Thomas.

Stedman's concise medical dictionary, 2nd ed. 1994. McDonough, J.T., ed. Baltimore: Williams & Wilkins.

ADDITIONAL READINGS

Baechle, T., ed. 1994. *Essentials of strength training and conditioning.* Champaign, IL: Human Kinetics.

Bompa, T.O., and L.J. Comacchia. 1998. *Serious strength training.* Champaign, IL: Human Kinetics.

Bryant, C.X., and J.A. Peterson. 1998. Accuracy of fitness test. *Fit Mgmt Mag* 14(12): 52-54.

Caill, B.R., and E.H. Griffith. 1978. Effects of preseason conditioning on the incidence and severity of high school football knee injuries. *Am J Spts Med* 6(4): 180-184.

Chu, D.A. 1992. *Jumping into plyometrics.* Champaign, IL: Human Kinetics.

Chu, D.A. 1996. *Explosive power and strength: Complex training for maximum results.* Champaign, IL: Human Kinetics.

Dinitiman, G.B., R.D. Ward, and T. Tellez. 1997. *Sport speed.* Champaign, IL: Human Kinetics.

Durstine, J.L., ed. 1997. *ACSM's exercise management for persons with chronic disease.* Champaign, IL: Human Kinetics.

Heywood, V.H. 1997. *Advanced fitness assessment and exercise prescription.* Champaign, IL: Human Kinetics.

Kenneth, W.L., R.H. Humphrey, and C.X. Bryant. 1995. *ACSM's guidelines for exercise testing and prescription*, 5th ed. Philadelphia: Lippincott, Williams & Wilkins.

McArdle, W.D., et al. 1972. Reliability and interrelationships between maximal oxygen uptake, physical work capacity and step test scores in college women. *Med Sci Spts* 4: 182-186.

Steinberg, J. 1996. Women and weightlifting. *First Aider* 66(2): 6-8.

Zatsiorsky, V.M. 1995. *Science and practice of strength training.* Champaign, IL: Human Kinetics.

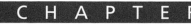

Pharmacology
in Athletic Medicine

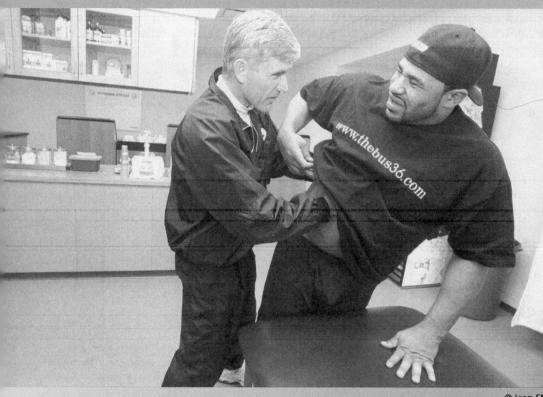

© Icon SMI

Objectives

After reading this chapter, the student should be able to do the following:

1. Define and list examples of generic versus trade-name drugs.

2. Discuss why drugs are classified as nonprescription, prescription, or controlled substances.

3. Identify the methods of administering medical drugs to the patient.

4. Define "agonist" and "antagonist" as related to medicinal drugs.

5. Identify the various sources one could use to find information on drugs.

6. Describe how to find information on the USOC or the NCAA banned drug lists.

7. Discuss the inflammatory process and describe how drugs may affect that process.

8. Identify the more common side effects of anti-inflammatory drugs and the steps that may be taken to reduce these unwanted outcomes.

9. Describe the effects of analgesics and discuss reasons to limit their use in sport participation.

10. Identify ways in which a fungal infection may be controlled with medicinal drugs.

11. Describe ways in which a laxative may be misused.

Kaitlyn, a swimmer on the university team, woke up with a splitting headache. After the first class of the day she decided to stop by the athletic training room and see if the team physician could help her. Danielle, a sophomore student athletic trainer, was available, but all the staff athletic trainers and the team physician were in a meeting. Kaitlyn's next class was in 15 minutes, and there was no telling how long it might be until the doctor would be back in the office.

"What can I do to help you?" Danielle asked.

"My head is killing me. I thought the doc could check me out. I can't stand it any longer," Kaitlyn said.

"We have some Tylenol—would that help?" Danielle said.

"No, I doubt it. When I get this kind of headache I really need strong stuff," Kaitlyn explained while she rubbed her forehead. "Doc gives me Darvocet and it works the best."

"I think I saw some of that in John's training bag. Let me look," suggested the ever-helpful Danielle.

The head athletic trainer's kit was neatly packed with little packages of pills. Danielle found the one marked Darvocet and removed it from the kit.

"Here's some!" she exclaimed as she offered it to the ailing swimmer.

"Great, thanks, Danielle. I'll take this right away and maybe I'll be able to concentrate in my next class. See ya later," Kaitlyn said as she headed off for the drinking fountain.

This scenario depicts an act that seems to be a harmless attempt to be helpful but is actually illegal. It has certainly taken place in athletic training rooms around the country many, many times over the history of the profession. The dispensing of prescription medication must occur only under the direct supervision of a licensed physician. Past practices of freely dispensing prescription and nonprescription drugs have led to very costly lawsuits involving the athletic department and employees that provided drugs to student-athletes.

UNDERSTANDING PHARMACOLOGY

It is critical to learn the basics of pharmacology, just as it is to understand the effects of any other treatment. With knowledge of what medicinals are used for specific problems, the way a drug works, and some of the mechanics of its action, the athletic trainer may better communicate with the individual taking the medicine, as well as with the prescribing physician, and thereby maximize the therapy for the individual.

In this chapter we focus on the application of pharmacology to specific problems frequently encountered in sports medicine settings. In no way should the reader construe this information to be comprehensive or infer that this bit of knowledge sufficiently prepares someone to prescribe or dispense medicinal drugs. This information will serve as a basis upon which to build an understanding of drug therapy and will allow the reader some understanding of how and why drugs work. In the Athletic Training Education Series text titled *Management Strategies in Athletic Training, Third Edition*, you will learn methods of organizing plans to legally and safely store medication within the sport treatment facility.

DRUG NOMENCLATURE AND CLASSIFICATION

Pharmacology can be quite confusing to athletic trainers because of the variety of names given to drugs. Each drug can be identified according to its chemical, **generic**, or trade name. The chemical name, usually a long and difficult one, refers to the specific chemical structure of the compound. The generic name, also called the "official" or **"nonproprietary"** name, is usually shorter and is often derived from the chemical name. The trade name is the name the manufacturing company assigns to the compound. You might accurately surmise that several companies may manufacture an identical generic product but assign different names to it. For instance, ibuprofen is the common name or generic name for the **analgesic** known by the trade names Advil, Nuprin, Motrin, and the less familiar trade name of Rufen.

One very important aspect of understanding drugs is understanding the drug classifications. There are two general classifications of medicinal drugs: prescription and nonprescription or over-the-counter (OTC) drugs.

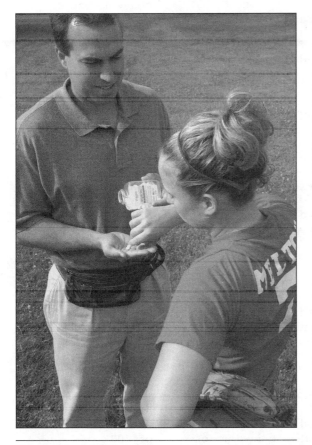

Figure 5.1 Athletic trainers need to remind people to follow dosage recommendations and to check with their physician or pharmacist before taking OTC medications.

Nonprescription or Over-the-Counter Drugs

Nonprescription drugs can be purchased by consumers directly from store shelves. In general, OTC medications are used for minor problems. These medications are judged to be safe or free of major side effects when taken in the recommended dosage. One must be careful when suggesting that an individual use an OTC medication. Always advise the person to follow the dosage recommendations on the product and to check with a pharmacist or physician before combining any medications (see figure 5.1). Too often, individuals self-medicate using OTC products that, if taken in combination with other compounds, can exert unwanted or even hazardous side effects.

Prescription Drugs

Classification as a prescription drug indicates that the individual will need a prescription for the medicine. The physician determines that the drug is necessary to treat an illness or condition. The physician also interviews the patient regarding the use of other drugs and provides information about drug interactions. In addition to the prescribing physician, the issuing pharmacist often reviews the effects, side effects, and precautions with the consumer at the time the medicine is issued.

Prescription drugs are further classified according to their potential for abuse. The government holds tight controls on the use of prescription drugs—hence the term "controlled substances." These drugs, with their potential for abuse, are further categorized into one of five schedules (schedules I-V). Schedule I drugs are the drugs with the highest potential for abuse and are approved for use in only a very limited number of patients; the schedule II, III, and IV drugs are successively less likely to be abused; and schedule V drugs have the lowest relative abuse potential. Table 5.1 gives examples of drugs on each schedule.

There are rules for prescribing, dispensing, and renewing prescriptions for all five types of controlled substances. The patient must have a written prescription for the controlled drug and must obtain the drug in person. These steps are necessary to prevent false ordering of these dangerous drugs as well as for ensuring that the drug is given to the proper person. If the team physician has drugs in his or her office, these drugs are kept under tight security in an area that is double-locked for added safety.

THE STUDY OF DRUGS

Pharmacology is the science of drugs. Researchers focus on two distinct areas when studying drugs: **pharmacotherapeutics** and **toxicology.** If we look at the roots of these two words we see a continuum, from therapeutic to toxic. We may all know cases in which a prescribed drug was used in excess of the dosage specified and there was a toxic effect. This toxic effect

Table 5.1

Controlled Substances by Schedule Classification

Schedule	Qualifications for designation	Drugs in schedule
Schedule I	(A) The drug or other substance has a high potential for abuse. (B) The drug or other substance has no currently accepted medical use in treatment in the United States. (C) There is a lack of accepted safety for use of the drug or other substance under medical supervision.	Opium Experimental opiate derivatives Hallucinogenic substances
Schedule II	(A) The drug or other substance has a high potential for abuse. (B) The drug or other substance has a currently accepted medical use in treatment in the United States or a currently accepted medical use with severe restrictions. (C) Abuse of the drug or other substance may lead to severe psychological or physical dependence.	Opiates (i.e., methadone, etc.) Methamphetamine
Schedule III	(A) The drug or other substance has a potential for abuse less than that of the drugs or other substances in schedules I and II. (B) The drug or other substance has a currently accepted medical use in treatment in the United States. (C) Abuse of the drug or other substance may lead to moderate or low physical dependence or high psychological dependence.	Stimulants Depressants Nalorphine Narcotic drugs Anabolic steroids
Schedule IV	(A) The drug or other substance has a low potential for abuse relative to the drugs or other substances in schedule III. (B) The drug or other substance has a currently accepted medical use in treatment in the United States. (C) Abuse of the drug or other substance may lead to limited physical dependence or psychological dependence relative to the drugs or other substances in schedule III.	Barbital Meprobamate Methylphenobarbital Phenobarbital
Schedule V	(A) The drug or other substance has a low potential for abuse relative to the drugs or other substances in schedule IV. (B) The drug or other substance has a currently accepted medical use in treatment in the United States. (C) Abuse of the drug or other substance may lead to limited physical dependence or psychological dependence relative to the drugs or other substances in schedule IV.	Not more than 200 mg codeine per 100 ml or per 100 g Not more than 100 mg opium per 100 ml or per 100 g

is usually not lethal (although sufficient dosages may cause a life-threatening condition), but the effect is not desirable and usually not therapeutic; it is thus called an unwanted effect. The subjects of toxicology and pharmacotherapeutics are extensive and are far beyond the scope of this chapter. Therefore the discussion here is limited to the major therapeutic effects, as well as some of the unwanted effects, of common drugs used in athletic health care.

Pharmacokinetics

As the word "kinetics" indicates, **pharmacokinetics** is the study of how the medicine moves (kinetic = movement). Pharmacokinetics can be broken down into four subcategories: absorption, distribution, metabolism, and elimination. Here we look briefly at the basis of each of these so that we may better understand specific medicinals later in this chapter.

Before absorption can occur, the drug must enter the body. There are two primary ways in which a drug is administered: enteral and non-enteral. The **enteral** route is termed **alimentary** or enteral because of its pathway into the body via the alimentary canal, or digestive system. Some of the routes of enteral administration are the oral, **sublingual,** and rectal. The non-enteral route is termed **parenteral** because entry into the body is through a pathway other than the alimentary canal. This method usually allows the drug to be delivered directly

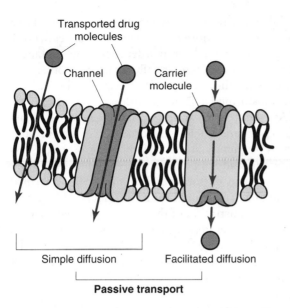

Figure 5.2 Some drugs are absorbed through the membrane by simple passive or facilitated passive diffusion.

to the target site, making the quantity of drug actually reaching the target more predictable. Routes of parenteral administration include inhalation, injection, and **topical** and **transdermal** application.

Drug Absorption

Absorption is the movement of the drug across a cell's membrane. Movement across a membrane is usually accomplished by some method of diffusion or transport (see figure 5.2). Generally, the smaller the drug compound, the more easily it moves across a cell membrane, thus allowing greater distribution. Additionally, if the drug is lipid soluble, this means that it breaks down or binds with fats and thus is able to gain access to more tissues, leading to greater distribution.

If there is a difference in chemical concentration on two sides of a permeable membrane, the chemical will move from the area of high concentration to the area of lower concentration. This is termed passive diffusion, a method of transporting substances across the cell membrane. "Passive" emphasizes the fact that the movement occurs without any energy expenditure; the driving force is the pressure difference on the two sides of the membrane.

Diffusion at cell junctions must occur if a compound is to be administered through the alimentary canal but needs to be distributed to an area outside the canal (i.e., the nervous system or muscular system). The diffusion of the compound occurs in the space between cells; this space may either allow or prohibit the passage of drugs, as in the case of the blood–brain barrier. The capillary walls in the brain produce a barrier to many water-soluble compounds, yet the barrier is permeable to lipid-soluble substances. This is one of the reasons that some drugs can affect the central nervous system quite readily (such as anesthetics) while others are rather ineffective in that role.

In general, the more lipid soluble the drug is, the more tissues will be affected (wider distribution) and the more potential the drug will have to exert an effect on the central nervous system.

Drug Distribution

Once the drug is absorbed from its point of entry, the circulatory system distributes the drug throughout the body, thus the "distribution." The extent to which the drug reaches the systemic circulation is termed **bioavailability**, which is expressed as the percentage of the drug that reaches the bloodstream. Once the drug is in the systemic circulation, further distribution into body tissues may be necessary to allow it to reach the target area. Furthermore, many drugs have to cross cell membranes and tissue barriers to reach the desired target.

Drug Transformation and Elimination

Basically, the process of drug transformation involves making substances soluble for excretion from the liver or urinary tract. The process that determines whether a compound is excreted in the bile (liver) or the urine is complicated and depends on the patient's internal physiology. Drugs that are processed through the kidneys will be excreted in the urine while drugs processed through the digestive tract are eliminated from the body into the stool. Most drugs, especially water-soluble drugs, are excreted into the urine. The acidity of the urine can affect the rate of elimination of a drug. The acidity of the urine can be changed by diet, drugs, or kidney disorders. This is an important concept in the treatment of poisoning or drug overdose. In these cases the acidity of the urine is changed if the patient is given other drugs (such as an antacid like sodium bicarbonate or an acid like ammonium chloride) to speed up the elimination of the toxic drug. The kidney, liver, lungs, and gastrointestinal tract all can help in the process of transformation, each with the task of making the substance soluble and ready for elimination.

The effectiveness of drugs that are fat soluble may be altered when they are converted to a water-soluble state in the liver. Some drugs may become more potent when they are converted in the liver. Other drugs may require transformation in the liver in order to become therapeutic. Some drugs are not metabolized at all and may be excreted totally intact. Still others are transformed into other compounds that have some other therapeutic or even a toxic effect.

Aspirin is among the drugs that must be transformed in order to produce any therapeutic value. Drugs like this are called prodrugs. Another particular drug (not to be named) is marketed in the United States as a muscle relaxant but undergoes a transformation in the liver into a potent and very addictive compound that is frequently abused. Many other drugs possess these metabolic characteristics, complicating the study of pharmacology even further.

The amount of time needed to reduce the drug concentration in the body to 50% is termed the drug half-life. Knowledge of the half-life of a drug is important for understanding how often the drug is administered. Usually, after administration of the drug for five half-lives, a steady state is achieved in which the amount administered is equal to the amount eliminated. The half-life and the steady state of a drug are the factors that lead a physician to prescribe a loading dose of a drug—a first dose that is twice the normal dose. The loading dose allows the concentration to reach effective levels more rapidly.

Pharmacodynamics: How the Drug Works

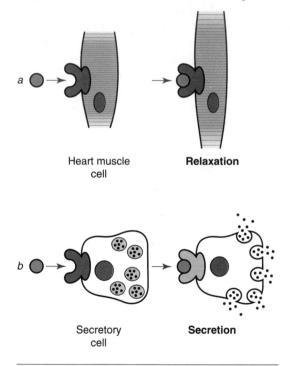

Heart muscle cell   **Relaxation**

Secretory cell   **Secretion**

Figure 5.3 Some drugs act by binding to specific target receptors in the cell's membrane.

From Alberts et al. 1993.

The word **pharmacodynamics** can be broken down into "pharmaco" and "dynamics." Dynamics relates to the Greek word "*dynamikos*," meaning powerful. Thus, pharmacodynamics refers to the power the drug has on the body, or the way it exerts its effect. Drugs act by binding to specific target receptors on the cell's exterior. When a drug binds to a receptor, it triggers a cellular process and thereby activates the therapeutic response (see figure 5.3).

Similarly to muscles, drugs have agonists and antagonists. Just as an agonistic muscle produces a change, the agonist drug acts with the receptor site to produce a change. There are also drugs that work in the opposite fashion. These, called antagonists, exert an inhibitory action on the receptor cell. This action suppresses the activity of the cell that is the cause of the patient's discomfort or disorder. For example, if you stepped into a patch of poison ivy you might break out in some allergic response like itching and hives. You could use a topical antihistamine like Benadryl cream that would block the histamine (allergic) reaction, and your itching and hives would go away quite quickly. The reason is that the Benadryl (diphenhydramine) binds with the body tissues that cause the allergic reaction, inhibiting the cell function.

Efficacy refers to how effectively a drug works. Certainly we would all prefer to take a drug if we could be assured of its efficacy in treating the condition. The ability of the drug to produce an effect is not always related to the drug's potency. The potency of a drug is a measure of the dose of the medicinal needed to produce a specific effect. A more potent drug is not a more effective drug; it would have the same effect as another drug, but with the more potent drug the effect can be achieved with a lower dose. Tolerance to a drug simply indicates that the body cells have built up a kind of resistance to the drug so that increased amounts are needed to achieve the same effect. This tolerance makes the drug appear less potent, but actually the drug has become less efficient because of the changes in the cell.

III Effects of Medications

To understand how and why particular drugs work, one must also consider the nondesired effects of a drug. Some of the nondesired effects are adverse or side effects, allergic (and anaphylactic) reactions, and drug interactions.

Therapeutic Side Effects

It may be interesting to note that an antihypertensive drug (drug used to reduce high blood pressure), minoxodil, has a side effect of causing hypertrichosis (the growth of body hair). Although it may seem odd to mention this, there's a reason. Minoxodil, marketed under the trade name Rogaine, is used topically to actually stimulate hair growth—an example of a drug that is used therapeutically for its side effects.

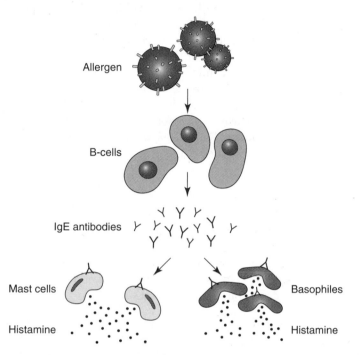

Figure 5.4 An allergic reaction mechanism in the body.

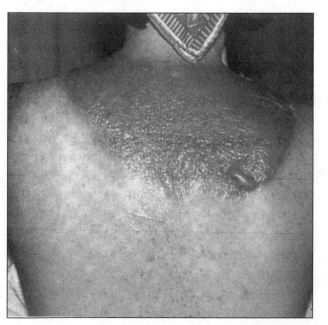

Drug Adverse Effects

Often drugs produce undesired effects or effects unrelated to the reason for taking the medication; these are called adverse effects. The adverse effects of a drug are often highly predictable, and most patients tolerate them quite easily. While a drug is being tested for Food and Drug Administration (FDA) approval, researchers record and track common adverse effects. If the drug is considered safe and is approved, then the drug manufacturer is required by law to list the adverse effects on the packaging material or on product inserts. Occasionally, however, adverse effects may not be anticipated or in individual cases may be different from the ones listed. Remind those you are working with to check the product inserts, call their physician, or talk to a pharmacist if they have any questions or concerns regarding adverse effects. Also, educate yourself about the unwanted side effects of medications your athletes or clients are taking.

Drug Allergies

Adverse drug reactions have become an increasingly common medical problem with the use of increasing numbers of therapeutic and diagnostic agents. In the United States, these reactions affect an estimated 1 to 2 million people a year. Adverse drug reactions are believed to be the most common cause of **iatrogenic** (caused by the treatment itself) illnesses, and up to 30% of hospitalized patients may experience such a reaction (see figures 5.4 and 5.5). These reactions can be divided into two broad categories: toxic and allergic. Most adverse reactions, including unwanted side effects, overdoses, and drug interactions, are toxic. Only 6% to 10% are allergic reactions, but these are the most serious. Death is reported in 1 of every 10,000 cases.

A patient is said to have a drug allergy when the medicine produces a response different from what is expected. For example, a product called Zomax was taken off the market a short time after it was introduced because many people who took this aspirin-like product developed severe itching and hives, signs of allergic response. Severe allergenic reactions may involve anaphylactic responses that include

Figure 5.5 Itching, burning skin rash is a common allergic response.

Reprinted from Bronner and Hood 1983.

bronchospasm, **hypotension,** shock, and death if not treated quickly. It is always important to know of any allergies in those you work with, and keeping that record on the individual's chart as well as on the preparticipation physical is recommended. The allergic response is much different from an unwanted side effect: The adverse effect is something that a majority of the people who take the medication will report, but an allergy is a definite contraindication to use of the medicine.

Drug Interactions

Drug interactions are also factors that play a big role in understanding drug effects. A drug interaction is just what the name implies: an interaction between two drugs. This happens when drugs that are metabolized serve to stimulate or depress the metabolism of other drugs. These interactions may be agonistic (compounding the effect of the medication, also termed synergistic) or antagonistic (canceling the effect of the medication). For example, alcohol is a drug and should not be consumed while the individual is taking a prescribed drug, because alcohol is agonistic with many drugs and will increase the potential for side effects of the medication. As an example of the opposite, or antagonistic, effect there have been reports—although the research has not been conclusive—that some antibiotics decrease the effectiveness of oral contraceptives in certain women. Thus the synergistic (agonistic) effect compounds the effect or side effects of a drug, while the antagonistic effect could reduce or even cancel the effect of the drug.

Sources of Drug Information

The idea of drug receptors and agonistic or antagonistic effects of drugs is much more complex than this very simplified description indicates. The student of pharmacology investigates the exact cells with which the drug interacts and the extent to which the action occurs. For our purposes, knowledge that the system exists will help us understand why a particular drug works the way it does; yet for additional information, there are places to turn.

- *Physician's Desk Reference. Physician's Desk Reference (PDR)* is a text commonly available in sports medicine departments. The *PDR* is an exhaustive reference for prescription drugs, classifying each drug by trade name and generic name as well as providing a pictorial guide to aid in the identification of medicinals. The information on each drug includes dosage parameters, effects, and side effects: all the information included in the product information provided by the manufacturer. One of the difficulties with this reference is that it does not list all generic drugs—and generic drugs are often the ones that the consumer chooses.

- *Facts and Comparisons. Facts and Comparisons* is a reference similar to the *PDR*, but it includes many of the generic drugs. One tremendous benefit of *Facts and Comparisons* is that it is published in a binder into which one can easily insert the monthly updates that are provided.

- Product information. The pharmacist preparing the prescription often supplies product information. Cooperation with a local pharmacist may allow the athletic trainer nearly immediate information on any drug of interest.

- United States Olympic Committee banned drug list. A wide variety of drugs have been found to be potentially dangerous to the athlete or to offer an unfair advantage in sport.

Clinical Pharmacology at Gold Standard Multimedia (www.gsm.com) is available to aid the practitioner in understanding various drugs. Just as with the printed drug references, this Web site includes product information, drug references, and a search function. The clinician may purchase a subscription to GSM's materials and receive up-to-date information that can even be downloaded to a personal data assistant (PDA).

The NCAA has a list of banned substances at www1.ncaa.org/membership/ed_outreach/health-safety/drug_testing/banned_drug_classes.pdf. An athlete or anyone else interested in finding out if a drug is banned can access the Resource Exchange Center (www.drugfreesport.com), a division of the National Center for Drug Free Sport. One can submit the name of a drug and receive information on the banned status of substances including dietary **supplements**.

Table 5.2
Abbreviations for Dosage As Used in Pharmacology

Abbreviation	Latin term	Meaning
bid	bis in die	Twice daily
tid	ter in die	Three times daily
qid	quater in die	Four times daily

Sport organizations have stepped forward to control the use of these drugs. Both the National Collegiate Athletic Association (NCAA) and the United States Olympic Committee (USOC) publish their own banned drug lists. In addition, both organizations make their drug-testing policy clear to competing athletes, including such aspects as the frequency of testing and the ramifications of positive tests.

Although the prescription and dispensation of medicinal drugs are out of the scope of practice of the athletic trainer, every health care practitioner should be aware of actions and side effects of the majority of drugs in categories commonly used in athletic medicine. In your investigation of medicinal drugs, dosage may be discussed. In medicine, abbreviations are used to denote the number of doses per day. Table 5.2 identifies the common abbreviations used to indicate dosage schedules.

DRUG-TESTING POLICIES AND PROCEDURES

As mentioned previously, each organization (USOC, NCAA, NFL, etc.) establishes its unique drug-testing policy under which all athletes on those teams are governed. Many individual schools and teams establish their own drug-testing programs.

In general, drug testing is done with a urine test. The urine is collected under same-sex observation of the void. Student-athletes are typically informed of the test and escorted immediately to the testing site. After the void, the urine is packaged, identified, and sent off to an analysis laboratory for testing. When athletes are unable to void, they are required to stay in the testing area and it is suggested that they drink the provided beverages until the urge to urinate occurs. All beverages provided in the testing center must be in individual, closed containers and should be free of caffeine.

Positive test findings are reported to the designated team authorities and the appropriate sanctions are levied. These sanctions vary according to the particular drug-testing policy of the group, school, team, or league.

The NCAA tests athletes at random times during the school year as well as at championship events. Event testing is usually done at the conclusion of the contest, whether it is the first or the final round of the tournament. The athlete(s) are met at the conclusion of the contest by a courier. This courier is responsible for staying with the athlete from the time the athlete is informed that he or she must report to the drug-testing area until the athlete is signed in by the NCAA-appointed drug-testing staff. Once the drug test is complete, the urine is analyzed and any positive findings are reported to the conference, to the person's coach, and often to the school athletic director. Positive drug-testing results obtained in championship events are often devastating to the individual as well as the team and school because the student-athlete has disobeyed conference rules, will forfeit the event if won, and will be stripped of eligibility to compete for the next 365 days.

DRUGS SPECIFIC TO ATHLETIC-RELATED CONDITIONS

As an athletic trainer, it may not be as important to understand pharmacology as deeply as you understand anatomy, yet some knowledge of each of the types of drugs you may encounter can prove beneficial in caring for athletes. The sections to follow present drugs according to a general classification of their action. Each subsection is a brief discussion of general information about the drug followed by detail on how the drug is administered, its adverse effects, and the implications for the athletic trainer. The other aspects of **pharmacokinetics** (absorption, distribution, transformation, and elimination), pharmacodynamics, and drug interactions are typically areas the athletic trainer depends on the physician to understand. These areas are not within the scope of this introductory unit.

Inflammation and Drug Treatment

As an athletic trainer, you will encounter individuals with inflammation, the most common effect of injury or overuse. This is a vascular response to physiological tissue damage. This vascular response prevents, or at least limits, the spread of injury-causing agents to the adjacent tissues. In addition, the process of inflammation serves to dispose of cellular debris and sets the stage for the repair process to begin (see figure 5.6). When trauma occurs, the offended tissue becomes an active inflammatory site. Initially there is a short period of vasoconstriction that occurs to prevent further bleeding. Shortly after this period is a release of chemical mediators (histamine, bradykinin, thromboxanes, leukotrienes, and prostaglandins) that cause a vasodilatation of the vessels in the area. With vasodilatation comes an increase in the permeability of the vessel walls, allowing white blood cells to enter the injury site. With increased membrane permeability, there is an increased flow of cellular fluid into the area, causing localized edema (swelling).

Drugs that are able to block or inhibit this series of events are classified as **anti-inflammatory** agents. Anti-inflammatory drugs can be classified as **nonsteroidal** or steroidal. Within the nonsteroidals is the category of salicylates.

Nonsteroidal Anti-Inflammatory Agents: Salicylates

Aspirin and other salicylates are, worldwide, the most frequently used drug in the treatment of pain, fever, and inflammation. Aspirin is the main member of the family of salicylates and the first nonsteroidal anti-inflammatory drug (NSAID) that was introduced. Aspirin remains the standard by which the other NSAIDs are compared. Aspirin is a **pro-drug**, which means that it is inactive until it is metabolized or broken down into its constituent parts. In the case of aspirin, this chemical breakdown process occurs in the liver.

One of the most distinct characteristics of aspirin is that it permanently binds to platelets (a type of small cell within the blood that helps it to clot), effectively terminating the platelet's synthesis of thromboxane. Since a platelet's life span is at least 7 days (8-10 days),

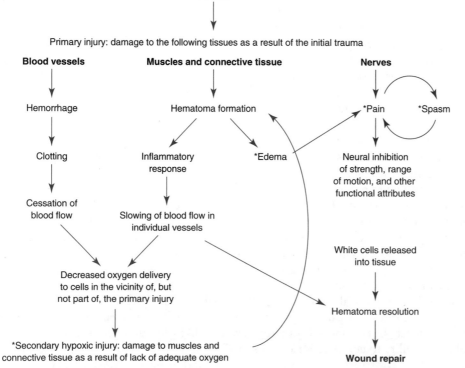

Figure 5.6 Inflammatory response to trauma.

the anticoagulant effects of aspirin continue for approximately one week to 10 days after the dosage is discontinued.

Aspirin is often combined with other ingredients to modify its effect. If aspirin is too harsh for the patient's intestinal **mucosa,** the salicylate may be buffered. The agent used to buffer the aspirin is usually an antacid product that serves to neutralize the stomach's acidity and thus decrease the potential for gastric irritation. Another additive is in the form of an external coating of the tablet that will slow down the rate at which the medicine dissolves, leading to a slower release of the aspirin's effect (delayed release). Caffeine added to aspirin products has become a staple on the market (Excedrin Migraine) for headache sufferers. The addition of caffeine acts to elevate mood as well as to constrict blood vessels that may be distended, causing the increased headache pain.

Many varied types of aspirin products are marketed, all with specific claims regarding their effectiveness against pain or their ability to reduce pain without stomach upset. People should fully evaluate each product for its actual effectiveness before subscribing to its claims.

Routes of Administration

Aspirin products are most commonly administered by mouth. This enteric administration may include tablets, capsules, chewable tablets, chewing gum, and even liquids. Think about an athlete who has incurred a broken jaw. Some forms of salicylates may be less desirable for this individual (especially if the jaw was wired shut); thus the liquid administration would be the best choice.

Another enteric administration is a suppository. A salicylate suppository may be chosen for an athlete who is vomiting and thus unable to ingest the aspirin.

Adverse Effects of Salicylates

As mentioned earlier, aspirin binds with blood platelets; this can be considered an adverse effect of the drug. In people who are elderly, aspirin is often used to thin the blood in an attempt to reduce the chance of blood clots in the brain or heart. In this case, the binding with platelets may be a desired effect and not an adverse effect; but in the young, athletic population, thinned blood could be problematic. Since trauma is associated with bleeding, and aspirin can decrease the availability of platelets, bleeding can be prolonged. Bruising and bleeding in the joints can be increased; thus it is not advisable to administer aspirin in the active population.

Gastrointestinal (GI) irritation as well as GI damage has long been recognized as the primary problem with aspirin. This GI effect may be attributable to irritation of the gastric mucosa caused by the drug, or to the inhibition of prostaglandins that protect the stomach from acidic conditions. Some patients have more difficulty than others with GI irritation when taking aspirin; people who have a history of ulcers are the most affected. Coating of the drug is sometimes employed in an attempt to delay dissolution of the drug until it reaches the small intestine. This coating, called enteric coating, not only delays dissolution and release, but also delays the therapeutic effects of the drug—and still does not preclude irritation of the duodenum (first part of the small intestine). Buffering of the tablet has also been used to blunt the drug's acidic effects on the gastric mucosa. Taking the aspirin with a meal will also buffer the acidic effect, but this too will delay the onset of desired effects. A last resort, or a choice for patients with known stomach ulcers, is to combine the aspirin therapy with a second drug designed to prevent or treat, or both prevent and treat, GI irritation. This dual therapy is certainly not required in all patients but may be the only alternative in some gastric-sensitive patients.

Hepatic (liver) and renal (kidney) disorders, although rare, can be produced in patients with preexisting diseases or in those using NSAIDs for prolonged periods or in high doses.

Aspirin overdose, known as aspirin intoxication or poisoning, may occur with doses of 10 to 30 g, but this figure remains highly patient specific and quite variable. The overdose is usually accompanied by headache, **tinnitus** (ringing in the ears), hearing difficulties, confusion, and GI irritation. Children are much more vulnerable than adults to aspirin overdose, especially if treated with adult doses of the drug.

Aspirin has also been associated with a rare condition known as Reye's syndrome. Reye's occurs in children and young teens, often after they have had chicken pox or influenza.

Symptoms associated with Reye's syndrome include high fever, vomiting, liver dysfunction, and a decreasing level of alertness that progresses rapidly and often leads to delirium, convulsions, and coma and has the potential to cause death. There is no definite link between aspirin and Reye's, but it is recommended that aspirin and other NSAIDs not be used to treat fever in children and teenagers.

A small percentage of the general population exhibits an aspirin intolerance or hypersensitivity. These individuals have allergic reactions of bronchospasm, **urticaria** (hives), and severe **rhinitis** (inflammation of the nasal mucosa) within a few hours of ingesting aspirin. A potential exists for cardiovascular shock in these people, so in this group the use of any NSAID is contraindicated.

Some studies have shown that aspirin and some common NSAIDs inhibit the synthesis of some of the components of connective tissue, with implications for the healing of cartilage, tendons, ligaments, and bone. These studies have not fully established this negative connection; therefore continued research is necessary.

Implications for the Athletic Trainer

The main concern about the use of aspirin and other salicylates in the physically active population is the effect on the blood's clotting mechanisms. Since activity is often associated with trauma (micro- and macro-), bleeding is not uncommon. If the salicylate drugs are being used and trauma occurs, the chance of excessive bleeding is increased.

Another concern one would have in the use of salicylates is irritation of the stomach. If a person were to take a salicylate immediately after a workout or competition, the natural buffers from a meal may not be present, thus increasing the likelihood of gastric upset.

It is always wise to fully evaluate the severity of the pain and the other treatment options available before recommending any anti-inflammatory drugs for the physically active individual.

Non-Salicylate, Nonsteroidal Anti-Inflammatory Drugs

All NSAIDs have the properties of analgesia, **antipyresis,** and anticoagulation as well as an ability to control inflammation. The level at which the NSAID exerts these effects is drug and dose dependent. There exists a plethora of NSAIDs, with more being introduced on a frequent basis. Most commonly NSAIDs are grouped according to their chemical similarities.

A relatively recent development in the treatment of inflammation occurred in the late 1990s. This development focused on the cyclooxygenase-2 (COX-2) inhibitors, medications that target prostaglandins, one of the main chemical mediators that cause inflammation. It has been established that the body produces two main types of prostaglandins: the COX-1 and -2 prostaglandins. The COX-1 prostaglandins are produced by the stomach and other body tissues. These prostaglandins are credited with protecting the gastric muscosa, thus preventing or limiting stomach upset. The COX-2 prostaglandins are those responsible in the inflammatory process. The traditional NSAIDs have some effect on both the COX-1 and the COX-2 pathways, while the newer NSAIDs, called the COX-2 inhibitors, primarily inhibit the inflammatory pathway without disturbing the protection of the gastric lining through the COX-1 pathway.

Many NSAIDs exist on the market, making the doctor's decision on which drug to use a bit more challenging. Few clinical differences are found among the various groups or families of NSAIDs, although some reports indicate that the side effects and adverse reactions are greatest with a family of NSAIDs called fenamic acid compounds. The therapeutic effect of any NSAID is patient specific and is based on the clinical response rather than some predetermined indication. Generally, if an individual is being treated with a compound from one group without improvement, the prescribing physician changes the medication to a compound in another family of NSAIDs. It is not unusual, in patients not responding to one compound, to try two or more drugs before finding an effective choice. Each NSAID family targets its effect on a specific part of the inflammatory process. Specific drugs within that family will act in the same way. The sports medicine professional should have easy reference to information on each NSAID family. See "Groups of Nonsteroidal Anti-Inflammatory Drugs" on page 175 for a listing of generic names for each NSAID classification.

Groups of Nonsteroidal Anti-Inflammatory Drugs

Acetic Acids
Diclofenac
Etodolac
Indomethacin
Ketoralac
Sulindac
Tolmetin
Enolic acids
Oxphenbutazone
Phenylbutazon
Piroxicam

Fenamic Acids
Meclofenamic acid
Mefenamic acid

Proprionic Acids
Fenoprofen
Flurbiprofen
Ibuprofen
Ketoprofen
Naproxen
Suprofen

Carboxylic Acids
Aspirin
Choline
Salicylate
Difunisal
Magnesium salicylate
Salicylamide
Salsalate
Sodium salicylate

COX-2 Inhibitors
Celecoxib
Rofecoxib
Meloxicam
Valdecoxib

Each classification of NSAID consists of a variety of products. This listing represents some of the many products available. Products are listed (by generic name) under the family or group name.

More differences have been reported in evaluation of the cyclooxygenase inhibition characteristics of the drug. The COX-2 inhibitors are much less apt to cause stomach upset and thus can exert their anti-inflammatory influence without the unwanted gastric effects. In future years, the COX-2 inhibitors will certainly come to be the NSAID of choice for most sport-related trauma.

Yet another way to classify the NSAID family of drugs is by their availability without a prescription. The NSAID groups available over the counter include ibuprofens (Advil, Motrin, and Nuprin), the ketoprofen group (Orudis and Actron), and the naproxen group (Aleve and Naprosyn).

Administration

NSAIDs are generally administered by mouth, in the form of a tablet, capsule, or liquid. Some anti-inflammatory drugs are available for use in the eye; these are called ophthalmic preparations. Some NSAID drugs, such as Toradol, are administered intramuscularly initially and then with oral doses.

Adverse Effects of Nonsteroidal Anti-Inflammatory Drugs

Similar to the salicylates, the NSAIDs in the COX-1 inhibitor group are often associated with gastric irritation, nausea, and vomiting. This unwanted effect of the drug can be virtually eliminated with the use of the COX-2 inhibitor NSAIDs. If GI disturbances are problematic, the patient may be able to reduce the symptoms by ingesting the drug only with a full meal and by ingesting large quantities of fluids.

Some drugs in the NSAID category are associated with central nervous system (CNS) effects such as frontal headache, dizziness, vertigo, and mental confusion.

The NSAID phenylbutazone (Butazolodin) has been reported to be poorly tolerated by many, with adverse effects occurring in approximately one-half of all patients treated with the drug (Mycek et al. 2000, 411). Aplastic anemia is the most significant and serious of the unwanted effects. Other adverse effects are similar to those with other NSAIDs.

Implications for the Athletic Trainer

Since inflammation is probably the most common complaint of the athlete, anti-inflammatory drugs use will be quite frequent. With that in mind, it is important for the athletic trainer to understand the adverse effects common to NSAID use and report those conditions to the prescribing physician. When an athlete is undergoing any treatment for a sport injury, it is wise to frequently reevaluate the signs and symptoms so that a change can be made (whether in medication or in the physical therapy plan) to attempt to produce some improvement.

Athletes should be reminded of the importance of taking the NSAID with a meal and of following the directions on the prescription. Failure to follow the directions often leads to adverse effects from the drug.

Anti-Inflammatory Drugs: Corticosteroids

Interest in developing adrenal steroids (corticosteroids) originated in the 1930s when scientists were investigating the function of the adrenal glands in an effort to develop synthetic compounds with the same effects as the normal adrenal function. Some but not all effects were reproduced, and research continued until investigators in 1949 observed a dramatic decrease in the symptoms of arthritic patients when the steroid cortisone (a glucocorticoid) was administered. Cortisone and corticotrophin were successful as anti-inflammatory agents, but interest in discovering other functions and products of the adrenal gland continued. In 1953, further research uncovered a drug named aldosterone, a mineralocorticoid produced by the adrenal gland, which was found to be a major factor in the maintenance of the body's fluid and electrolyte balance.

Adrenal steroids have proven to be quite successful (although the effect is temporary) in the management of **rheumatoid arthritis,** but the drugs are not without side effects. The number and severity of the side effects are the primary reason behind the limited use of the drug. In most medical communities, oral steroid anti-inflammatory agents are used only when the NSAIDs fail, or in occasional cases in which immediate results are required, but then only for the short term and usually in the form of a dose pack. The dose pack allows an immediate loading of the drug into the person's system; a gradual decrease in the amount of steroid taken then follows until the dose pack is finished (about five days to one week).

There are two adrenal steroid compounds: glucocorticoids and mineralocorticoids. The mineralocorticoids are most commonly used to supplement a patient's deficient adrenal production. The glucocorticoids are the compounds most frequently used in athletics, mainly because of their excellent anti-inflammatory action. The effect on the patient's inflammatory symptoms include reduction of tissue heat, reduction of **erythema,** control of swelling, and decrease in local tenderness. The glucocorticoids are also effective in suppressing immune responses in some diseases like asthma.

The way the glucocorticoids affect the inflammatory process is through inhibition of prostaglandin and leukotriene production as well as by impairing the function of macrophages and leukocytes. Both functions, and others like them, effectively suppress the body's inflammatory response.

The glucocorticoids used most commonly in athletics are cortisone, hydrocortisone (Cortaid), prednisone, methylprednisolone (Medrol), and dexamethasone (Decadron). Usually, the exact drug is chosen due to its duration of action (see table 5.3).

Glucocorticoid Adverse Effects

Among the adverse effects of glucocorticoids is the common ill effect associated with gluco-

Table 5.3
Common Injectable Glucocorticoids Used in Athletics

Generic name	Trade name (if any)
Cortisone	
Dexamethasone	Decadron
Hydrocortisone	Cortaid
Methylprednisolone	Medrol
Prednisone	

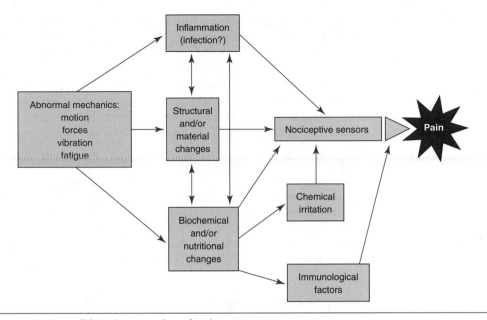

Figure 5.7   A possible pain control mechanism.
Adapted from White 1989.

corticoid injection in and around a joint. The strong catabolic effect of a glucocorticoid is not limited to the target structure and has been implicated as the cause of actual tendon rupture.

Implications for the Athletic Trainer

Although the athletic trainer will not prescribe corticosteroids, it is essential that you understand what they are and their intended effects. It should not be a surprise if an athlete reports to you that the doctor gave him or her "steroids" if the physician has failed to explain the drug therapy well. It would be wise to educate the athlete regarding the difference between anabolic (muscle building) steroids and corticosteroids (anti-inflammatory drugs).

In all cases of adrenal steroid use in and around joints, the sport trainer should keep a record of the area of injection, the strength of the steroid, and the patient's response. Always consult the physician when an individual reports having received a "cortisone" injection so that you can establish all the facts of the treatment provided.

It is also important to keep excellent records in the patient chart when you know that a corticosteroid has been prescribed, especially if more conclusive evidence is found to relate corticosteroids with soft-tissue (especially muscle) injury.

Pain and Analgesics

Pain is one of the more common complaints heard in athletic medicine. The pain may be the result of acute trauma or chronic irritation or may be iatrogenic (caused by the treatment) following surgery. Regardless of the cause, the first concern should always be to alleviate the offending factor.

If the causal factor of pain is inflammation, an anti-inflammatory agent may affect the pain at the same time that it decreases the inflammation. In some cases, however, the pain must be controlled in order to allow the individual to function more freely or allow the healing process to continue, or both. Understanding pain and the physiological processing of noxious (painful) stimuli, as seen in figure 5.7, will be an asset when the time comes to study the therapeutic treatment of pain, a topic of prime concern in both *Therapeutic Exercise for Musculoskeletal Injuries* and *Therapeutic Modalities for Musculoskeletal Injuries* in this Athletic Training Education Series. For now, we concentrate only on the control of pain using pharmaceutical medications; the other texts discuss the complex nature of the physiology of pain.

It is important for the reader to understand the difference between medicating people to allow them to function normally in life, and perhaps even in rehabilitation, and medicating individuals to allow them to continue to participate in the activity that caused the injury. It is important to realize that pain is a signal. Pain usually prevents an individual from continuing in a harmful activity. Masking this signal through the use of analgesics is not only risky; it may be strictly contraindicated in some conditions. Additionally, every participant, coach, and sports medicine professional should be aware of the potential dangers associated with the misuse of analgesics. No game or contest should be more important than the individual's health and well-being.

Pain medications run the gamut from the OTC products available in the local drugstore and supermarket to the strictly controlled narcotic drugs that are highly regulated and quite potent. Certainly we all recognize the difference between the analgesic needed for a mild headache and the medication that may be required after reconstructive surgery. This wide range of products provides the physician with many choices in the pharmaceutical management of pain. Most physicians would agree that pain should be managed with the least harmful, least addictive drug possible. Here we consider two main types of analgesics: non-narcotics and narcotics.

Narcotic Analgesics

The two main types of analgesics are both used for pain, yet the stronger, more addictive narcotic pain relievers are reserved for severe pain such as postoperative pain or pain from serious tissue damage.

Narcotic pain relievers have a limited use for most sport injuries. Moderate to severe pain, such as acute pain following a significant injury or surgery, is often treated with prescription drugs rather than the OTC agents. Narcotic analgesics of the opioid family provide excellent relief from this more severe pain because of their ability to bind within the central nervous system and interrupt **nociceptive** (pain) transmission. Opioid analgesics, however, have a negative side: They can cause physical as well as psychological addiction. This fear of addiction is typically not a concern in the treatment of acute traumatic injury because the duration of use of the narcotic drug is very short. Long-term use of narcotic painkillers, on the other hand, should be avoided because of the increased risk of drug dependence. In the mid-90s a very prominent National Football League star openly admitted to having become addicted to pain medications taken during the football season. Following this public announcement, most individuals and sports medicine specialists began looking more critically at their use of pain medications. Masking pain to allow someone to participate is certainly not condoned by the medical community and should never be done without careful protection of the injured area to avoid exacerbation of the problem.

Among the opiates, three specific drugs are familiar to the general public: morphine, codeine, and heroin. Heroin is not used for sports medicine needs and is not discussed here. Morphine is used to relieve moderate to severe pain and is often used as the standard with which other prescription analgesics are compared. Codeine is frequently the analgesic of choice for oral preparations of medicinals to control postsurgical or severe pain.

Endogenous opioids are a group of opioids that are produced in the human body and are often referred to generically as endorphins, yet there are actually three groups of endogenous opioids: endorphins, dynorphins, and enkephalins. Endogenous opioids are manufactured in the brain and released as the body attempts to control pain. They have specific receptors in the central and peripheral nervous system, giving them a very direct avenue of action; yet endogenous opioids are not as potent as the exogenous opioids. Exogenous opioids such as morphine, codeine, and heroin are either natural (from a plant), semisynthetic (from a plant and also manufactured), or synthetic (manufactured).

Opioid receptors have been the subject of much detailed research since their discovery. That there is more than one type of opioid receptor has been well documented. It has also been documented that the different receptors allow different effects to occur. Not only are the effects of the opioids controlled by the receptors, but the side effects also vary according to the particular receptor.

Non-Narcotic Analgesics

Generally, the non-narcotic analgesics are the same drugs as the NSAIDs (including aspirin and salicylates), since the NSAIDs are able to work in both capacities (analgesic and anti-inflammatory). Salicylates, ibuprofen, and acetaminophen are the most common names associated with OTC analgesics. Salicylates and ibuprofen products are NSAIDs; acetaminophen is the only non-narcotic that is not also an NSAID.

Both the analgesic and the anti-inflammatory actions of salicylates are believed to be caused by peripheral inhibition of prostaglandin synthesis as with the other NSAIDs. However, in contrast to other NSAIDs, aspirin may also inhibit the action and synthesis of other mediators of inflammation.

Antipyretic effects of salicylates are a result of inhibition of prostaglandin synthesis in the **hypothalamus** rather than at the local site as in its other actions. Aspirin also may increase the blood flow to the skin and cause sweating, thus dissipating heat associated with a fever.

Another analgesic that is not an anti-inflammatory is acetaminophen (Tylenol, Datril, Pamprin, and Panadol). Acetaminophen is a weak prostaglandin inhibitor in the peripheral tissues. Its effect is similar to that of aspirin in diminishing pain or fever, but it is not at all helpful in the reduction of inflammation. Acetaminophen is the analgesic of choice when the patient is allergic to aspirin or has intolerance to salicylates. Children with viral infections may be treated with acetaminophen without the risk of Reye's syndrome associated with use of aspirin products.

Acetaminophen is very useful in the treatment of mild to moderate pain and is provided in OTC strengths of 325 and 500 mg in tablet, capsule, and liquid-preparation forms. In Europe, paracetamol is the equivalent to acetaminophen and is quite readily available. Liquid acetaminophen preparations are also available, which is quite helpful when acetaminophen is needed for intraoral injury or for surgery involving the jaw or mouth.

A narcotic agent to increase the drug's potency may supplement acetaminophen. This combination, such as Tylenol III or Tylenol IV, is often used for the treatment of severe pain associated with fractures, dislocations, or other trauma, including surgery. The narcotic (usually codeine) adds the analgesic effect of the narcotic pain reliever to that of the acetaminophen; the narcotic-supplemented acetaminophen is therefore a high-level analgesic limited in its use to patients with severe pain. Acetaminophen with codeine (Tylenol III, Tylenol IV) is a controlled prescription drug because of the narcotic; thus use will be strictly monitored.

Administration of Analgesics

Analgesics have a wide variety of routes of administration, probably because of the wide variety of situations in which pain is the dominant complaint.

Analgesics are most commonly taken by mouth in either a pill, capsule, or liquid form, but may also be given transdermally by **iontophoresis** or a specialized patch; by injection into a muscle; or **intravenously.** You may hear of a patient having an analgesic "pump" following surgery. This most often involves one of the narcotic pain relievers, and the pump allows the patient to administer small doses of the drug as the pain dictates, always with the machine preventing an overdose of the medicine.

Adverse Effects of Analgesic Therapy

The most common unwanted effects of opioids include drowsiness, dizziness, blurred vision, nausea, vomiting, and constipation. Addiction to opioid drugs, as previously stated, is also a risk from both a physical and a psychological point of view. There is clear, documented evidence that morphine causes a physical addiction—as evident in the severe withdrawal symptoms experienced by addicts when the drug is no longer available. At first the patient feels uneasy or nervous and may experience depression. Physical signs of addiction occur during withdrawal and include sweating, nausea, and vomiting. Muscle tremors and twitching are also associated with narcotic withdrawal. Withdrawal symptoms can last anywhere from 36 hr to five days. After this withdrawal period the person may still have a strong psychological addiction to the drug, such as a strong desire or craving for a "fix." Psychological addiction can last for years and is often thought to be the most difficult part of the addiction/withdrawal process.

As we discussed earlier, aspirin inhibits platelet function, but the body's blood-clotting mechanisms usually begin to return to normal within 36 hr after the last dose of the drug. Other salicylates have minimal effect on platelets, and acetaminophen has no effect on the platelets.

Gastrointestinal irritation is fairly common with the use of many of the NSAIDs and salicylates but less common with the COX-2 inhibitor classes. Aspirin and buffered aspirin products have approximately the same absorption rate; however, the incidence of bleeding is reported to be higher with plain aspirin tablets than with the buffered products. Gastrointestinal mucosa injury is seen less often with coated aspirin than with plain aspirin or buffered aspirin. Patients with erosive gastritis or peptic ulcer should avoid salicylates because of the possibility of exacerbating the condition.

Tinnitus and hearing loss associated with salicylate therapy are dose related and usually completely reversible, typically subsiding within 24 to 48 hr after the dose is reduced or discontinued.

Implications for the Athletic Trainer

It is important to understand the types of analgesics available for the treatment of pain. Although you will not prescribe drugs, you should be able to inform the athlete regarding the type of analgesic prescribed or what might be expected following a surgical procedure. Additionally, understanding of the various alternative choices of pain medication may prove to be beneficial in helping athletes decide wisely when selecting an OTC analgesic for minor pain.

Anesthetics: General and Local

It is probably obvious that a surgical patient will most likely need both sensory sedation and full muscle relaxation in order for the surgeon to perform the needed procedure. This is accomplished by the use of general anesthesia. The vast area of general anesthetics is quite complex and beyond the scope of this book, yet a simple explanation is that a combination of drugs is needed to prepare for, achieve, and bring the patient back from anesthesia. General anesthetics are drugs that are very general in their action; they cause the patient to become unconscious, amnesic, and totally relaxed muscularly. Because of the multiple systems involved in sedating a patient for surgery, several drugs are combined to achieve and maintain the specific anesthetic goal.

From time to time the surgeon may elect to use a local anesthetic rather than a general anesthetic. Local anesthetics are capable of blocking all nerves, thus acting on both sensory and motor functions. Although motor paralysis may at times be desirable, it may limit the ability of the patient to cooperate, as in obstetric delivery and in some surgeries of the nervous system (when the motor function of the nerve must remain intact but the sensory fibers are being cut). In most cases of local anesthesia used in athletic medicine, both the sensory and motor functions are affected. Minor surgery or suturing of open wounds is usually accomplished under a local anesthesia. Only the area of concern needs to be affected, and the local anesthetic provides just sufficient results. An individual in need of dental work typically receives a local anesthetic to decrease the associated pain. This anesthesia is not limited to the sensory nerve, and the person often returns from the appointment showing signs of facial muscle paralysis.

The choice of a local anesthetic for a specific procedure is typically based on the duration of the action needed. Procaine (Novocain) and chloroprocaine are short acting; lidocaine (Xylocaine, etc.), mepivacaine (Carbocaine, Isocaine), and prilocaine (Citanest) have an intermediate duration of action; and tetracaine (Pontocaine), bupivacaine (Marcaine), and etidocaine (Duranest) are long-acting drugs (see table 5.4).

In the treatment of superficial abrasions, several preparations are available to reduce the sensitivity of the exposed nerve endings. Some of the topical preparations on the market include Benzocaine, Nupercainal, and Xylocaine (available in ointment, cream, jelly, and solution forms).

Table 5.4
Pharmacokinetic Properties of Local Anesthetics

Anesthetic agent	Rate of onset of anesthesia	Duration of action
Novocain	Rapid	Short
Xylocaine	Slow	Moderate
Carbocaine, Isocaine		
Citanest		
Marcaine	Rapid	Long
Pontocaine		
Duranest		

Table 5.5
Skeletal Muscle Relaxants Used in Surgery

Drug	Main effects	Side effects
Depolarizing drugs (succinylcholine)	Skeletal muscle paralysis following muscle fasciculations. All skeletal muscles will be involved, including respiratory muscles.	Cardiac arrhythmia Hyperkalemia with a possibility of cardiac arrest Increased intraocular pressure Increased intragastric pressure and potential of vomiting Postoperative muscle pain
Non-depolarizing drugs (tubocurarine)	Skeletal muscle paralysis with small muscle paralysis first and respiratory paralysis last.	Hypotension (low blood pressure)

Administration of Anesthetics

General anesthetics are administered either by inhalation or as an intravenous preparation; local anesthetics can be administered via injection or applied topically (iontophoresis or **cutaneous** application without a driving current).

Adverse Effects

Knowledge of the adverse effects (see table 5.5) associated with anesthesia can help us understand the reason behind many of the operative precautions that are exercised. The anesthesiologist has several duties in keeping the individual sedated during a surgical procedure; this function, although often noticed but given relatively little attention by the untrained observer, is actually extremely critical to a safe and comfortable sedation during surgery. The adverse effects are numerous, but are clearly understood, allowing steps to be taken to avoid problems during surgery. Specific adverse effects include cardiovascular effects (hypotension and arrhythmia), increased **intragastric** pressure, intraorbital pressure, postoperative muscle pain, and histamine responses (itching and hives).

Implications for the Athletic Trainer

Rest assured, without specialized training, you will not find yourself administering general anesthetics, yet it is good to understand both the things you may observe when attending surgery and the things the patient is undergoing during the operative procedure.

In many college and professional athletic facilities, the team physicians keep at least two injectable local anesthetics on hand, typically one shorter-acting (Xylocaine) and one longer-acting (Marcaine) anesthetic. In these settings you may be asked to set up the physician's area with the injectables; thus an understanding of the various types of anesthetics may be critical if the physician asks you to set out short- or long-acting supplies only. The addition of a vasoconstrictor (epinephrine) to the local anesthetic will decrease the rate of absorption of the anesthetic and thus increase the duration of action.

Central-Acting Muscle Relaxants

A variety of compounds are available to reduce muscle spasm associated with local injury. Some of the numerous generic names (and trade names) are carisoprodol (Soma), chlorzoxazone (Parafon Forte; chlorzoxazone and acetaminophen), cyclobenzaprine hydrochloride (Flexeril), diazepam (Valium), methocarbamol (Robaxin), and orphenadrine (Norgesic; orphenadrine with aspirin and caffeine).

Often the drug treatment of muscle spasm involves a muscle relaxant with an analgesic that is added in an effort to provide pain relief. Regardless of the type of skeletal muscle relaxant used, the mechanism of action is not well understood; yet the overall effect is sedation. All the drugs have some general depressant activity on the central nervous system, and the ability of the compound to selectively relax skeletal muscle has not been proven.

Administration of Muscle Relaxants

Most muscle relaxants are administered orally or by injection.

Adverse Effects of Muscle Relaxants

Because of the sedative action of these drugs, the primary side effect is drowsiness with the addition of some dizziness. Nausea, light-headedness, vertigo, ataxia, and headache may occur depending on the patient and the specific muscle relaxant used. Some physicians feel that the side effects and central action of the skeletal muscle relaxant are sufficient reason not to prescribe them for the student-athlete. In cases in which the muscle spasm is severe and must be blocked to allow the athlete to sleep comfortably, the physician may prescribe a relaxant to be taken at bedtime.

Implications for the Athletic Trainer

It is wise to understand the effect of skeletal muscle relaxants and to advise the individual accordingly. The sedative effect—although not the specific effect one might want—often reduces local muscle spasm associated with athletic injury. It is important to remind someone taking a muscle relaxant that the drug has a strong sedative effect and that use during the day might interfere with normal daily activities. Because of the specific nature of physical therapy and the general effects of the drug therapy treatment, it is also important to emphasize the need for compliance with any physical therapy prescribed.

NON-ORTHOPEDIC MEDICINALS

The general group of non-orthopedic medicinals is truly open-ended. The number of drugs available equals the variety of medical problems that one might encounter. Some categorization is obviously necessary. We will examine some of the drugs used for common, non-orthopedic problems that affect all individuals, namely, drugs for upper-respiratory system problems, drugs to combat infections, and drugs for digestive tract disturbances.

Medications for Upper Respiratory Tract Conditions

Unfortunately, the common cold is very tenacious, lasting about a week regardless of the therapeutic measures taken. Among the few things one can do is to reduce or control the symptoms: runny nose, congestion, sore throat, and the like. Two types of drugs are available to help with the congestion or runny nose effects: decongestants and antihistamines. A persistent cough can present an irritating problem both in daily life generally and in sport activity. Suppression of the cough reflex has long been a recognized action of opioids, particularly codeine; but this is not a favored drug to use because of its addictive potential and also because it often leaves the patient with a feeling of euphoria or drowsiness. Four main non-narcotic preparations are prescribed for management of the congestion or cough (or both) associated with an upper respiratory illness or allergies: decongestants, antihistamines, **antitussives,** and expectorants.

Decongestants

Decongestants are used when there is sinus congestion with or without nasal discharge. Allergies and the common cold are often seasonal; they also vary with area of the country. Decongestants used to treat these symptoms are members of the alpha-1-adrenergic agonist family of medicines.

Some of the more common decongestants are pseudoephedrine, ephedrine, epinephrine, and oxymetazoline. Each drug is manufactured by various companies under different trade names (see table 5.6).

Administration of Decongestants

The alpha-1-agonists may be taken systematically (oral forms) or applied locally to the nasal mucosa via aerosols.

Adverse Effects

The primary adverse effects of decongestants include headache, dizziness, nervousness, nausea, and cardiovascular irregularities, all of which become more apparent with continued use. The decongestant usually does not make the person feel tired or lethargic; on the contrary, some individuals feel that the alpha-1-agonist actually produces a feeling of heightened arousal or a "buzz."

Implications for the Athletic Trainer

Since it is within the law to provide a single dose of an OTC medication, you may find that this is within the scope of your job. If it is, and athletes see you for a decongestant, it is very important that you record the drug and dosage provided. Situations have happened in which the athlete finds that the decongestant gives him or her a "buzz," and soon the athlete is depending on the sports medicine staff to provide the dose. Without a good record system, the athlete may see several different people on the health care staff and from each obtain a single dose. This multiple dosing is certainly dangerous and a bad situation to allow to develop.

Antihistamines

Antihistamines are used for a number of problems in athletics. Not only are they helpful in the management of allergic responses to hay fever, they are often used for their strong secondary effect, sedation. The antihistamines can be used to produce a mild sedation helpful in management of the restless individual who is unable to fall asleep.

Table 5.6
Grouping Decongestants Used in Athletics

Generic grouping	Common trade names	Dosage form
Pseudoephedrine	Actifed, Sudafed, and others	Oral: tablets and liquid
Ephedrine	Primatene Tablets	Oral: tablets and liquid
Epinephrine	Primatene Mist	Nasal spray
Oxymetazoline (or phenylephrine)	Neo-Synephrine, Afrin	Nasal spray and tablets

Table 5.7
Common Antihistamines

Generic name	Trade name(s)	Sedative effect
Brompheniramine	Dimetane	Low
Chlorpheniramine	Chlor-Trimeton	Low
Clemastine	Tavist	Low
Loratadine	Claritin	Low
Terfenadine	Seldane	Low
Diphenhydramine	Benadryl, others	High
Dimenhydrinate	Dramamine	High
Doxylamine	Unisom	High

The numerous antihistamines vary in the degree of sedation they cause, which is often the adverse effect that limits the use of this type of drug. Newer antihistamines do not cross the blood–brain barrier and thus exert less of the sedative effect but are quite effective in producing the desired effects of drying up the mucosal vasculature and decreasing congestion. Table 5.7 shows some of the more commonly used antihistamines; as you may notice, some of the trade names are those associated with preparations to help you sleep. As noted earlier, this is a side effect of the antihistamine; but because the effect is so strong, the drugs are marketed for their secondary effect. One might regard an antihistamine as actually two drugs in one, although caution is warranted if sleep or drowsiness is not a wanted effect.

Administration of Antihistamines

Antihistamines are usually taken orally, either by pill or as a liquid.

Adverse Effects

Although antihistamines often produce drowsiness, this may not be classified as an "unwanted" or adverse effect. Nonetheless, one must include drowsiness in the classification of adverse effects when discussing medications for the upper respiratory tract.

Reports of dry mouth, decreased coordination, tightness in the chest, dizziness, and blood pressure changes are additional adverse effects of antihistamines.

Implications for the Athletic Trainer

When suggesting an OTC product for the athlete to purchase, it is prudent to inform the person of the potential drowsiness that could occur. If the athlete needs to study, drive, or otherwise be alert, the choice of antihistamine becomes more important.

Antitussives

Antitussives are used to suppress coughing, but usually only for the short term. With the exception of the opioids, as mentioned previously, use of the antitussives varies according to the physician's and pharmacist's personal preferences. Frequently the patient or parent searching for something to control a cough is met with such an array of choices that the decision becomes quite difficult. Some of the more common of these drugs are listed in table 5.8.

Table 5.8
Common Antitussives (Cough Suppressants)

Generic name	Trade name(s)	Action
Codeine	Many	Direct inhibitory effect on brainstem cough center
Hydrocodone	Triaminic Expectorant DH	Similar to action of codeine
Dextromethorphan	Many	Similar to action of codeine
Caramiphen	Tuss-Ornade	Antihistamine
Benzonatate	Tessalon Perle	Anesthetic to respiratory mucosa

Administration of Antitussives

The oral route of administration of antitussives is well known to most people. Cough syrups, lozenges, and pills are all commonly used in an attempt to reduce a cough.

Adverse Effects

Antitussives may cause drowsiness or a feeling of dizziness in some people, while in others the antitussive may cause restlessness and nervousness. Additionally, they may cause constipation, especially if taken for several weeks.

Implications for the Athletic Trainer

Many athletes do not realize the difference between cough and cold medications such as expectorants, cough suppressants, or decongestants. Educating athletes about the antitussives will help them make the best purchase for their symptoms. When an athlete has a cough for weeks on end, it may be important to help the person find a health care provider who will be able to prescribe stronger medication than what is available for general, OTC purchase.

Expectorants and Mucolytics

The substances called expectorants and mucolytics are grouped together pharmacologically but are quite different in effect. The mucolytic drugs help to decrease the viscosity of respiratory excretions, while expectorants serve to facilitate the production and ejection of the mucus. Typically these types of agents are used to decrease the accumulation of thick, viscous secretions that clog respiratory passages. Often the expectorants and mucolytics are used in conjunction with antitussives and decongestants. Some physicians feel that the effects of the drugs are no better than that provided by a household humidifier. The only mucolytic drug currently in use is acetylcysteine, yet the number of products known as expectorants is great. The most common expectorant, guaifenesin, is used in many OTC preparations. The way guaifenesin works is unclear, yet the FDA recognizes its positive effects.

Administration

Most expectorants and mucolytics are provided in the oral forms. Cough syrups are well labeled with the word "expectorant."

Adverse Effects

The primary adverse effect is GI upset, and this is exacerbated if the syrup is taken on an empty stomach. Other unwanted effects include insomnia, headache, vertigo, skin rash, and breathing problems.

Implications for the Athletic Trainer

Expectorants and mucolytics have a special role in the management of the common cold. When evaluating the types of medicinals to help abate the symptoms of cough and congestion, one must pay attention to the type of cough. Coughs that sound as if they are producing movement of phlegm from the lungs are called productive coughs. These types of coughs may benefit from the use of mucolytic and expectorants, while the harsh, raspy cough that sounds dry will usually not benefit from this type of therapy.

Bronchodilators (Beta-Adrenergic Agonists)

There are a number of bronchodilators on the market; most, if used by persons with asthma, are in the form of an inhaler (see figure 5.8). Bronchodilators are often beta-adrenergic agonists, and they cause smooth-muscle relaxation, effectively opening the constricted airways. Albuterol is the most common product used in athletic health care; two trade names of albuterol are Proventil and Ventolin (inhalers). Following inhalation, the effects are seen within 5 to 15 min and last from 3 to 6 hr.

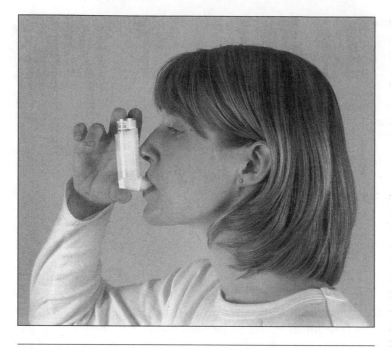

Figure 5.8 Inhalers are used to deliver drugs to treat asthmatic symptoms.

The use of inhalants is intended for those who have asthma, yet some physicians prescribe an inhaler when mucus is plugging the respiratory airways. The active agent in the inhaler is actually the critical factor, yet the method of administration (inhalation) allows the drug to be delivered directly to the respiratory tissues with minimal side effects. A person who has asthma may be prescribed anti-inflammatory agents as well as bronchodilators to reverse the bronchial constriction associated with the condition.

The classification "asthmatic" encompasses a wide range of involvement. Some people experience bronchoconstriction only when exercising (exercise-induced bronchospasm), while others experience constriction of the air passageway day in and day out. Changes in environmental conditions and minor colds affect the person with asthma much more than people without this condition. Patients experiencing more severe forms of asthma, or those in an acute episode, may be given the anti-inflammatory drugs (cortisone preparations) in an effort to control the swelling in the bronchioles once the bronchodilator opens the passages sufficiently. Products such as Azmacort and Flovent are steroid preparations that either prevent the narrowing or relax the smooth muscle of the air passages. These preparations may be on the banned drug list for college and Olympic sports, and it is prudent to investigate the legality of such a drug prior to use in a competitive individual.

Administration of Bronchodilators

Most often the drug is provided in a metered-dose inhaler: Each time the canister is activated it emits a metered dose. For severe breathing problems a "breathing treatment" is employed in which a **nebulizer** mixes the drug into a fine mist; the drug is then dispensed over a period of about 10 min, providing improved distribution of the drug into the bronchioles.

Adverse Effects of Bronchodilators

One of the most disconcerting side effects with use of inhalers involves its effects on the heart. After a breathing treatment, people often experience a "racing heart" or other cardiac irregularities. Inhaler treatment may also be followed by a central nervous system effect that gives the individual a sense of nervousness. Long-term use of bronchodilators may cause inflammatory conditions of the pharynx due to the medicine's coming into contact with the back of the throat.

Implications for the Athletic Trainer:

The major problem with the use of bronchodilators is the patient's hand–breath coordination. The individual must maximally exhale and then time the depression of the canister with an inhalation. Too often, however, the timing is good but the inhaler is aimed so that the drug is placed at the back of the throat. Occasionally a breathing treatment may be needed and may be administered in the team physician's office by the physician or local paramedics.

Infections and Antibiotics

When we talk about infection we should certainly stop for a moment and ask ourselves why an infection has occurred. A small amount of prevention may be all that is needed to avoid the use of medicinal drugs. A good rule is that all open wounds must be well cleansed with soap and warm water. Some irritants or bacteria enter the skin or other tissues, and no outward sign of injury is noticed until infection is present. When infection develops, medicinal drugs may be needed.

There is some confusion surrounding the terminology used with reference to drugs for treating infections. It helps to think of the infection in terms of the cause and to know that the name of a drug for treating infection will have the prefix "anti-" followed by the term for the offending element—that is, antibacterials, antifungals, and so on. The term antibiotic denotes an agent used to kill an organism. We will discuss the antibiotics in terms of their specific function—either antibacterial or antifungal.

Antibacterial Agents

Topical antibacterial agents are often used in athletics after cleansing of an open wound. Although use of the antibacterial in this situation is mostly prophylactic, the agent can be effective for treating some superficial wound infections. The most proper way to deal with an infection is to take a culture and employ sensitivity studies to determine what type of bacterium is causing the infection. Since some bacteria are resistant to specific agents, treatment with these agents will be ineffective. Unless the infection is full-blown, the athletic trainer may adequately treat superficial wounds with one or more of the products commonly available over the counter.

Antibacterial agents used topically usually contain a mixture of antibacterial agents and include a variety of trade-name products—the more common being Neosporin, Polysporin, and Bacitracin, among many others with similar names.

An interesting side note concerns a "trainer's trick" to care for the superficial wounds caused by artificial turf. Obviously, with all turf burns, the most critical factor in preventing infection is thorough cleaning of the wound. This very often is extremely difficult because of the irritation of many nerve endings on the abraded skin. Reducing the sensitivity of the skin prior to cleaning the wound often allows one to fully cleanse the skin surface. This is easy to do during the competition at the same time that one covers the open wound. Simple application of a topical anesthetic in lieu of an antibiotic will allow the anesthetic to desensitize the area while the athlete completes the contest; afterward, the person can shower and clean the wound with less discomfort. The products used to aid in the anesthetic action include the true anesthetics available in cream or ointment form and the anesthetic creams designed for hemorrhoid treatment, which provide both the antibacterial and the anesthetic effect.

Antibacterial agents, regardless of the tissue infected, are classified according to their effect, whether it be via inhibition of the bacterial cell's wall and its function (penicillins and cephalosporins), via inhibition of bacterial protein synthesis (aminoglycosides, erythromycin, and tetracycline), or, finally, via inhibition of the bacterial DNA/RNA function (sulfanilamides). Some of the trade names associated with the antibacterials are listed in table 5.9.

Table 5.9
Common Antibacterial Agents

Action	Generic name	Trade name(s)
Cell membrane synthesis inhibition	Penicillin	V-Cillin, Amoxil, many others
	Cephalosporin	Keflex, Keflin, Ultrace, Suprax, many others
	Bacitracin	Bacitracin ointment
Protein synthesis inhibition	Erythromycin	E-Mycin, EES, Erythrocin, others
	Tetracycline	Achromycin V, Vibramycin, others
DNA/RNA inhibition	Fluoroquinolone	Cipro
	Sulfanilamide	Gantrisin, Silvadene

Administration of Antibacterials

Topical applications are the most familiar form of application of antibacterials used in athletics. Systemic infections may be treated with oral antibacterials, and severe infections may be treated with injectable forms of the medicines.

Adverse Effects of Antibacterials

Medical professionals have warned against the overprescribing of antibacterials in the young patient due to the potential of an increased resistance to the drug. Other unwanted effects include diarrhea, nausea and vomiting, rash, injection site inflammation, and seizures.

Implications for the Athletic Trainer

The antibacterial agents often used by the athletic trainer are those administered topically. Rarely will drugs administered topically cause systemic intolerance; thus there are no precautions to their use, short of an allergic response. In the case of treatment of superficial abrasions such as turf burns, thorough cleansing of the wound and application of a topical antibacterial agent are strongly recommended.

Antifungals

Fungal infections are much like bacterial infections; however, the agents used to treat bacteria will not affect fungi, and agents effective against fungi are not effective against bacteria. Primarily, the antifungal agents work by disrupting fungal membrane functions. Most healthy individuals do not develop the fungal infections that are associated with people whose immune system has been suppressed.

When oral antifungal medications are used for tenacious infections such as those under the nail bed (toenails are especially prone to fungal infections), the physician may advise the person to take the medication just prior to exercise. The reason is that the antifungal medication is distributed to the nail bed through perspiration, so the more the person perspires the more effective the treatment can be. Unfortunately, these nail bed infections are usually quite tough, and eradication using oral antifungals can take months.

Not infrequently, people are bothered by fungal infections in areas of high moisture such as the groin, feet, and hands. The individual should be educated regarding good hygiene to control or prevent fungal infections. Control entails keeping the area as dry as possible, taking care to use only clean garments over the affected tissues, and, if necessary, beginning the application of an antifungal agent.

The person with a fungal infection needs to apply the antifungal medication to the affected area two to three times daily. With regular application of an antifungal cream or ointment, the fungus can be brought under control within two or three weeks, after which time the person may be able to switch to a powder form. Too often people notice the problem and self-treat it with the powder antifungal, only to minimally control the spread rather than effectively treat the fungus. Some products are prescription drugs and others are over the counter; some products are combined with a topical corticosteroid that may provide more rapid improvement than is possible with the antifungal alone. Some of the topical antifungals are listed in table 5.10.

Administration of Antifungals

Antifungal agents are of two varieties: oral medication (pills) and topical medication (cream, ointment, and powder). The oral medications are used for subcutaneous (below the skin) and systemic mycoses (diseases caused by fungi), whereas superficial mycoses are easily treated using topical agents.

Table 5.10
Common Topical Antifungal Preparations

Generic name	Trade name(s)
Clortrimazole	Clotrimazole Cream 1% (prescription), Lotrimin
Miconazole	Micatine, Monistat
Naftifine	Naftin (not good against yeasts)
Tolnaftate	Tinactin

Adverse Effects of Antifungals

The topical antifungals are fairly free of adverse effects, yet the oral form of the drug suffers from a variety of unwanted effects such as headache, neurological changes, liver disorders, and some degree of photosensitivity.

Implications for the Athletic Trainer

Careful observation of the skin and nail beds of the athlete may be the first step in caring for fungal infections. Refer the athlete to a physician for diagnosis and proper medical care, especially when topical antifungal OTC medications do not seem to manage the problem. Sub-ungual (under the nail) infections and infections that appear to be spreading must be treated by a physician. Educating athletes about the treatment measures may help them to make the proper decision in consulting a physician.

Drugs for Treatment of Gastrointestinal Problems

Athletes have problems similar to those of the population in general; GI disturbances are not uncommon. The athlete may be under great stress, resulting in diarrhea or upset stomach. Travel and changes in eating habits may cause constipation, or, conversely, loose stools or actual diarrhea. All digestive system problems are manageable if they are recognized; it is just a matter of having the athlete report the problem.

Antidiarrheals

Two classes of drugs are used to treat diarrhea: opioids (Lomotil, Imodium) and non-opioids (Donnagel). Both effectively slow the movement of food through the GI tract. One aspect to note, however, is that antidiarrheals produce bowel "paralysis"; and if the diarrhea is associated with an infection, the infection may continue to proliferate, creating a potential for bowel rupture secondary to the expanding infection. Caution is always in order when one is treating diarrhea with no known etiology.

Some of the products used to treat diarrhea are also adsorbents (not "absorbents"). These products will adsorb (attach other substances to their surface without any chemical action) the harmful substances (bacteria and other toxins), but there is question about how effective they are in decreasing stool production and water. Kaopectate and Pepto-Bismol are among these products (bismuth salicylate), which also decrease gastric acid secretion and may aid in quieting an upset stomach.

Administration of Antidiarrheals

Antidiarrheals are available for oral consumption in the liquid form as well as tablets or capsules.

Adverse Effects

In addition to the effect of bowel paralysis, the antidiarrheals often cause constipation if taken for a prolonged period. The opioid antidiarrheals, like other opioids, may cause drowsiness and dizziness as an unwanted side effect.

Implications for the Athletic Trainer

Often the athlete is quite shy about reporting bouts of diarrhea, so it becomes important to understand the seriousness of the condition if and when the athlete confides in you. Not only should you understand the treatment and precautions regarding diarrhea; you also need to understand the sequelae of the condition. Whenever excess water is lost through the bowel, the body quickly enters a state of fluid depletion. Care must be taken to replenish fluids and electrolytes in the athlete who is experiencing diarrhea.

Laxatives

Although a less frequent problem in the young, healthy population, constipation may be a problem in the athletic arena (more among the coaches and administrators than the athletes!). The two main products used to reduce constipation are bulk-forming laxatives and bowel stimulants.

Bulk-forming laxatives (Metamucil and the hyperosmotic agents) absorb water in the lower GI tract and stretch the bowel, stimulating peristalsis. Most of these products contain dietary fiber to aid in more regular action of the bowel. Bowel stimulants act to irritate the intestinal mucosa or the **splanchnic** nerves serving the bowel. This type of laxative includes Dulcolax, Ex-Lax, and other commonly available products.

Administration

The bulk-forming laxatives are for oral consumption, coming in convenient wafer form or a powder that one would mix with water or another beverage. The bowel stimulants are usually administered rectally via suppository or enema application methods.

Adverse Effects of Laxative Use

The unwelcome effects of oral laxatives include feelings of bloating or cramping of the bowel. Some reversal of the constipation can occur, resulting in diarrhea. Other reports of nausea, flatulence (intestinal gas), and an increased thirst have been noted. The rectally administered laxatives have been known to cause rectal area discomfort including bleeding, blistering, burning, itching, or pain.

Implications for the Athletic Trainer

Unfortunately, the laxatives are a group of drugs that may be misused by some. College athletic trainers have found gymnasts and wrestlers using laxatives to clear the bowel in an attempt to decrease body weight. This practice is dangerous because the medication interrupts the body's normal physiology. The large intestine is responsible for removing fluids from the waste material, and with a bowel stimulant or laxative the large intestine is so irritated that fluid absorption is aborted and the waste expelled. Dehydration can result from the misuse of a laxative, predisposing the individual to additional harm especially if exercising in a warm environment such as a wrestling room. Those responsible need to exercise care in both drug inventory and dispensation procedures so that it is easier to recognize any misuse of these medications.

Antiemetics

Emesis, or vomiting, is sometimes troublesome for individuals with pregame anxiety or motion sickness. The antiemetics most often used for this type of problem include dimenhydrinate (Dramamine) and meclizine (Antivert, Bonine). Some antacids and adsorbents also help in soothing the gastric mucosa and decreasing the irritation that is causing the vomiting.

Administration

Except in the case of a medical condition causing frequent vomiting (such as with chemotherapy), emesis can be controlled with oral medications.

Adverse Effects

The typical products used for emesis, unfortunately, are apt to cause drowsiness or a headache, neither of which would be welcome during an athletic competition.

Implications for the Athletic Trainer

Medical conditions unrelated to simple anxiety can also cause vomiting. Early stages of pregnancy, for example, may cause vomiting as well as medical problems such as heat exhaustion, appendicitis, food poisoning, head injury, and various diseases. The underlying cause of vomiting must be understood and evaluated, and caution must be exercised in treating athletes who have recurrent bouts of vomiting.

Pharmacology in Athletic Medicine   191

Antacids

Some people experience occasional minor gastric upset due to their eating habits. The drugs used to decrease the stomach irritation will actually neutralize stomach acids. Antacids contain a combination of a carbonate or hydroxide and an aluminum, magnesium, or calcium that work together to control the gastric pH.

Others have gastric ulcers or irritable bowel syndrome (IBS) that may require medications designed to block the release of gastric acid. Such preparations include Tagamet, Pepcid, and Zantac.

Administration of Antacids

The most common form of antacid is the chewable tablet, many of these being readily available without a prescription. Other oral forms include powders or tablets that are to be dissolved in water or other fluid, liquid forms, and chewing gum. Medications for IBS are most often in tablet or liquid form, but can be administered by injection or intravenously for severe medical conditions.

Adverse Effects

When antacids are taken as directed, very few adverse effects are noted. If the medicine is taken in large doses or over a long time, minor unwanted effects occur, including a chalky taste, mild constipation or diarrhea, thirst, stomach cramps, and whitish or speckled stools. Unwanted effects such as those that may accompany Tagamet, Pepcid, and Zantac administration include headache, dizziness and diarrhea, or nausea and vomiting.

Implications for the Athletic Trainer

Products to settle the stomach are sometimes used in an attempt to counteract poor eating habits, and the health care specialist should educate the patient to attack the problem at the cause, that is, nutritional habits, and not depend on the quick-fix antacid. Chronic use of antacids has a potential to contribute to kidney stones. There is insufficient evidence to establish a causal relationship, but this is still reason enough to convince a person to stop using these products if at all possible.

SUMMARY

1. *Define and list examples of generic versus trade-name drugs.*

   By generic drug, we mean a drug that is referred to by its "official" or nonproprietary name. This name is often derived from the chemical name but is much shorter and simpler. An example of a generic drug is acetaminophen; a trade name of acetaminophen is Tylenol. There can be as many trade names (proprietary names) as there are companies that make the product.

2. *Discuss why drugs are classified as nonprescription, prescription, or controlled substances.*

   Nonprescription (OTC) drugs can be obtained right from the store shelf. Taking the OTC drug as indicated on the label should pose no difficulties for most patients (unless the patient has an allergy to that medication). Over-the-counter drugs are usually sufficient for minor problems. Prescription drugs are more powerful drugs that must be selected by the physician (or other certified professional such as a physician's assistant). In order to avoid adverse drug interactions, the prescribing health care practitioner will interview the patient about allergies and other medications being taken. Prescription medications can be refilled with the permission of the physician. Controlled substances are those drugs that have a high potential for abuse. There are rules for prescribing, dispensing, and renewing prescriptions for the five types of controlled substances. These drugs must be kept in a secure area of the facility, and those responsible must keep thorough records of any controlled drugs dispensed.

3. *Identify the methods of administering medicinal drugs to the patient.*

Drugs can be administered via the digestive system (enteral), meaning that the drug is taken in (by mouth, under the tongue [sublingually], or rectally) and the drug then enters the appropriate organ or system from that point of origin. Non-enteral methods of administration include delivery by injection (including IV, intra-articular, intramuscular), application to the skin (topical), inhalation, and transport through the skin (transdermal).

4. *Define agonist and antagonist as related to medicinal drugs.*

An agonist to a drug will assist with the same function as the drug does. The effect of taking two agonistic drugs would be an enhancement of the primary effect. The antagonist is opposite in its effect or counterproductive to the primary medication. Taking both the drug and an antagonist to it would cancel or decrease the effectiveness of the primary drug.

5. *Identify the various sources one could use to find information on drugs.*

One can obtain information about a particular drug by asking a pharmacist for patient information on the drug. Other sources include various books containing drug information such as the *PDR* and *Facts and Comparisons*.

6. *Describe how one might find information on the USOC or the NCAA banned drug lists.*

Information on policies on the use of various drugs can usually be obtained from the governing body for the athletic group. For instance, to find out what drugs are banned for Olympic athletes you would contact the USOC and request its banned drug list; for information regarding banned drugs in college athletics you can contact the NCAA. The Internet is an excellent way to obtain contact information for these organizations.

7. *Discuss the inflammatory process and describe how drugs may affect that process.*

Prostaglandins and thromboxanes are implicated in the production of pain, inflammation, fever, and excessive blood clotting. Prostaglandins are produced by the synthesis of arachidonic acid that is ingested in our normal diet. The pathway by which the prostaglandins are produced is called the cyclooxygenase pathway. Nonsteroidal anti-inflammatory drugs act by blocking the cyclooxygenase pathway, which affects the production of prostaglandins and thus decreases inflammation, pain, fever, and excessive blood clotting.

8. *Identify the more common side effects of anti-inflammatory drugs and the steps that may be taken to reduce these unwanted outcomes.*

In general, the major side effect of NSAIDs is stomach upset. Some agents are less irritating to the stomach mucosa or do not cause as much bleeding from the irritation. The best method of prohibiting or limiting this side effect is to always take the NSAID with food or milk. Some people insist that an antacid taken in conjunction with the NSAID will reduce gastric upset, but this has not be proven scientifically. The patient should always be cautioned not to take the anti-inflammatory drug on an empty stomach.

9. *Describe the effects of analgesics and discuss reasons to limit their use in sport participation.*

Analgesics work on the same basis as the anti-inflammatory drugs, by blocking the cyclooxygenase pathway—effectively blocking the production of prostaglandins. The main reason for not using analgesics during sport participation is that pain is often the signal of structural damage. Without the nociceptive input (pain), the participant may continue to stress the injured tissues, exacerbating the condition.

10. *Identify ways in which a fungal infection may be controlled with medicinal drugs.*

    Fungal infections may present a superficial problem (skin fungus) or a subcutaneous problem (under skin layers). Fungal infections that are not superficial are difficult to treat with the standard OTC antifungals that are effective for the superficial problems. Systemic fungal infections are treated with an oral antifungal. In addition, superficial fungal infections are resistant to the powder form of many OTC antifungals. It is important to educate infected participants about use of the antifungal creams and ointments in order to eradicate the fungus, and then to suggest use of the powder to keep the environment unfavorable for the fungus to return.

11. *Describe ways in which a laxative may be misused.*

    Loss of body weight is very important to some participants. Unfortunately, laxatives can help people artificially reduce their weight. This misuse of laxatives can lead to serious health concerns and should be avoided.

CRITICAL THINKING QUESTIONS

1. Your softball coach has recently been coming to the athletic treatment area to obtain a dose of Tums. You have noticed him on occasion, but never really paid attention to how frequently he asks for the antacid. Explain how you might approach the coach to learn more about his antacid use.

2. One of your swimmers has been having shoulder impingement symptoms. You evaluated the athlete and offered some exercises to help balance the shoulder muscles. The athlete was also referred to the physician for evaluation. In that evaluation, the doctor mentioned that the exercises were very important and that the athlete should begin a course of anti-inflammatory medication. You know that the athlete has had an irritable stomach in the past. Explain what adjustments may be made in the prescribing of an anti-inflammatory drug for this athlete.

3. The athletic director at your high school has asked you to develop a drug-testing program for the athletic teams. He wants to make the testing random with regard to who is tested and when people are tested, but other than that, he has no limitations on the cost of the program. Design an ideal drug-testing program for your high school athletic department.

4. A freshman soccer player has been doing strengthening exercises for her previously sprained ankle. One day you notice that she tossed her backpack in a corner of the exercise area and some bottles fell out. Concerned about her knowledge of drugs, you ask what the bottles contain. She answers by showing you three bottles: Bayer aspirin, Tylenol, and Orudis. You ask her if she is taking all three of the pills and how much of each, and she says only that it depends on the day. Explain the appropriate use of each of these in an active athlete and give recommendations for which one(s) this player might want to use to help in controlling the ankle inflammation and pain.

5. Several members of your college track team come to you asking how they can find information on "banned drugs." They explain that they came to you because they didn't want the head athletic trainer to think they were "doing drugs." They say they just want to be sure they are not doing anything that might disqualify them from the upcoming track meet sponsored by "TAC" (The Athletic Conference). Explain how you could help these athletes.

CITED SOURCES

Mycek, M.K, R.A. Harvey, and P.C. Champe. 2000. *Pharmacology: Lippincott's Illustrated Reviews.* Baltimore: Lippincott, Williams and Wilkins.

ADDITIONAL READINGS

Colgan, M. 1993. *Optimum sports nutrition.* New York: Advanced Research Press.

Colgan, M. 1996. *Hormonal health.* Vancouver: Apple.

Faigenbaum, A.D., L.D. Zaichkowsky, D.E. Gardner, and L.J. Micheli. 1998. Anabolic steroid use by male and female middle school students. *Pediatrics* 101(5): E6.

Kochakian, C.D. 1990. Metabolites of testosterone: Significance in the vital economy. *Steroids* 55: 92-97.

Kochakian, C.D., and J.R. Murlin. 1936. The relationship of synthetic male hormone androstenedione to the protein and energy metabolism of castrated dogs and the protein metabolism of a normal dog. *Am J Physiol* 117: 642-657.

Mahesh, V.B., and R.B. Greenblatt. 1962. The in-vivo conversion of dehydroepiandrosterone and androstenedione to testosterone in the human. *Acta Endocrinol* 41: 400-406.

Stryer, L. 1981. *Biochemistry*, 2nd ed. New York: Freeman.

Yarasheski, K.E., J.A. Campbell, K. Smith, M.J. Rennie, J.O. Hollosky, and D.M. Bier. 1992. Effect of growth hormone and resistance exercise on muscle growth in young men. *Am J Physiol* 262: E261-E267.

Yesalis, C.E., ed. 1993. *Anabolic steroids in sport and exercise.* Champaign, IL: Human Kinetics.

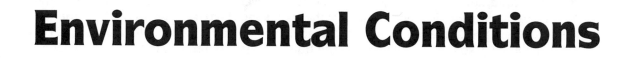

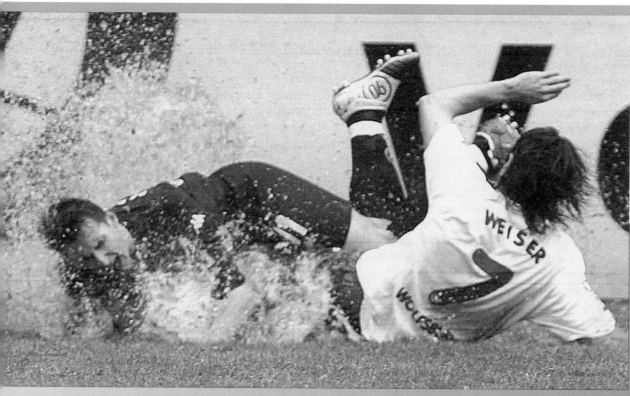

CHAPTER **6**

Environmental Conditions

© Bongarts/SportsChrome

Objectives

After reading this chapter, the student should be able to do the following:

1. List and give examples of the four cooling methods used to rid a body of excess heat.

2. Identify steps a person should take to lessen the risks of exercising in very hot and humid conditions.

3. List and explain three ways in which a physically active person could determine the heat and humidity in a climate he or she is visiting.

4. List the major symptoms associated with heat exhaustion.

5. Identify two major problems associated with exercise in a very cold environment and explain how these problems might be avoided.

6. Explain the concept of windchill and how it may affect the physically active individual exercising in a cold environment.

7. Identify several factors that should raise concern if one is exercising outdoors during a thunderstorm.

8. List things one should observe when inspecting a playing environment for safety.

Jake enjoyed doing as much running as he could, given his work schedule. After work he would change into his running clothes and hit the trail along the river near his office in the suburbs of Rochester, New York. Jake was a native of Philadelphia and had gone to college at Temple University. Another runner Jake would often see on the trail was also from the Philadelphia area. One day this runner, Paul, mentioned starting training for a 20K race on the Fourth of July. Paul thought it was going to be great—the Liberty Race, set in the middle of Philadelphia on July 4, 1999. Jake got to thinking of doing that race too.

"July 4th—that gives me just over three weeks to prepare," Jake kept thinking. "Monday I'll start my program!" he said to himself. He spent the weekend researching training programs for distance races. He realized quickly that he would need to increase his mileage and that this would require longer workout periods.

Jake dedicated every evening to his training program. He increased his mileage and began to feel that everything was falling into place. He had his flight arrangements to go to Philadelphia on July 3; he'd stay with a college buddy that night, and the race was to begin at noon at the Liberty Bell. Everything was right.

Before he knew it, there he was, right in the middle of the pack of runners. Then he heard, "Runners, take your marks. . . ." They were off.

Jake was running well at the 5K mark, but thinking, "15K to go, only a quarter of the way there." By the halfway mark he began feeling really tired. The air was closing in around him as he ran. "Boy, it's humid here," he muttered to himself. He attempted to grab water at each of the aid stations along the route. "Dang, I never could get the hang of drinking while I'm running," he thought as he spilled more water than he drank and tossed the cup to the ground.

By the 15K mark, Jake was in trouble. "Come on, push!"—he was starting to get mad at himself. His calf muscles were tightening; his back was beginning to feel sore. "Just 5K more . . . don't be so soft," he told himself.

The next thing Jake knew was that paramedics were standing over him. He had a tube in his arm and cold cloths all over his body.

"What. . . ?" he said as he attempted to raise his head.

"Relax, you're okay," said one of the medics. "You suffered heatstroke. Are you from this area?"

"No, I'm from upstate New York," Jake responded, still exhausted.

"Well, the temperature and humidity are extremely high today—lots of people are having trouble," the medic said as he took Jake's blood pressure. "You're stabilizing now; I think you're over the hump."

They helped Jake sit up, and everything started to go black.

"Steady there," the medic said, seeing Jake's response. "You're very dehydrated; we're putting some fluids back into your body now. You'll feel better in no time."

"Hey, thanks. Where did I fall out?" Jake asked, not remembering finishing the race.

"You made it across the line, but collapsed right there," the medic said, pointing to a spot just beyond the finish line. "You must have run right through heat exhaustion all the way to heatstroke! Your internal temperature was so high, you may have just lost a little of your memory during those last couple of miles."

"Wow. I guess last night really took it out of me," Jake confessed as his buddies finally found him, still sitting in a pool of water that had accumulated from the fluids the medics had used.

"Dude, sorry about keeping you up so late!" his buddy said apologetically. "I'm amazed you still ran the race!"

"Perhaps he shouldn't have, but he did. You guys need to take Jake over to urgent care and have him checked over thoroughly. Here's a copy of our paperwork to give the physician," said the paramedic as he excused himself to help other runners still having difficulties. "Take care!"

Jake was lucky this time. All he did on the flight back to New York was drink water and think how fortunate he had been that the paramedics had been there. He had never even considered that the environment in Philadelphia wasn't the same as in upstate New York.

This chapter addresses those aspects of the environment that we cannot change but can prepare to deal with effectively. As seen in the opening scenario, weather conditions are among those factors that can have a great influence on sport participation.

When speaking of the environment, we refer not only to the temperature and humidity of the surrounding air, but also to weather conditions such as storms. Beyond the natural environment, the local environment of the court, field, or facility may also pose a threat to safe participation.

TEMPERATURE REGULATION AND HEAT EXCHANGE

A person's perception of heat may occur internally or externally. The human body has an extremely efficient mechanism for maintaining the internal body temperature, making it difficult for the individual to detect small changes. External perception of heat may occur much more rapidly because of the sensory organs located in the skin.

Although heat is a good thing when it is cold outside and you decide to go for a run or workout, heat in the middle of summer may not be so welcome. Actually, when the temperature of your environment is between 70° and 80° (neutral environmental temperature) or is higher, the heat that your body produces (metabolic heat) can place a huge load on your ability to regulate internal heat. The "normal" body temperature is 98.6°. This may be misleading, however, if an individual's normal body temperature (normal meaning that the person is free of illness) is 99°. Every person has his or her own "normal" body temperature, and even that temperature will fluctuate up and down throughout the day; 98.6° signifies the average normal body temperature for humans, and the normal range is from 97° to 100° F.

Core Temperature and Basal Metabolism

Core temperature, or the temperature of the internal systems, is regulated in the brain via the hypothalamus (see figure 6.1). Core temperature can be affected by increasing the heat production (warming the body) or increasing the heat dissipation (cooling the body). Core temperatures are very precise, so that small deviations from the normal core temperature (called the set point) are offset by large adjustments in the body.

There are two major internal sources of heat: basal metabolism and exercise metabolism. Basal metabolism is the caloric expenditure of an individual at rest. Since caloric expenditure is energy, it represents the minimum amount of energy required to maintain life at normal body temperature. When you start exercising, a second heat source is applied; the heat from exercise (heat is the by-product of metabolism) is exercise metabolism. Strenuous-exercise metabolism may produce 15 to 18 times the amount of heat of basal metabolism, depending on your level of fitness. The human body can also absorb heat from external sources, such as the sun, a fire, and hot drinks. You can end up with far more heat than you need, and in this situation if you were not able to shed the excess, you would experience heat illnesses and even risk death.

Core Temperature Changes During Illness

Usually the healthy individual can manage the internal temperature quite well, but a person's core temperature may be disturbed by illness that is accompanied by a fever. When a person has a fever, the set point of the core temperature changes. With this change, the range of acceptable temperatures is shifted and the individual often complains of feeling chilled, especially at the onset of the fever. A simplified explanation is that this shift in set point causes the body to perceive itself to be below the proper temperature, and the sensation of a chill results. This occurs because the core temperature is below the set point. As the body produces and conserves heat, the core temperature rises; but in a short time, the core temperature extends beyond the range of the accepted temperatures because of the shift in the set point. As the core temperature remains at the level above and beyond the set point,

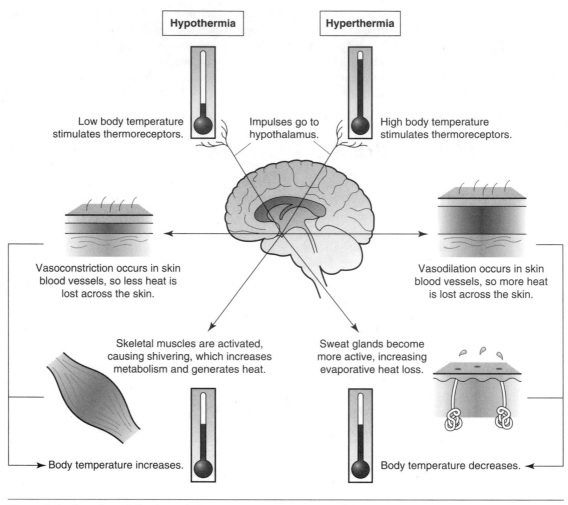

Figure 6.1 Function of the hypothalamus.
Adapted from Wilmore and Costill 1994.

the patient complains of feeling too hot. The delicate balance is still within control, yet the range of acceptance is shifted.

Altering Body Temperature

Whether it is hot or cold in your environment, your body attempts to stay at its normal temperature. To do this, it can use four mechanisms: sweat glands (to keep your skin moist and assist with cooling), smooth muscle of the blood vessels (which constrict or dilate the arterioles as needed to control blood flow to the skin), skeletal muscles (which generate heat by working or shivering), and some of the internal organs called endocrine glands (hormones produced by these glands cause cells to increase their metabolic rate). Together, these four systems effectively regulate the internal temperature of your body to keep you in a safe zone.

PHYSIOLOGICAL RESPONSES TO EXERCISE IN THE HEAT

When we exercise in the heat, our body continually attempts to control its internal temperature. The body burns glycogen for energy, and that process produces heat. As exercise in the warm environment continues, several adaptations occur: The heart rate increases, energy levels decline, and sweating increases.

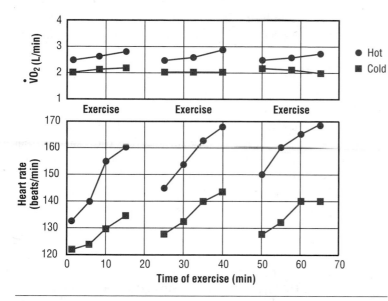

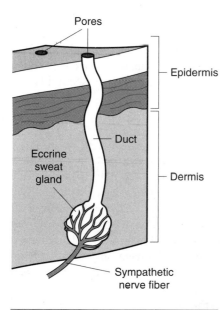

Figure 6.2 Oxygen uptake and heart rate responses during exercise in hot (40° C, 15% humidity) and cold (9° C, 55% humidity) conditions.

Reprinted from Fink et al. 1975.

Increased Heart Rate

The cardiovascular system works to supply muscles with sufficient blood to sustain performance. Unfortunately, when working in a warm or hot environment, the cardiovascular system has an additional, and sometimes competing, function: to pump blood to the skin for cooling. Blood cannot go both places at once, so the cardiovascular system makes an adjustment: It decreases the amount of blood returned to the heart (because so much is shunted to the skin and the muscles). As you might imagine, with less blood available per stroke (called the stroke volume), the heart will have to beat more frequently. This adjustment in the heart rate is usually an obvious sign of exercise, but the increase in heart rate is even greater during exercise in the heat (see figure 6.2). Unfortunately, there is a limit to the amount of compensation the cardiovascular system can make.

Decreased Energy Levels

As you exercise in the heat, your heart rate increases, as does your need for oxygen. This seems only logical when you realize that the purpose of the blood is to carry oxygen. This increase in the need for oxygen is called oxygen consumption. With the increased oxygen consumption, your muscles use more glycogen and produce more lactate. As glycogen in the muscles is used up and lactate builds up, you begin to experience an increased feeling of fatigue. Your energy level is dropping.

Increased Sweating Leading to Decreased Blood Volume

The hypothalamus controls the rate of sweating. As the temperature of the blood rises, the hypothalamus is signaled to start the mechanisms to increase sweating (done through the sympathetic nervous system [see figure 6.3]). When working in a hot environment, you can lose more than 1 L of sweat per hour of work per square meter of your body surface. This translates to a loss of 1.5 to 2.5 L of sweat per hour for an average-sized person (110-165 lb [50-75 kg]). At this sweat rate, the person is losing 2% to 4% of his or her body weight during each hour of work. As fluid (essentially water) is lost from the body, the blood also loses fluid. Since blood is about 80% water, a loss of water in the blood causes a decreased blood volume.

Temperature regulation is a critical function for every human being and only increases in importance for the physically active individual. Cooling mechanisms, conditioning in the particular environment, and fluid replacement are essential for risk-free physical performance.

Figure 6.3 Anatomy of a sweat gland that is innervated by a sympathetic nerve.

COOLING MECHANISMS

During exercise, the human body produces heat. This internal heat must be transferred to the environment, or dangerous levels of heat will accumulate inside the body. Under normal conditions, the body is capable of managing this heat, but in extreme conditions even the best-conditioned athlete may be taxed. In the attempt to dissipate heat, the body may utilize

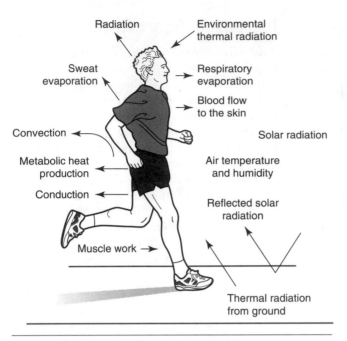

Figure 6.4   Normal methods of heat transfer.

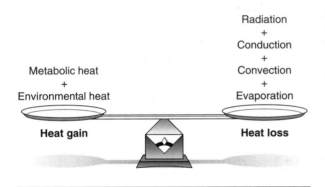

Figure 6.5   Methods of heat gain and heat loss.
Adapted from Wilmore and Costill 2004.

one of four heat transfer methods shown in figures 6.4 and 6.5: conduction, convection, evaporation, and radiation.

Conduction

Conduction as a method of transfer of heat from the human body to the surrounding environment may take two steps. First there is a transfer of heat from the core of the body to the body surface. We can visualize that mechanism by thinking of blood at normal temperatures. As the blood moves into the muscles, the heat is transferred by conduction to the blood from the hot muscle; thus the temperature of the blood rises. The warmed blood is now taken to the body surface, where the heat is transferred to the skin. Step two in the conduction of heat to the environment is very minimal. As you might surmise, contact between the skin surface and a cooler object must occur in order for heat to be dissipated through conduction. You may observe this scenario readily while watching your dog on a hot summer day. Dogs dig holes in the ground to provide a cooler point of contact; or if in the house, they may lie on a tile floor with all their limbs spread. The animal is attempting to maximize conduction cooling effects. On the other side of the spectrum, if the air or contact surface is warmer than your skin, the heat will be conducted to your skin, thereby warming it. Heat will move only from the warmer toward the cooler surface or object (second law of thermodynamics).

Convection

Convection is more complex than conduction because it depends on movement of molecules in contact with the body surface. Natural convection occurs when the air that is in direct contact with the body grows warmer. The warming of the air causes it to expand, and this decreases its density. As the density decreases, the air rises and is replaced by unwarmed, cooler air, and the process starts again. Forced convection occurs not from a difference in temperature but from a difference in external pressure exerted on the air as it flows past the body. If an athlete is outside on a hot day with a breeze, the air movement past the body allows forced convection to occur, and the air in the personal air space is warmed and pushed on, replaced by new air to be warmed. On a very windy day the cooling by convection occurs in the same way, but the efficiency of cooling does not increase. Without wind, convective heat loss practically stops when you are not moving. It is important to realize that the dissipation of heat by convection is often combined with the effects of evaporation and really cannot be viewed by itself when the situation is a person exercising in a natural environment (see figure 6.6). In fact, in the exercising person, convection makes an extremely small contribution to the total heat loss.

Evaporation

Evaporation occurs between the skin and the environment as well as between the respiratory tract and the outside environment. The loss of heat from evaporation is our major method of dissipating core temperature to the surrounding environment. We are often quite cognizant of the moisture on our skin after exertion, or even after a shower. How quickly the skin dries is proportional to the rate of evaporation and in turn related to heat being transferred to the

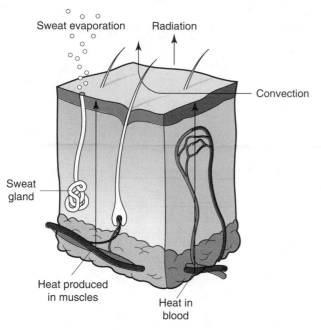

Sweat evaporation   Radiation

Convection

Sweat gland

Heat produced in muscles

Heat in blood

Figure 6.6   Convection.

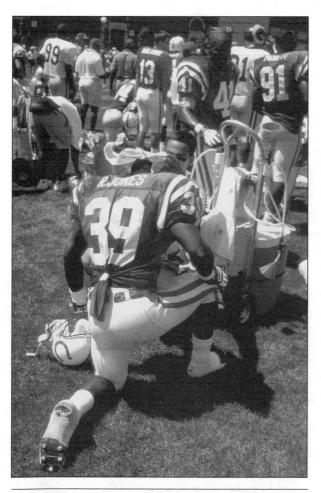

Figure 6.7   A person must adapt to temperature and humidity.

environment or the amount of cooling effect. When we are in a very humid climate we may notice that this dampness on our skin lasts longer. The dampness occurs because the rate of evaporation is low. The vapor pressure (the partial pressure of water vapor in the air) and the air temperature are important factors for understanding how much evaporation will be possible. When working with the physically active, one should always consider temperature and humidity and how they relate to the body's heat-response mechanisms. If the air is saturated (high humidity), the body will no longer effectively cool by evaporation.

Radiation

Radiation is the exchange of heat energy by electromagnetic waves, a process that occurs at the speed of light. The proportion of the total body heat loss by radiation depends on the temperature difference between the body surface and the environment, but also on the effective radiating area. Some areas of the body, the underarms and the digital web spaces, radiate to other body surfaces and do not contribute to overall heat loss. In a fully extended position, only about 75% of the total body surface is available for radiation. Radiation, in the true sense of the term, requires a very wide difference between the temperature of the object (individual) and that of the environment. Radiation can actually cause absorption of heat from the environment rather than dissipating body heat to the environment. For example, if someone exercises in direct sunlight, significant heat may be transferred to the body.

ADAPTING TO ENVIRONMENTAL HEAT

In addition to a person's cooling mechanisms, other factors contribute to the body's ability to adjust to exercise in the hot environment: acclimatization and hydration. When people pay close attention to preventive measures, prevention of heat illness seems simple (see figure 6.7).

Acclimatization

People can gradually adapt to a temperature difference by planning the training program so that their body has the opportunity to adapt to the heat and humidity present as the training intensity increases; this is called **acclimatization** (see table 6.1). Without time to acclimatize, a sudden increase in exercise intensity at the same time as a sudden change in environmental conditions could prove too much for the body to handle, resulting in some form of heat illness.

As one might guess, when the air temperature is near or above the body's temperature, cooling is required or performance will deteriorate. Cooling of the exercising body is achieved by various means, depending on the level of activity and the environmental humidity. If the air temperature is above body temperature, cooling will not be possible through

Steps to Remember When Adjusting to a Hot Environment

- If the temperature is 80° to 90° F and the humidity is less than 70%, just monitor athletes prone to heat illness.
- If the temperature is 80° to 90° F and the humidity is greater than 70%, include a 10-min rest every hour. Change wet clothes frequently.
- If the temperature is 90° to 100° F and the humidity is less than 70%, have a 10-min rest every hour. Change wet clothes frequently.
- If the temperature is 90° to 100° F and the humidity is greater than 70%, schedule short practices in the evenings or early morning. Require only T-shirts and shorts.

Table 6.1
Steps to Remember When Adjusting to the Hot Environment

Time considerations	Fluid intake
Acclimatization usually takes 2 to 3 weeks.	
Exercise in the early morning and late evening for the first week.	Drink at least 3 L of water every day.
Work your way gradually toward midday exercise.	Drink .25 L of cold water every 15 min during intense exercise.
On very hot or hot/humid days, exercise early and late in the day only.	

conduction or convection; the body must depend solely on evaporative cooling. Environmental humidity reduces the ability of the body to cool by the evaporative mechanism, and core temperature may reach dangerous levels. Fortunately, adaptation of the human body can occur when the individual is given sufficient time to adjust to exercise in a hot or humid climate or one that is both hot and humid.

High school and college athletic conferences impose regulations on football teams to allow the athletes to adjust to exercise in the particular climate prior to participating in full football attire. The addition of the heavy pads required in football and other contact sports acts to further reduce the body's ability to dissipate heat.

Different geographic locations throughout the world present specific challenges. Unless you train in the same environmental conditions as those you expect to perform in, serious **thermoregulatory** difficulties could be associated with strenuous exercise. A college-bound student who lives in a cool climate will find football practice much more difficult if he moves to a hot climate and begins working out in 100° temperatures. This difference in climates will be even greater should the player move to campus during a very humid period of the summer.

Hydration

One method of decreasing the risk of problems from the heat is to keep the athlete well hydrated (see figure 6.8). Exercise accelerates the body's loss of water, making **rehydration** essential. Coaches must be cooperative in allowing athletes to take frequent drinks of water during activity. Athletes should be educated regarding the need for water and should be encouraged to drink often during practices and games. People can avoid the feeling of being waterlogged by taking more frequent, small drinks of water rather than less frequent breaks

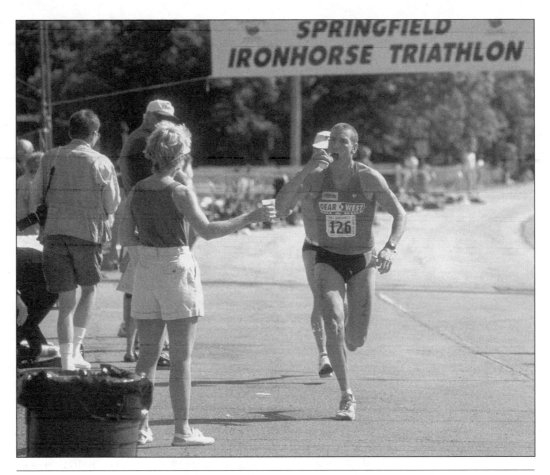

Figure 6.8 It is critical to take frequent, small water breaks throughout a workout or event.

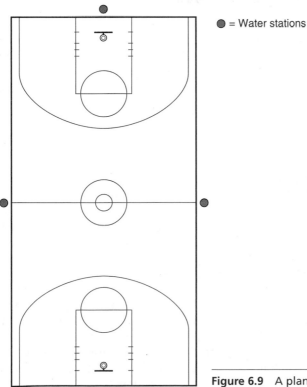

● = Water stations

during which they gulp down large quantities. We must remember that the feeling of thirst is not a good indication of the body's need for fluid. Usually, thirst is perceived long after the need for water has become critical. Generally, a person does not rehydrate to the full extent needed by the body; thus it is necessary to make a conscious effort to hydrate even when thirst is not perceived.

Maintaining Body Fluids

An ideal plan for fluid replacement would allow water (or electrolyte drink) consumption at convenient stopping points during drills and scrimmage. A plan for a basketball practice, as seen in figure 6.9, would position fluid-replacement stations at center court on each side of the gymnasium floor, as well as one station located under one of the basketball goals at a sufficient distance to ensure safety for any participating team members. This plan allows players who are waiting their turn in drills (at end line) to consume additional fluids; it also provides central locations for fluid replacement for players during periodic breaks as well as for substitutes during scrimmage sessions.

Figure 6.9 A plan for water replacement in basketball.

Team policies should be established regarding the frequency and length of rest breaks during practices in high heat and humidity. Rest breaks should allow time for the athlete to sit down, preferably in a cool location (or if outdoors, in a shaded area), and to consume several cups of water or electrolyte drink or both. Some teams use other methods of cooling the athlete, including water misters for increased cooling via evaporation and cooling vests that the athlete may don to help with conductive cooling.

Monitoring Hydration by Weight

Hydration status can be monitored, although roughly, by doing something as simple as recording the individual's body weight. Weight should be taken and recorded before exercise and then after exercise, with the participant wearing the same clothes both times. The process is easier if participants weigh in street clothes before changing into the exercise gear. After they have showered and put on their street clothes, they weigh again. When practice occurs twice in a day, the weight lost during the first practice should be replaced before the second workout begins. The rapid loss of body weight is almost exclusively water loss, which can have a serious effect on the individual's ability to adapt to the heat during exercise. A very small amount (1-2%) of dehydration can compromise performance, and weight loss of more than 3% puts the exercising individual at a much greater risk of heat illness.

An athletic trainer is usually able to observe many participants during practices and workouts. Athletic trainers may spot various warning signs that heat illness is imminent. Individuals who carry extra weight are more prone to heat-related problems than are thinner individuals; extremely hard-working athletes who hustle on every play may experience heat problems more quickly than others; and people who just don't like to drink water during a workout will often be the first to experience heat cramps or other heat illnesses. Watching each of these types of players, monitoring their fluid replacement by checking their body weight each practice, and urging them to drink cool sips of water on a frequent basis will aid in the prevention of heat problems. The National Athletic Trainers' Association (NATA) has published a position statement on the prevention of dehydration in the athlete, and your plan should be established on the basis of this information.

Monitoring Hydration Status by Urine Color

The National Research Council's fluid recommendations are individualized based on how many calories are burned each day. Adult women, who may expend 1,600 to 2,200 calories each day, need 6 1/2 to 9 cups of fluid; men, who often need 2,200 to 2,800 calories each day, are advised to drink 9 to 12 cups. To make things a little simpler, studies show that adequate fluid consumption is indicated by a pale yellow or straw-colored urine whereas dark urine suggests dehydration.

HEAT ILLNESS

As already outlined, human heat is lost in four ways: conduction, radiation, convection, and evaporation. Conduction, or heat loss through direct contact with something cooler than you, does not help much on a hot day. On a very hot afternoon, you may actually take in heat from a hot environment through radiation. Convection is heat loss through the movement of air around your body. Without wind, convective heat loss practically stops when you are not moving. That leaves evaporation, the vaporization of sweat from the skin, as the primary source of heat loss for the athlete. As your skin heats up, pores dilate and sweat floods out. Evaporation of the sweat cools your skin; heat is drawn from your blood near the surface of your body; and the cooler blood circulates to keep the body's core maintained at an acceptable temperature. Sweat comes from your circulatory system, and it is not uncommon to sweat out a liter of water in an hour during periods of exercise in a hot environment. This water loss may reach 2.5 L/hr with prolonged exercise. Sweat contains salt, a critical component of normal body function. It is this—the combined water and electrolyte depletion—that forms the basis of a spectrum of problems with one general name: heat illness.

Heat Syncope and Exertional Hypotension

A decrease in blood pressure can cause fainting. Two main situations in which an athlete may faint due to exercise or heat are heat syncope and exertional hypotension. Heat syncope occurs when the blood volume decreases and the body is unable to pump sufficient blood to the brain. The brain wants oxygen, and without blood flow it cannot get what is needed and will cause the individual to collapse or faint. The collapse allows the brain to receive more blood since the heart is now at the same level as the brain. Blood volume must be restored as soon as possible.

The second cause of fainting is **exertional** hypotension. This most often occurs when the athlete is exercising the large muscle groups in the legs and suddenly stops. The exercising muscles are engorged with blood, and without the pumping action of the leg muscles, the blood pools in the extremities. This in turn causes a decreased blood flow to the brain, and, again, the body collapses to bring the brain to the same level as the heart. This scenario is often seen at the finish line of a long race. The athlete finishes the race and in the finish area comes to a stop, and shortly thereafter collapses. Frequently this collapse is thought to be due to heat illness whereas in fact the victim's body fluid levels and core temperature are within safe limits.

Heat Cramps

When we exercise, if the body heat production becomes greater than body heat loss, we are heading toward heat illness. One of the harmful effects of this exercise and heat is painful spasm of major muscles that are being exercised, called heat cramps. Those who experience cramps are most often people unacclimatized to heat who are sweating profusely. Heat cramps are poorly understood; but they probably result not only from the water lost in sweat, but also from the imbalance between sodium (salt) and potassium once the level of body fluids decreases. That is, as the body's internal water level decreases, the concentrations of sodium and potassium increase, and small imbalances create much bigger problems. Gentle massage of the cramping muscles may provide some relief from the pain associated with the spasm and may even be enough to induce muscle relaxation, especially when combined with gentle stretching of the involved muscle (see figure 6.10). Drinking water is critical during this time of heat cramps. Heat cramps do not often occur in someone who is adequately hydrated.

Once the pain and spasm are gone, exercise may be continued if necessary, but rest is better. Often people experiencing heat cramps rest just long enough to allow the symptoms to abate; as soon as they return to play, the heat cramps also return.

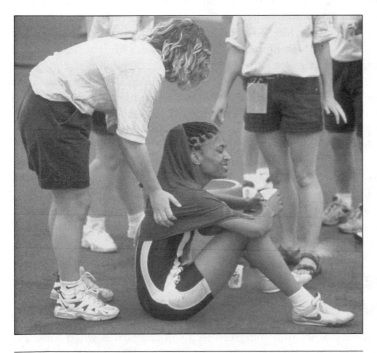

Figure 6.10 Heat cramps go away with gentle massage and lots of rest and water.

Heat Exhaustion

Prolonged sweating, without proper rehydration, can decrease the body's ability to dissipate heat. A buildup of body heat can lead to heat exhaustion, a condition characterized by headache, dizziness, nausea, rapid breathing, and, of course, exhaustion (see figure 6.11). People experiencing heat exhaustion are so sweaty that often they feel cool; they may have goose bumps and often complain of chills. Treatment should include moving the exhausted person to a shady spot if outdoors, or to a cooler location indoors, and giving the individual fluids. Some experts prefer using an electrolyte-balanced drink, but the drink should be watered down three or

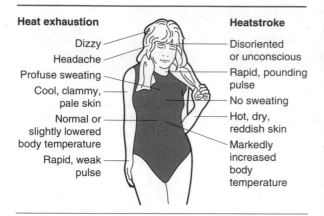

Heat exhaustion

Dizzy
Headache
Profuse sweating
Cool, clammy, pale skin
Normal or slightly lowered body temperature
Rapid, weak pulse

Heatstroke

Disoriented or unconscious
Rapid, pounding pulse
No sweating
Hot, dry, reddish skin
Markedly increased body temperature

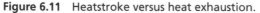

Figure 6.11   Heatstroke versus heat exhaustion.

four times for more rapid absorption in an exercising person. Maximum absorption ranges from 150 to 250 ml/15 min, so it takes about an hour to get a liter of fluid back into circulation. Heat exhaustion is not physiologically damaging, but it should be treated aggressively and signs and symptoms monitored to protect the athlete from core temperature rise.

Heatstroke

The most serious of heat-related illnesses is heatstroke, a problem that kills approximately 4,000 people in the United States every year. Heatstroke occurs when the body's thermoregulatory system stops working. Many of the symptoms of heatstroke are the same as for heat exhaustion. However, other indications of heatstroke are cessation of sweating, disorientation, and fainting or unconsciousness. Individuals experiencing heatstroke may be too disoriented to help themselves. There are two varieties of heatstroke: typical heatstroke and exertional heatstroke.

Typical Heatstroke

In typical heatstroke, the patient is usually elderly or sick, or both. Usually, environmental temperature and humidity have been high for several days, and people become dehydrated to the point where their heat-loss mechanisms are overwhelmed. It is as if they have run out of sweat; the skin gets hot, red, and dry. They lapse into a coma and, if untreated, will usually die.

Exertional Heatstroke

More and more people are succumbing to the second variety of heatstroke, exertional heatstroke. The person is usually young, fit, and unaccustomed to the heat. This patient is actively sweating but producing heat faster than it can be dissipated. Signs include, primarily, a sudden and very noticeable alteration in normal mental function: disorientation, irritability, combativeness, bizarre delusions, and incoherent speech. The skin is hot and red, but may be quite wet with sweat. Rapid breathing and rapid heart rates are often observed. Collapse is imminent. Quick cooling may be required to save this person's life; the best method includes submerging the individual in an ice bath. If total body submersion is not possible, removal of heavy clothing and covering the person with wet cloths, placing ice packs near major arteries such as those in the neck, groin, and axilla, and vigorous fanning will help to increase evaporative heat loss. A physician should see anyone who has experienced heatstroke as soon as possible, even if the person seems to have recovered. Too much internal heat can cause breakdowns in some body systems that show up later.

It is important to thoroughly evaluate the athlete suspected to have a heat illness. Core temperature is the only true measure of the extent of internal body heat and should be used as an emergency evaluation measure. This core temperature is best taken using a rectal thermometer, since other measurements of body temperature fail to adequately reflect the temperature of the body's core (Binkley et al. 2002, 334). Frequent questioning of the athlete to assess the level of consciousness and mental status is very important.

Factors Contributing to Heat Illness

It is always important to be familiar with factors that could predispose the physically active person to heat illness. When any one of these factors is combined with another, the risk of heat injury increases dramatically. Care must be taken to avoid heat stress when someone with a risk factor is exercising in a hot environment (see table 6.2). It is important to recognize and understand any limitations so that one can make appropriate adjustments in the exercise routine.

Table 6.2
Factors Contributing to the Risk of Heat Illness

Avoidable	Possibly avoidable	Unavoidable
Dehydration	Drug usage such as amphetamines, phenothiazines, and anticholinergics	Cardiovascular disease
Lack of acclimatization	Prolonged or excessive exercise (increased exercise demands)	Sweat gland dysfunction
Alcohol use		
Inappropriate clothing		

PREVENTION OF HEAT-RELATED ILLNESS

Heat illnesses can be preventable, but we must take the necessary steps. Children, people who are elderly, and those who are obese are particularly at risk of developing heat illness. However, even top athletes in superb condition can succumb to heat illness if they ignore the warning signs.

Several preventive measures can be taken to avoid problems due to heat illness: monitoring environmental conditions and adjusting practice sessions; monitoring athletes' weight loss/replacement between practices; and promoting good hydration habits in athletes. In addition, acclimatization must take place prior to the start of competitive drills and practices. If an athlete fails to acclimatize prior to the season, risks of heat illness can be much greater. Pay close attention to individuals who have moved from another climate, those who tend to sweat excessively, and those who have been ill or for any reason are not eating well. Understanding the individual's limitations is more important than the practice, test, or drill on any given day. Although you may understand this concept, it is equally important for you to help the athlete and coach understand and agree with this concept.

Monitoring Environmental Conditions

Taking temperature and humidity readings using a sling **psychrometer**, as seen in figure 6.12, or other heat and humidity device is an important procedure that should be conducted prior to every practice and contest for which there is the potential of temperature or humidity extremes. Taking the readings at the location of the contest is better than assuming that conditions there are the same as at the local weather station, airport, or other weather-forecasting facility. Use Web sources of heat and humidity readings only after you establish the validity and reliability of those data in comparison to the data collected on the field. Only after determining the validity of Web data should you assume that this is a good source for field conditions. Always be aware of special circumstances affecting the field, such as irrigation of the field itself or surrounding areas and local weather patterns. It is wise to fully understand the environmental conditions under which you are participating.

Steps to Take When Exercising in a Hot Environment

- Wear loose-fitting, lightweight clothing.
- Avoid headwear or remove it frequently for cooling.
- Take frequent rest breaks to drink fluids.
- Drink abundant fluids prior to, during, and after the workout.
- Avoid overheating if you are taking drugs that impair heat regulation or if you have a fever.

To get local weather, weather conditions at another location, or radar reports, check out www.intellicast.com, www.weatherunderground.com, or www.weather.com.

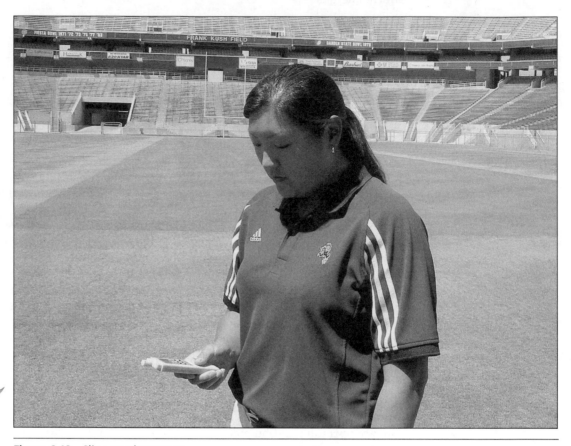

Figure 6.12   Sling psychrometer.
Photo courtesy of Edward Orr, ATC.

Heat Index

Physically active people sometimes wish to exercise in an area of the country they are visiting. Since they probably do not have access to a sling psychrometer, they can use local weather data to find out about the local heat and humidity. The heat index table (see table 6.3) shows how the temperature and dew point combine to produce the heat index value. Exercisers can use the heat index to determine adjustments for workout plans. When heat index reports are 95° to 105°, people fatigue more quickly while exercising and are more susceptible to heat cramps and heat exhaustion. Above 105°, there is a risk of heatstroke with prolonged activity, warranting appropriate modification of activity. In general, the higher the heat index, the less efficient evaporative cooling will be. Whenever possible, practices should be scheduled during cooler times of the day. If a scheduled practice must occur in high heat or humidity, it is wise to provide frequent fluid breaks during which athletes can take several (5-10) minutes' rest in a shaded area.

Local Relative Humidity Readings

Although not recommended if more accurate measurements are available, another method of determining the effect of the hot environment on exercise is to use local relative humidity

Table 6.3
Heat Index: Air Temperature and Dew Point = Heat Index

Temperature (°F)	Dew point (°F)							
	50	55	60	65	70	75	80	85
65	60.8	62.0	63.3	64.8				
70	70.5	71.4	72.5	73.8	75.3			
75	75.7	76.3	76.8	77.2	77.8	79.3		
80	78.3	79.2	80.2	81.4	83.0	85.5	89.5	
85	82.0	83.2	84.7	86.6	89.1	92.5	97.6	105.2
90	86.5	87.9	89.8	92.2	95.4	99.8	105.8	114.2
95	91.4	93.1	95.3	98.1	101.9	107.0	113.7	122.9
100	96.6	98.5	101.0	104.2	108.4	113.9	121.2	130.9
105	101.9	104.0	106.7	110.2	114.7	120.6	128.3	138.0
110	107.2	109.5	112.4	116.1	120.9	127.0	134.9	145.1
115	112.4	114.8	117.9	121.8	126.8	133.1	141.2	151.4
120	117.4	120.0	123.2	127.3	132.4	138.9	147.0	157.3

■ Only fit and heat-acclimatized athletes can participate safely.

▨ Heat-sensitive and unacclimatized athletes may suffer.

□ Little danger of heat stress for acclimatized athletes.

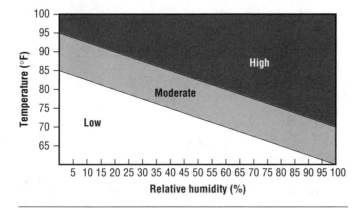

Figure 6.13 Temperature–humidity activity index.
Reprinted from NCAA 1999.

readings (see figure 6.13). Exercise should be modified when the apparent temperature becomes higher, especially if the person is unconditioned or unacclimatized (see table 6.4).

Table 6.5 gives apparent temperature (another form of the heat index chart), showing a combination of heat and humidity measures.

Monitoring Athlete's Weight Loss

Weight is a commonly used measure of an athlete's hydration. It is easy to monitor athletes' weight by weighing them prior to and following each practice. Obviously, the weight should be taken with the athlete in the same type of clothing at both weighing sessions. Weight lost during a practice should be replaced prior to the athlete's next participation. If an athlete fails to replace the weight lost by the time of weigh-in prior to the next session, caution is necessary. This ranges from merely providing additional fluids during the practice session to reducing the length of the practice session should the athlete show any signs of heat difficulties (cramps, confusion, etc.).

Promoting Good Hydration Habits

Hydration is an extremely important aspect of preventing heat illness, but also for general good nutrition. Many options exist regarding the "best" fluid: water or sport drink. The question then is, if a sport drink, which one? Water is an excellent source of fluid replacement, yet when the body is depleted of sodium and potassium (electrolytes), those too must be replenished. A condition called **"hyponatremia"** occurs when the level of sodium in the

Table 6.4
Suggested Exercise Adjustments Relative to Apparent Temperature Levels

Apparent temperature	Exercise plan
Below 90° F	No need to modify activity plan.
91-104° F	Increase fluid and rest breaks. Monitor athletes for heat cramps and signs of heat exhaustion.
105-129° F	Decrease exercise intensity unless well acclimatized. Be aware of danger signs.
130° F and up	Change time of practice or intensity of workout. Exercise with caution. High risk of heat illness exists.

Table 6.5
Apparent Temperature Calculations

Relative humidity (percent)	Air temperature (°F)							
	75	80	85	90	95	100	105	110
0	69	73	78	83	87	91	95	99
10	70	75	80	85	90	95	100	105
20	72	77	82	87	93	99	105	112
30	73	78	84	90	96	104	113	123
40	74	79	86	93	101	110	123	137
50	75	81	88	96	107	120	135	150
60	76	82	90	100	114	132	149	
70	77	85	93	106	124	144		
80	78	86	97	113	136			
90	79	88	102	122				
100	80	91	108					

Find the air temperature (°F) across the top of the chart; then read down the column until you find the row of the relative humidity reading (to the nearest 10%). That number is the apparent temperature.

body falls too low. This can actually be a result of replenishing fluids with water only, especially if the athlete is on a low-sodium diet.

Sport drinks are the common choice of active individuals concerned with fluids and electrolyte replacement. Making a choice between the various sport drinks is quite difficult. Two important factors to consider are carbohydrate (CHO) and sodium concentrations of the beverage. According to the NATA position statement on fluid replacement in athletics, "Consuming CHOs during the pre-exercise hydration session (2 to 3 hours pre-exercise), as in item 5, along with a normal daily diet increases glycogen stores. If exercise is intense, then consuming CHOs about 30 minutes pre-exercise may also be beneficial. Include CHOs in the rehydration beverage during exercise if the session lasts longer than 45 to 50 minutes or is intense. An ingestion rate of about 1 g/min (0.04 oz/min) maintains optimal carbohydrate metabolism: for example, 1 L of a 6% CHO drink per hour of exercise. CHO concentrations greater than 8% increase the rate of CHO delivery to the body but compromise the rate of fluid emptying from the stomach and absorbed from the intestine" (Casa et al. 2000, 213).

Although the sodium in the sport drink is not required in most sporting events, the addition of the sodium makes the drink taste much better. Athletes often admit that they would drink more if the fluid tasted good. Part of the battle of hydration is finding a fluid that the athlete likes and thus will drink sufficiently.

To further understand the differences among sport drinks, one would merely need to calculate the content of CHO by dividing the total CHO by the volume of fluid (converted to milliliters, which is equivalent to grams). The following are three of the more popular sport drinks, listed with their CHO content:

Sport Drink	*CHO Concentration*
Allsport	8% CHO (20 g CHO in 240 ml)
Gatorade	6% CHO (14 g CHO in 240 ml)
PowerAide	8% CHO (19 g CHO in 240 ml)

CARING FOR HEAT ILLNESS

Most people think that it is normal to experience some level of discomfort as exercise intensity increases. People may not recognize the degree of this discomfort until they can push no more and the body is compromised by some form of heat illness. It is essential that everyone associated with physically active individuals understand the symptoms associated with heat illness so that proper measures may be taken. Always remember that heat will continue to build up and that in the absence of the proper measures, conditions can quickly move from minor to more and more severe.

Heat Cramps

The initial sign of heat illness is typically heat cramps. These cramps are difficult to ignore. Often the person experiences such severe cramping that any muscle activity causes another muscle group to go into spasm. A severe cramp in a muscle may actually damage some of the muscle fibers, producing soreness in the muscle(s) that may last for days. Heat cramps are often a sign of excessive exposure to a hot environment and may signal that other more serious problems are to follow if proper care is not forthcoming. The cramps typically related to heat exposure involve the legs and the abdomen. Sometimes athletes continue to practice despite feeling tightness and cramping in the legs. They may not realize that the feeling is anything serious and may dismiss it as just fatigue. The cramps may intensify by the time the athlete returns to the locker room, or even as the person sits in an air-conditioned room or automobile.

It is important to render care as soon as muscle cramps are detected. Since people who are cramping are usually suffering from a low fluid level in the body, they need to ingest water and electrolyte replacements, if available.

Mild stretching of the cramping muscles may help relieve the spasm and associated pain. In some cases the cramping is so severe that most of the major muscles become involved. In this situation people may be so dehydrated that it is not possible to provide the fluids quickly enough through the gastrointestinal tract (oral consumption). Sometimes a trained medical professional decides to provide intravenous fluids to help rehydrate the person's body more quickly. Usually, given appropriate care, the cramping muscles will relax; but with a severe case of heat cramps, the likelihood of soreness the next day is very high.

Heat Exhaustion

The individual may enter into more serious stages of heat illness with little outward signs of trouble. Heat exhaustion can occur in anyone working or exercising in a hot, humid environment. Warning signs of heat exhaustion include heavy sweating, paleness, muscle cramps, tiredness, weakness, dizziness, headache, nausea or vomiting, and fainting. The skin may be cool and moist. The person's pulse rate will be fast and weak, and breathing will be fast and shallow. If heat exhaustion is untreated, it may progress to heatstroke. You should get the person medical attention immediately if symptoms are severe or if he or she has heart problems or high blood pressure.

Immediately, the individual needs cooling since the body is not doing a good enough job. The most immediate way to obtain massive body cooling is to submerge the athlete in a cold pool of water. If that is not available, get the patient into a cool area, loosen clothing, and allow the skin to be exposed to the cool air. Packing ice in the groin area and axilla can help in the cooling effort. You may help cool the body by fanning, or you may want to wipe the person's body with a cool cloth. Just as with the person who is having heat cramps, anyone experiencing heat exhaustion needs fluid replacement. If a person faints or becomes unconscious, you will not be able to get him or her to drink and must get medical help. To get more oxygen to the brain, you'll want to increase the blood available to the head. Elevation of the feet will help to get the blood from the extremities back to the heart for pumping up to the head. Remember: This problem may become worse in the absence of proper care.

Heatstroke

Heatstroke occurs when the signs of heat exhaustion are ignored. The body is overwhelmed by the heat, and the internal systems stop functioning. Heatstroke is life threatening, and one can usually recognize it by the presence of significant symptoms such as those listed here. The extreme confusion and hot skin will call attention to the presence of heatstroke. Skin moisture (sweating) is the significant difference between typical and exertional heatstroke: Typical heatstroke means that the person ran out of water and can't cool himself or herself, whereas people experiencing exertional heatstroke have enough water to allow them to sweat but not enough to keep up with the amount of heat they are producing. Don't be confused if you find all the signs of heatstroke with your healthy athlete but see that the skin is wet with perspiration. That just may be exertional heatstroke. If you feel you may be prone to errors in judgment in cases of heat illness, it would be better to err on the side of caution (see figure 6.14).

Although heatstroke is less common than other heat illnesses, it is a medical emergency. Proper care of an affected patient involves immediate cooling and transport to a hospital or other emergency care service. Send someone for help while you get the person into a cold pool or at least a shady area to provide external cooling. Fan the person with cool air; use wet, cool sponges to keep the skin moist; apply cool, wet towels to the major arteries (groin, armpits, neck). Do whatever you can to provide cool airflow over the damp skin to help the person dissipate heat. Because of the decreasing level of consciousness, making the person drink is usually not possible. Monitoring the vital signs is important to provide assurance that the airway remains open and the heart continues pumping. This information, as well as knowing the oral temperature, can be a great help to the medical specialists who will assist with the care of the patient in the ambulance and at the hospital or clinic. Additionally, blood pressure should be monitored, and if possible a comparison of blood pressure in supine versus pressure taken immediately upon standing should be recorded. This comparison of blood pressures allows one to see if the pressure is lower in standing than in supine. This drop in pressure is termed "orthostatic hypotension" and may indicate an athlete's dehydration.

Ultimately all physically active individuals must take responsibility for their own health and safety, because someone else may not always be around during workouts. The individual, the coach, and parents should be educated about the warning signs of heat stress and

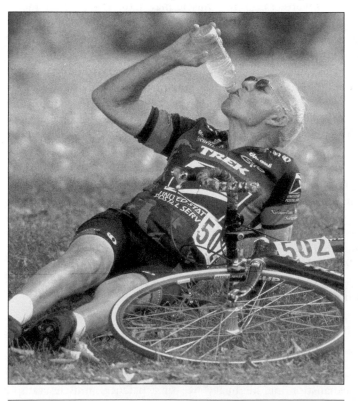

Figure 6.14 Be smart and take regular breaks to prevent heat exhaustion and the more serious heatstroke.

Symptoms of Heat Exhaustion

Late Symptoms

- Cool, moist skin
- Dilated pupils
- Headache
- Irrational behavior
- Pale skin
- Nausea and vomiting
- Unconsciousness

Early Symptoms

- Dizziness
- Fatigue
- Muscle cramps
- Nausea
- Profuse sweating
- Thirst
- Weakness and light-headedness

Caring for Heat Illness

What to Do

- Get the victim out of the heat and have him or her lie down in a cool place with feet elevated about 12 in. (30 cm).
- Apply cool, wet cloths (or cool water directly) to the skin; use a fan to lower temperature. Place cold compresses on the victim's neck, groin, and armpits. Submerge victim in a cool pool of water If available.
- Give the victim sport beverages or cool/cold water to sip. Give a half cup every 15 min.
- For muscle cramps, massage affected muscles gently but firmly until they relax. But do not withhold rehydration to provide massage.
- If the victim shows signs of shock (bluish lips and fingernails and decreased alertness), administer first aid for shock. If the victim starts having seizures, protect him or her from injury and give convulsion first aid.
- If the person loses consciousness, apply first aid for unconsciousness.
- For serious heat illness, keep the person cool until you get medical help.

What Not to Do

- Do not underestimate the seriousness of heat illness, especially if the person is a child, is elderly, or is injured.
- Do not give the person medications that are used to treat fever (such as aspirin). They will not help, and they may be harmful.
- Do not give salt tablets.
- Do not overlook possible complications resulting from the person's other medical problems (such as high blood pressure).
- Do not give liquids that contain alcohol or caffeine. They will interfere with the body's ability to control its internal temperature.
- Do not hesitate to get medical assistance.

taught to take prudent and wise steps to avoid serious problems. Adapting to new or changed environmental temperatures, adjusting the length or intensity of workouts, taking a cooler of water to the workout site, and drinking frequently are all essential practices. For monitoring hydration status, it is important to encourage participants to weigh before and after every workout as well as to be observant of the color of the urine. Physically active individuals must develop a healthy habit of hydrating before, during, and after every workout.

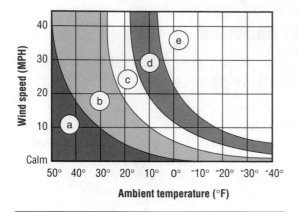

Figure 6.15 Ambient temperatures: *(a)* comfortable—requires normal precautions; *(b)* very cold—travel becomes uncomfortable; *(c)* bitterly cold—travel becomes uncomfortable even on clear, sunny days; *(d)* freezing of human flesh begins, depending upon degree of activity, amount of solar radiation, and character of skin and circulation; *(e)* survival efforts are required. Exposed flesh will freeze in less than 1 min.

Reprinted from NCAA 1999.

COLD ENVIRONMENTS

Although exercise in the cold is not as detrimental to the physiology of the human body as extreme heat can be, cold environments do create performance issues. Exercise in air temperatures below 60° F may lengthen reaction time and reduce manual dexterity and tactile sensitivity. Usually, people participating in a cold environment dress to retain body heat production and thus reduce the ill effects of low temperatures. The body's natural heat production through muscle activity, as well as sympathetic nervous system activation, is supplemented by the added insulation of clothing (see figure 6.15).

Hypothermia

Hypothermia occurs when the core temperature gets too low. Factors that increase the ill effects of cold include the patient's age, the patient's medical condition, and the ingestion of drugs or poisons. Wet conditions intensify the effects of cold. This is not the dampness from normal sweating during exercise, but a situation in which the participant's shoes are soaked from the moisture on the ground and from water spilled when taking drinks. The wet shoes and cold exposure can increase the likelihood of a local cold injury.

Hypothermia can be local or general, mild or severe. The patient's core temperature drops to between 90° and 95° (normal core temperature is 98.6°). This patient is alert, is shivering, and is maybe moving around in an attempt to produce heat. The key to knowing that the individual is experiencing mild hypothermia and not just feeling cold is increased heart rate and respiration. The skin is typically red, but will progress to cyanotic (showing blueness of the lips and under the nails). As the core temperature drops lower than 90°, the shivering stops and muscle activity decreases. Small muscles of the fingers stop first, and as the core temperature falls more, all muscle activity stops. As the core temperature reaches 85° the patient becomes lethargic and uncoordinated, and mental functions become disturbed.

Other Cold-Related Injuries

Cold-related injuries usually affect the extremities, especially the nose and ears, the hands, and the feet and toes (see figure 6.16). The factors that influence the severity of cold injury include length of exposure time, the combination of temperature and wind effects, previous cold injury, impaired circulation, and wet garments.

In most sporting events, athletes have sufficient time to cover exposed fingers between plays or series. Rewarming the hands in gloves or with the use of commercial hand warmers is usually sufficient to prevent frostbite; however, recognition of the condition is important for times when prevention has been inadequate. The signs of frostbite are hard, pale, and cold skin and a reduction in tactile sensation. People with **atherosclerosis** or those taking beta-blocker drugs are particularly susceptible to frostbite because of the decrease in the flow of blood to the skin.

In superficial cold injuries, the affected skin becomes pale (blanches), and normal color fails to return when the skin is palpated. The patient may experience a loss of feeling and sensation, and during rewarming may feel tingling of the affected part.

Deep cold injury, which is much more serious, occurs when tissues are actually frozen. Less severe deep cold injury is called frostbite. In frostbite the exposed part is damaged, but not as severely. Following frostbite, the skin may remain red, tender, and very sensi-

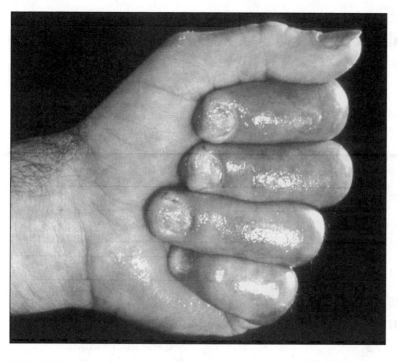

Figure 6.16 Superficial cold injuries.
© Bruce Coleman, Inc.

tive to the cold. Deep cold injuries are rare in athletics and should be easy to prevent. The published National Collegiate Athletic Association (NCAA) guidelines for preventing cold injuries are presented here, as are the steps in caring for an athlete who has experienced overexposure to the cold. Remember, human tissue damages very easily when cold, so take extreme care when touching cold or frostbitten areas of the body.

Windchill

It is necessary to monitor all exposure to cold and to take precautions to avoid cold injury. With good common sense and wise selection of athletic apparel, cold injury should be preventable.

When people engage in sport in very cold environments, the wind may present an even greater risk for hypothermia. Table 6.6 depicts the **windchill** factor, a parameter associated with wind in cold environments. To read the chart you need to know the wind speed (obtained from the local radio station, weather bureau, or airport) and the air temperature. Read down the left margin for the wind speed and then across the top for the air temperature. A wind speed of 15 mph (24 km/hr) in combination with an air temperature of 10° F is equal to an air temperature of –21° F. Wind increases the cooling effect of the temperature and can make a cool day feel quite cold.

Table 6.6
Windchill Factor: Temperature and Wind = Relative Temperature

Wind (knots)	Temperature (°F)														
	40	35	30	25	20	15	10	5	0	–5	–10	–15	–20	–25	–30
0	36	30	25	19	14	8	3	–2	–8	–13	–19	–24	–30	–35	–40
10	26	20	13	7	1	–6	–12	–18	–25	–31	–37	–44	–50	–56	–63
15	20	13	6	–1	–7	–14	–21	–28	–35	–42	–49	–56	–63	–70	–77
20	16	9	2	–6	–13	–20	–28	–35	–42	–50	–57	–64	–72	–79	–86
25	13	6	–2	–9	–17	–25	–32	–40	–47	–55	–63	–70	–78	–85	–93
30	11	4	–4	–12	–20	–28	–35	–43	–51	–59	–66	–74	–82	–90	–98
35	10	2	–6	–14	–22	–30	–37	–45	–53	–61	–69	–77	–85	–93	–101
40	9	1	–7	–15	–23	–31	–39	–47	–55	–63	–71	–79	–87	–95	–103

To read this chart, find the air temperature (°F) in the top row of numbers. Read the column downward until you find the row containing the wind velocity. That reading is the windchill factor.

National Collegiate Athletic Association Recommendations for Preventing Cold Injuries

- Layer clothing: Use several thin layers rather than a single heavy garment.
- Cover the head: As much as 50% of an individual's total heat loss is from the head and neck region.
- Protect the hands: Cover the hands if there is any chance of frostbite; mittens are warmer than gloves.
- Stay dry: Water increases body heat loss. Use a vapor barrier next to the skin or a material that will wick moisture away from the skin surface.
- Stay hydrated: Dehydration alters the body's ability to regulate heat.
- Warm up thoroughly: Generate body heat through muscle activity before and throughout the exercise period. Stay warm even after the workout, and cool down gradually once finished with the workout.
- Warm incoming air: Use a scarf over the nose and mouth to help prevent bronchospasm from exposing the airways to severe cold.

Steps in Caring for Cold Injury

- Move the athlete out of the cold environment.
- Remove any wet or restrictive clothing.
- Do not allow the athlete to use the injured part.
- Avoid handling the injured part.
- Do not rub or massage the area.

Adapted from NCAA 1999.

OTHER WEATHER CONDITIONS

Other weather conditions that pose a threat to the health and safety of physically active people include thunderstorms and lightning storms. The blowing, gusting winds of a thunderstorm may injure the eyes if dust or dirt is blown about. Lightning storms are nature's deadliest force and are potentially very dangerous. A summer storm may travel very quickly, placing the entire team at risk of injury in the event of a lightning strike. Tornados are usually born out of severe thunderstorms.

Lightning Strikes

Athletic fields are often very large, open areas where the nearest structures are the light poles or, on an athletic club field, the raised stand for the filming of practice. These tall, typically metal structures are more likely targets for lightning than are many other types of structures; yet if a bolt of lightning hits such a structure, the arc of the electricity has the potential to injure anyone nearby. If a thunderstorm is occurring in the area, team camera crew members should be advised to stay off any metal towers. The appearance of a lightning bolt is usually followed by a clap of thunder. The delay between sight and sound occurs as a result of the speed of light versus the speed of sound. An easy and very practical way to figure out your distance from a lightning bolt is to count the number of seconds (one one thousand, two

The National Lightning Safety Institute is an independent, nonprofit consulting, education, and research organization that advocates a risk management approach to lightning hazard mitigation. Visit the organization's Web site at www.lightningsafety.com.

Decision Tree for Personal Lightning Safety

The National Lightning Safety Institute (NLSI) recommends that all organizations prepare a Lightning Safety Plan and inform all personnel of its contents. Briefly, lightning safety is "anticipating a high-risk situation and moving to a low-risk location." Lightning Safety Plans should be site specific, but they all share a common outline:

1. Advanced warning of the hazard. Some options:
   - "If you can see it, flee it. If you can hear it, clear it."
   - TV Weather Channel; NOAA Weather Radio.
   - Fancy lightning detectors; off-site meteorological services.
2. Make decision to suspend activities and notify people.
   - The 30/30 rule says to shut down when lightning is 6 miles away. Use a "flash to bang" (lightning to thunder) count: Five seconds equals 1 mile (10 = 2 miles; 20 = 4 miles; 30 = 6 miles).
   - Notify people via radio, siren, or other means.
3. Move to safe location.
   - A large permanent building or metal vehicle is best.
   - Unsafe places are near metal or water; under trees; on hills; near electrical and electronics equipment.
4. Reassess the hazard.
   - It's usually safe after no thunder and no lightning have been observed for 30 min. Be conservative here.
5. Inform people to resume activities.

National Lightning Safety Institute 1999.

Information regarding severe storms can be obtained though the National Severe Storm Laboratory, National Oceanic and Atmospheric Administration, at www.nssl.noaa.gov.

---

one thousand . . .) between when you see the lightning bolt and when you hear the clap of thunder. Divide this number by five, and that should tell you approximately how many miles away the storm is.

Depending on the speed with which the storm is traveling and the direction of its movement, the team may need to clear the field. The team should remain under cover until about 30 min have passed without lightning. Teams should develop a policy for postponing practice or games in the event of a lightning storm. The NCAA has published guidelines for member institutions regarding athletics during a lightning storm. All teams should have a person on the staff responsible for watching any approaching storms and for notifying team members when it is time to take cover. Remember: Electricity can be conducted through metal (think of all the things around the field that are metal, including the pipes for the water!), and the electricity from a bolt of lightning that strikes the ground may travel along those pathways. Also, don't assume that lightning doesn't strike twice in the same place; it does.

Tornados

Other types of foul weather are characteristic of specific areas of the country and particular months of the year. People living in "Tornado Alley" (which includes Texas, Oklahoma, Florida, Kansas, Nebraska, Iowa, and Missouri), for example, know the devastation that such violent storms can produce. Tornados can be stationary or can travel at speeds of up to 70 mph (113 km/hr). Although most tornado damage is caused by the violent winds, most tornado injuries and deaths result from flying debris. Clues that a tornado could develop are a dark, often greenish-looking sky, large hail, and a loud roar similar to the sound of a freight train. No matter what area of the country you live in, there is the potential for severe weather. Know the types of weather that are approaching your area, and pay attention to weather reports and to what you see outside. Be wise when subjecting an entire team to bad weather; it's not just you who will be affected.

OTHER ENVIRONMENTAL FACTORS INFLUENCING SPORT PARTICIPATION

The word "environment" may create in your mind an image of weather conditions—and that's what we have focused on up to now. True, weather is a component of our environment, and weather conditions have been the cause of athletic-related deaths in the United States. But weather is not the only factor within the environment that can pose a threat to safe athletic performance. Other important types of environmental risk factors include altitude, the physical characteristics of the facilities and equipment, and potential disease-transmitting organisms in the athletic environment.

Altitude

Just as important as acclimatizing to heat and humidity is the acclimatization to altitude. When an athlete changes training or competition venues and begins working out at high altitude (>2,000 m or 6,550 ft), the body must adapt to the thinner air and less partial pressure of oxygen. The immediate changes observed are an increase in heart rate and respiration. This occurs both at rest and during submaximal exercise, in an attempt to overcome the lower levels of oxygen. Due to this lower oxygen level, top performances will be impossible until acclimation occurs.

Acclimatization to the new altitude requires sufficient time for the red blood cells to accommodate to the low partial pressures of oxygen, as they both increase in number and acquire the ability to absorb and release oxygen more efficiently. The length of time needed for this and other adaptations varies depending on the level of fitness of the individual.

When faced with a change in altitude, the athlete must recognize that the physiological requirements of working at the higher altitude will take a toll on the level of performance. Time for acclimatization is necessary to allow high-level performance.

Facilities and Equipment

Any sport activity may take place in a physical environment that has unsafe or unhealthful characteristics. For each sport with which you are involved, it is wise to spend time analyzing the potential risks in this regard.

Inspecting the Area

Although it may be true that most schools and universities have an office responsible for managing the risks on campus, it is still essential that everyone associated with the institution be alert and observant. Reporting playing field hazards to the risk-management department or the facilities manager in the athletic department (or both) usually ensures that the hazard will be corrected.

A careful survey of the playing court or field should be conducted prior to any practice or game. Anticipation of obstructions to safe play such as unpadded supports or walls, fences, and bleachers too close to the area of play will help avoid problems. Goal supports should be padded before the first practice if the posts are in a position that may cause a collision. Observe the field for potholes, sprinkler heads, or other obstacles. Make sure the court is free of wet spots or other surface hazards. Be very observant and use a critical eye when walking over your practice area.

Physical Obstructions on the Field

It is always crucial to take care to provide as risk free a playing area as possible. Walking over the field or court before a practice or competition gives the coach or athletic trainer the opportunity to recognize any potentially hazardous conditions. Objects to check include posts and standards, building walls, and field-surface obstructions.

Goalposts, standards, and all immovable objects located within the area of play must have sufficient padding that players will not incur serious injury upon contact with them. Building walls are another type of structure that may present risk. Occasionally sport activity takes place on a court or field that was constructed without proper attention to the distance required for an athlete to stop prior to contacting a wall. Obviously the wall cannot be moved, but the court lines may be adjusted to allow a safe stopping distance. Regardless of the potential to adjust the distance from the end line to the wall, walls that may limit the safe deceleration of an athlete at full speed must have padding to help absorb the force of the contact.

There also may be obstructions on the field surface itself. Potholes and sprinkler heads in the field of play are common. A careful inspection of the entire field and the 10 ft (3 m) surrounding the field boundary should be undertaken at frequent intervals during the sport season. Sprinkler heads should be flush with or slightly below the level of the playing surface. If at all possible, the athletic field should be designed with watering needs taken into account so that it is possible to provide adequate water coverage with a minimum number of sprinklers within the area of play.

Other Obstructions

Just as a wall that is too close to a sideline or end line may increase the risk of injury, bleachers, benches, and other seating structures may be placed too close to the area of play. The placement of any permanent structure should be considered and thoroughly evaluated before a final location is selected. Movable benches, tables, and seats should be evaluated and repositioned if necessary before the start of every sport session and every practice.

Backyard Courts

Although backyard courts are seldom used for official contests, many athletes do train on such surfaces. It would seem that common sense should prevail when people build a sport court, yet many backyards are the sites of athletic injuries. Courts with physical elements that are hazardous to play must be used only for practice in specific skills of the sport that one can perform while still safely avoiding the obstacle. For example, a basketball hoop attached to the garage may be unsafe for doing layups. Rather than using that court for a pickup game, people should use it for shooting practice in which they are not apt to collide with the garage.

Disease-Transmitting Organisms in Facilities and on Equipment

As a final type of environmental hazard we consider disease-transmitting organisms in facilities and on equipment. The element of the facility most commonly associated with the risk of disease transmission is the wrestling mat. Because of the physical contact between an athlete and the mat, bacteria and fungi may be transferred to the mat surface. With the high temperatures typically maintained in most wrestling rooms, the environment becomes conducive to bacterial growth. Disinfecting the mat after every practice should be a priority for every wrestling program. With proper care of the facility, bacterial and fungal growth can be controlled and the risk of transmission of bacteria and viruses between athletes greatly reduced.

In addition to appearing on "community" items such as the wrestling mat, contact dermatoses may occur on one individual but not spread to other members of the team. Rashes, boils, or other skin conditions may erupt as a result of contact between an athlete's skin and some part of the protective equipment. When this is the case, the first step to the "cure" is finding the cause and making the appropriate changes. Treatment of the skin condition without changing the offending equipment will only prolong the course of the ailment.

It is important for those responsible to understand how to reduce the likelihood of spreading bacteria via equipment. If skin irritation occurs on a body part that comes into contact with sport equipment, that equipment should be treated to reduce its potential to harbor bacteria. Sometimes it is more effective to dispose of equipment than to attempt disinfection. Items that may harbor bacteria and that should be disposed of if a skin irritation erupts include knee pads used in basketball and volleyball, shin pads used in soccer, and plastic pads used inside the helmet in football. Items that should be cleaned include the larger, more costly items: shoulder pads such as those used in football, the shoes used in any sport. These items should be thoroughly cleaned, and athletes should not wear them next to the skin; instead, for skin protection, they should wear T-shirts under the pads and should wear clean, white socks with the shoes.

Finally, and above all else, coaches and athletic trainers must remember that following Universal Precautions is the best means of reducing the risk of transmission of bloodborne pathogens in athletics. The extra time it takes people to perform Universal Precautions and use proper procedures, such as pulling on a pair of gloves, is quite small compared to the time they would lose as a result of contracting a virus.

SUMMARY

1. *List and give examples of the four cooling methods used to rid a body of excess heat.*

   Evaporation occurs when water is heated and vaporizes into the atmosphere. This takes place when a person sweats: That moisture evaporates, allowing heat to escape and cooling to occur. Conduction takes place when a hot surface is in contact with a cooler surface. Heat moves from the warmer to the cooler area, as when your dog lies on the kitchen floor with all four limbs spread. The contact area of the hotter object (the dog) allows heat to transfer to the cooler area (the floor). Convection occurs when the air surrounding the individual is warmed. The warm air expands and its density decreases, making it lighter, and it then rises. When that warm air moves upward, it is replaced by cooler air. This is what is happening to the football player who is playing on a very cold day. If he removes his helmet you can see the convection currents as the warm air rises off his head. Radiation comes from a heat source that is not in direct contact with the body; it warms the air by virtue of its temperature. This happens constantly when the sun is shining. The radiant energy of the sun warms us and everything around us.

2. *Identify steps a person should take to lessen the risks of exercising in very hot and humid conditions.*

   To allow yourself to tolerate high heat and humidity, you should always take sufficient time to acclimatize to the environmental temperatures by starting with moderate to light levels of activity and working up to your current levels. If the day is unusually hot or humid, you may need to adjust your workout by increasing the number of rest periods, or decreasing the length of the exercise session, or both. To allow your body to dissipate heat well, a high level of hydration is essential. Monitoring hydration status is very important for decreasing the ill effects of working out in a hot and humid climate.

3. *List and explain three ways in which a physically active person could determine the heat and humidity in a climate he or she is visiting.*

   If equipment is available, you should take measurements at the exact location of the workout. If not, you could use the heat index or the relative humidity readings from the local weather service. Because areas of a town are under different environmental conditions, the use of data from some other area is usually less accurate. For instance, measurements at the airport are taken in a very dry area (the runway and tarmac), but data from the golf course are from a shady area that is often high in moisture. These two readings in the same town are often quite different.

4. *List the major symptoms associated with heat exhaustion.*

   People experiencing heat exhaustion are usually becoming dehydrated. They often have headache, dizziness, nausea, rapid breathing, and fatigue. They are usually actively sweating, and their skin is cool and pale.

5. *Identify two major problems associated with exercise in a very cold environment and explain how those problems might be avoided.*

   The two major illnesses resulting from cold exposure are hypothermia and frostbite. Hypothermia, a drop in the core temperature, affects the entire body. Wet clothing or shoes cause a person to lose heat more quickly; other factors are the person's age, medical conditions, and the ingestion of drugs or poisons. The NCAA recommends that people minimize the ill effects of cold temperatures by wearing several lighter layers of clothing rather than one heavy garment; wearing wicking fabric next to the skin to avoid moisture accumulation; remaining well hydrated to aid the body in maintaining internal temperature; covering the head to retain as much heat as possible; warming up thoroughly and attempting to retain that heat; and covering the hands to avoid frostbite and warming the incoming air by wearing a scarf or other cloth over the nose and mouth. Frostbite, a type of cold injury, affects exposed areas of the skin. Cold injuries are negatively affected by length of time the parts are exposed, the windchill, previous cold injury, impaired circulation, and wearing of wet garments. To avoid cold injuries like frostbite, individuals should understand how cold it is and make necessary adjustments in such factors as clothing and length of time they will be outdoors; they should also avoid wearing clothes that become wet. Persons who have had a previous cold injury or have impaired circulation should take additional care to avoid long exposure and to wear protective layers if they will be out for extended periods.

6. *Explain the concept of windchill and how it may affect the physically active individual exercising in a cold environment.*

   Windchill refers to the effects of wind as it combines with cold temperatures. A cold wind is much colder than cold temperature alone. If people consider only the temperature of the air when deciding how to dress or how long to exercise, they may be prone to cold injury if it is also windy.

7. *Identify several factors that should raise concern if one is exercising outdoors during a thunderstorm.*

   Thunderstorms are often associated with other factors, and it is those other factors that raise concern for the individual exercising outdoors. First, the wind can blow sand or dust into the eyes. This is especially important on ball fields, where the infield dirt is almost always loosely packed and apt to be blown around by gusts of wind. Secondly, the thunderstorm is an indication that lightning is nearby, and lightning is attracted to metal objects that sit high in an open field. The final concern, especially in some parts of the country, is the potential for tornados. Although not all thunderstorms spawn tornados, when tornados occur they always follow a thunderstorm.

8. *List things one should observe when inspecting a playing environment for safety.*

   The playing area should be inspected on a routine basis. The inspection should include all areas where potential for injury exists. Observe the condition of the playing surface to ensure that there are no dangerous holes, projecting sprinkler heads, or problems with the floor and that all goalposts or other standards are well padded. Observe the boundaries of the playing area to ensure that all benches and other equipment are well removed from the sideline. If any equipment or parts of the facility appear to be within the path of an errant participant, pad that obstacle to ensure that any contact with the object will be cushioned.

CRITICAL THINKING QUESTIONS

1. You have just been hired to coordinate the sport teams for all middle schools in a school district. The district has five schools, and each school has boys' and girls' soccer, basketball, tennis, and track, as well as girls' volleyball and boys' football. One of your job responsibilities is to review the playing areas and make recommendations for any safety measures that may be needed. Visit a middle school in your neighborhood and evaluate each field or court to be used. Write up a summary of each area with recommendations for increased safety.

2. One of your high school student-athletes is going to spend the summer with his father, who lives in North Dakota, and will not return to Houston (Texas) until the first day of football. Discuss potential areas of concern and give recommendations for the athlete to follow to limit the potential problems.

3. You are the coach/athletic trainer for a small high school. There is no physician available to the team, and the school nurse is in only on Thursdays. One of your wrestlers reports to you saying that he has been feeling "hot and cold" since Monday (this is Tuesday). Overall he admits he is not feeling real well, but the biggest complaint is the chills and fever. Discuss the steps you would take in evaluating this athlete for participation. Explain why the athlete may be complaining of "chills."

4. One of your college defensive backs has been wearing a bandana over his head, under his football helmet. He has been complaining of having heat cramps near the end of practice and wants to know what to do to prevent them. Explain the common reason for the heat cramps. Do you see any reason to advise him *not* to wear the bandana? Discuss this.

5. You are working for a college football team during the preseason camp. The athletes are practicing twice a day. You are asked to organize a system for monitoring the athletes' hydration status. Explain how you might accomplish this. Discuss the personnel you would need to institute this plan.

6. After a tough soccer practice in the heat, one of your strikers lay down, exhausted, on the field. When you arrive to help him, you fear his body temperature may be a problem because you notice that his shirt is soaking wet but he is quite dry and warm to the touch. Since he is a black athlete you are unable to detect a skin color change, but you think he seems hot. Explain what you can do to help him. Be thorough in your explanation (i.e., tell who will help him and how it will be done).

CITED SOURCES

Binkley, H.M., J Beckett, D.J. Casa, D.M. Kleiner, et al. 2002. National Athletic Trainers' Association position statement: Exertional heat illnesses. *J Athl Trng* 37(3): 329–343.

Casa, D.J., L.E. Armstrong, S.K. Hillman, et al. 2000. National Athletic Trainers' Association position statement: Fluid replacement for athletes. *J Athl Trng* 35(2): 212–224.

National Lightning Safety Institute. 2004. Decision tree for personal lightning safety. www.lightningsafety.com/nlsi_pls/decision_tree_people.html (accessed June 15, 2004).

NCAA. 2002. Guideline 2c: Prevention of heat illness. http://ncaa.org/library/sports_sciences/sports_med_handbook/2003-04/index.html (accessed June 15, 2004).

Wilmore, J.H., and D.L. Costill. 2004. *Physiology of Sport and Exercise*, 3rd ed. Champaign, IL: Human Kinetics.

ADDITIONAL READINGS

Backer, H.D., and S. Collins. 1999. Use of a handheld, battery-operated chemistry analyzer for evaluation of heat-related symptoms in the backcountry of Grand Canyon National Park: A brief report. *Ann Emerg Med* 33(4): 418-422.

Barrow, M.W., and K.A. Clark. 1998. Heat-related illnesses. *Am Fam Physician* 58(3): 749-756, 759.

Bergeron, M.F., C.M. Maresh, L.E. Armstrong, J.F. Signorile, J.W. Castellani, R.W. Kenefick, K.E. LaGasse, and D.A. Riebe. 1995. Fluid-electrolyte balance associated with tennis match play in a hot environment. *Int J Spt Nutr* 5(3): 180-193.

Eichner, E.R. 1998. Treatment of suspected heat illness. *Int J Spts Med Suppl* 2: S150-S153.

Franklin, Q.J., and M. Compeggie. 1999. Splenic syndrome in sickle cell trait: Four case presentations and a review of the literature. *Mil Med* 164(3): 230-233.

Hsieh, M., R. Roth, D.L. Davis, H. Larrabee, and C.W. Callaway. 2002. Hyponatremia in runners requiring on-site medical treatment at a single marathon. *Med Sci Spts Exerc* 34: 185-189.

Maughan, R.J., and J.B. Leiper. 1999. Limitations to fluid replacement during exercise. *Can J Appl Physiol* 24(2): 173-187.

Murray, R. 1998. Rehydration strategies—balancing substrate, fluid, and electrolyte provision. *Int J Spts Med Suppl* 2: S133-S135.

Noakes, T.D. 1998. Fluid and electrolyte disturbances in heat illness. *Int J Spts Med Suppl* 2: S146-S149.

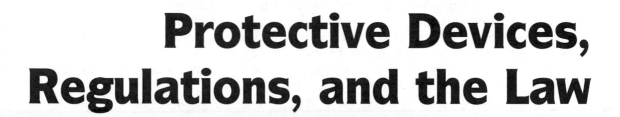

Protective Devices, Regulations, and the Law

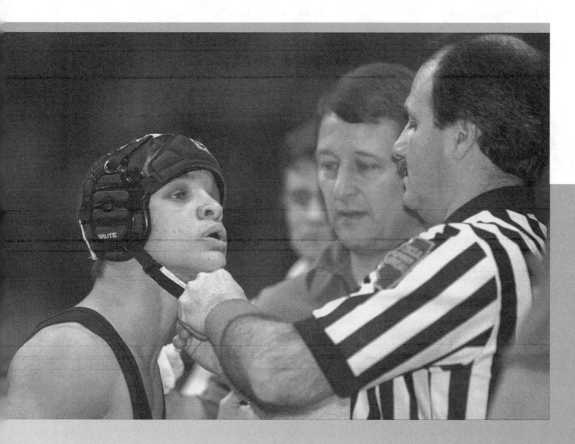

Objectives

After reading this chapter, the student will be able to do the following:

1. Identify the eight factors to consider in fabricating a protective splint for a physically active individual; present examples of times when each of those factors would become critical.

2. Explain the various types of materials according to their requirement for heat in the molding process.

3. Explain the function of a voluntary standards organization and describe how such an organization might impact sport equipment.

4. Explain the significance of the National Operating Committee on Standards for Athletic Equipment seal on protective headgear and discuss ways in which that seal would serve to protect the wearer.

5. Identify the factors considered in determining legal liability for an injury that occurred after alteration of protective equipment.

Charles, a sophomore trying out for the soccer team, was extremely close to making the varsity squad when, one day at practice, he lost his footing in a drill and slam!—down on his left hip he went. The good news was that nothing was broken; the bad news was that any little tap to the area caused so much pain that Charles didn't think he could stand it.

Jill, the athletic trainer for the team, suggested that Charles use a pad over the sore area. Charles thought that idea was crazy. Run with a pad on his hip?

"Let me make a custom pad for you, Charles; I'll put it into a special pocket sewn into a pair of spandex shorts like you wear under your workout shorts."

"Okay, but if it doesn't feel right I don't have to wear it, do I?" asked Charles.

"No. If you don't like it, you won't play well. I want you to have the best chance you can of making this team," said Jill with empathy for the athlete in this difficult situation.

The pad was made, and Charles tried it on.

"Hey, this feels pretty good next to my bruise! Why doesn't the pressure of the pad hurt?" queried Charles.

"I cut a hole out of the foam material, right where the sore area is. All the pressure is absorbed into the pad and dispersed onto parts of your hip that can take the pressure. The bruised area is within the donut hole," Jill responded.

Charles was happy and headed off to try out a couple "bumps" against a fellow player.

"How's it feel?" Jill asked when Charles came jogging by her on the field.

"Excellent! I can't even tell it's sore. I can really take a hit on it and I feel nothing! Thanks. See ya after practice."

Charles hustled, ran, fell, and collided with others during that afternoon's practice. After practice he dropped into the athletic training room for his ice treatment and reevaluation. There was no further injury—and even better, the soreness was going away.

Prevention of sport injuries depends to a great extent on properly designed and properly fitting protective equipment. Sometimes, as in Charles' case, specialty pads are fabricated to protect injured areas so that they will not be further aggravated by participation. Athletes also wear many other types of protective devices. Players need to know about the protective devices recommended for their sport. The coach and athletic trainer should be aware of the options for using fabricated and purchased protective devices and of issues concerning the proper fitting of equipment. In this chapter we consider these equipment issues and also look at the development of sport safety rules, legal concerns about equipment use in sport, and concepts of **liability**.

ENERGY ABSORPTION AND FORCE DISSIPATION

Careful evaluation of an injury may indicate that the athlete can return to play provided there is sufficient protection. Often a commercially available pad, brace, or other device is available, but sometimes a custom fit or application is required. These pads or splints may be used to immobilize an area to allow healing to continue without disruption, as well as to dissipate the force of contact in the area onto other parts of the surrounding anatomy.

Protective Splints

The goal of the protective **splint** is to protect, stabilize, or immobilize the injured area. When fabricating splints, the clinician should follow basic splinting principles of immobilizing above and below the injured area. Yet when the splint is supporting a limb for return to play, immobilization of the joint above and below the site of injury may be quite restrictive (see figure 7.1). The major goal in providing rigid fixation for an area is twofold: to limit the motion occurring in the area and to dissipate forces away from the site of injury.

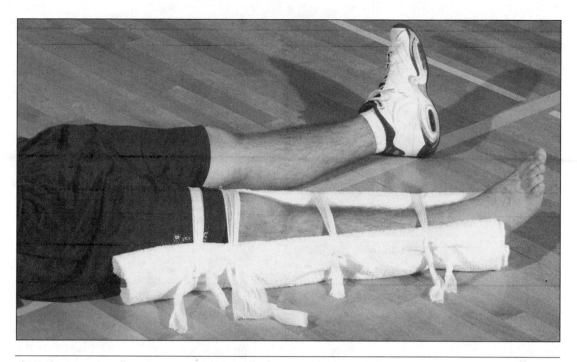

Figure 7.1   Basic splinting principles involve immobilizing above and below the injured area.

In determining the type and style of a protective splint, one must have a basic knowledge of the anatomy involved. Often, a soft-tissue injury can be splinted so that direct contact is avoided, but activation of the bruised muscle causes as much pain as direct contact, or even more. If one is familiar with the structures underlying the area of trauma, one can manually test the muscles to determine underlying pathology or irritability. Additionally we must be aware of the actions at the involved joint to avoid interfering with or changing normal joint mechanics. Obstruction of normal joint motion can cause compensatory motor patterns to develop, which in turn may produce secondary syndromes of overuse.

Finally, before fabricating a custom splint, the clinician must understand the properties of the splinting materials available for use.

Material Properties

The clinician has eight properties to consider in order to determine the suitability of a material for fabricating a protective playing splint. In this section we look briefly at each of these factors:

1. Density
2. Strength
3. Rigidity or stiffness
4. Conformability
5. Self-adherence
6. Durability
7. Ease of fabrication
8. Availability and cost

Density

Density refers to the weight of the material in relation to the volume or amount that will be used. For example, if a player experiences a contusion (bruise) to the forearm, a protective pad may be indicated to prevent repeated blows to the area. If you decide to use a sleeve lined with a pad of a dense, viscoelastic material (like Sorbothane), the weight of the arm with the pad may be significant. This may not be a problem in a sport such as football, but think about the forearm of a gymnast. The additional weight of the forearm may produce an imbalance between the right and left sides, resulting in a much different feeling during performance of gymnastics stunts and rotational movements. For a gymnast, you would probably use a

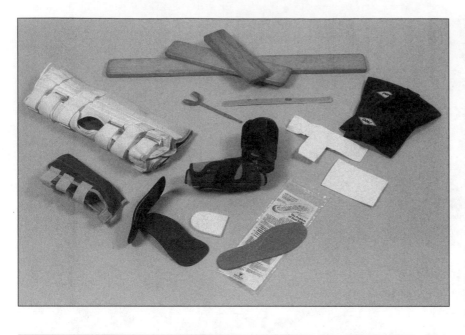

Figure 7.2 In choosing a particular density, consider the type and velocity of contact a participant may experience and match these to the level of protection needed.

sleeve with a lightweight, open-cell foam pad to protect the area from repeated blows.

When choosing between materials of differing density, you must bear in mind the type and velocity of contact from which you are attempting to protect the participant (see figure 7.2). Dense materials offer very good protection, but that protection often comes at the price of bulk and weight. Sleeves or pads made of a viscoelastic material really provide excellent shock disruption to the area that they cover or come into contact with, but they may not be suitable for a physically active person. See table 7.1 for a listing of materials, their densities, and some brand names for products of each type. Various foam materials are often employed as padding under a hard shell designed to distribute forces.

The foams come in a variety of densities and also differ on a number of properties. Some foams offer great resistance to impact because of their high density. Others offer more compression with contact (lower-density foams) but respond from the contact with a "memory" of the previous dimensions. Foam products are numerous, and the variety can become overwhelming. It is always wise to request a sample of the material so that you may fully understand possible applications to your needs. Because of the number of products on the market, knowing what materials are available is a tremendous task. Table 7.1 lists some of the various products according to density.

It should be obvious that for a protective splint, the best choice is a material that has as low a density as possible while still performing the protective function needed. Your decision should take into consideration the participant's freedom of movement with the protective material in place. Avoid materials and splints that cause unusual patterns of movement.

Table 7.1
Protective Materials and Their Densities

Density	Type of material	Examples of products
High density	Silicone elastomer "casting" material, viscoelastic materials, some foams	Silicone: various vendors' silicone elastomer liquid Viscoelastic: Smith and Nephew, Akton, and others Felts and foams: open-cell foams such as Smith and Nephew Carve-It or Sorbothane, Langer Biomechanics PPT, various orthopedic felts
Medium density	Fiberglass splinting materials, polyethylene and other thermoplastic moldable plastics, most orthopedic felt, some foams	Fiberglass: 3M Scotch-cast, Smith and Nephew Dynacast Thermoplastics: J & J Orthoplast, Smith and Nephew Polyform, Polyflex II, Air Thru, Ezeform, Aquaplast, and many others Felts and foams: Spenco silicone pads, various felts and foams
Low density	Some foams, cotton padding, neoprene rubber	Foams: Smith and Nephew Polycushion or Contour Foam

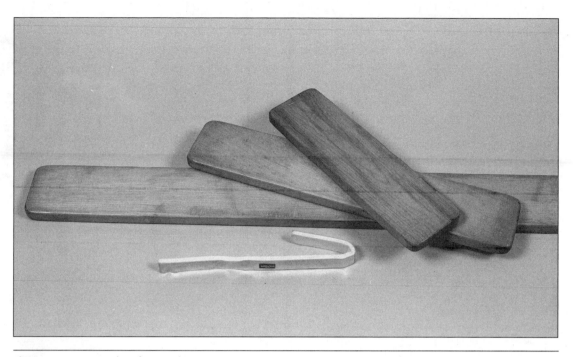

Figure 7.3 Strength refers to the maximum external stress or load that a material can withstand.

Strength

Strength refers to the maximum external stress or load that a material can withstand. The strength of a material is important to ensuring that the splint will function as intended (see figure 7.3). Some materials may be strong enough for normal daily activity but not capable of withstanding the stresses of high-impact athletic participation. If you wanted to provide a splint or support to help prevent inversion ankle sprains, you could select an elastic sleeve, a formed plastic stirrup with air bladder, a lace-up ankle brace, or even a custom-formed hard plastic ankle brace. If the individual had a sedentary job and did not intend to participate in physical activities, the elastic sleeve might provide sufficient support and protection. However, if the person wanted to continue going to basketball practice after work, you might need to consider one of the other devices. The elastic provides compression, but the strength of the material is too low to prevent the ankle from inverting during physical activity.

Rigidity

Rigidity or stiffness refers to the amount of bending or compression that occurs in response to a measured amount of applied stress. Stiffness is measured and evaluated using the concept of "modulus of elasticity." A product with a high modulus is of a stiffer material, while a product with a low modulus gives greater flexibility (less stiffness) and has an ability to absorb shock better (see figure 7.4). A fiberglass splint has a high modulus of elasticity; once "set," the fiberglass is very rigid and nonbending. A splint made of aluminum is an example of a splint with a low modulus. To protect the broken hand of a person who is highly physically active, the fiberglass splint or cast might be the best choice; for someone whose activity level is less apt to lead to contact with the healing hand, an aluminum hand splint may be sufficient. The high-modulus fiberglass will not yield and will provide rigid immobilization, whereas the aluminum splint can actually be bent if that is desired. Strength becomes an important factor in working with the physically active when one is attempting to limit the movement of a joint or area.

Rigidity depends on the type of material used as well as on the thickness and shape of the material once it is formed into the protective device. Again, the bulk of the finished product may be the limiting factor, requiring use of a stiffer or more rigid material.

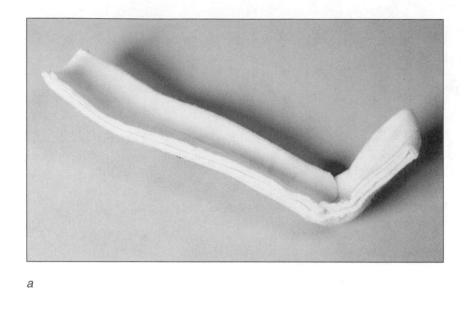

a

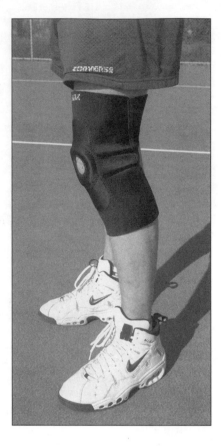

Figure 7.4 *(a)* A product classified as high modulus; *(b)* material with a low modulus.

b

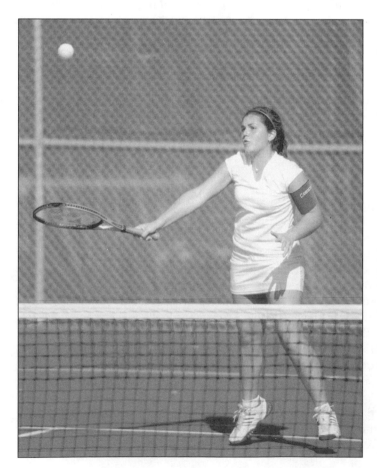

Conformability

Conformability is the ease with which material forms to fit the body part. Most athletes in most sports want to wear a well-fitting uniform, and they have the same attitude about any protective device they may need to wear. If the product is sufficiently strong, dense, and stiff, it may still fail to provide the proper protection if it will not bend or conform to the body part to be protected. For example, a dense foam that is 0.5 in. (1.27 cm) thick may be an excellent choice for its ability to disperse the force of contact; yet when you try to adapt that foam to fit snugly around a bruised knee, you find that it is too inflexible to conform. A nylon or Lycra sleeve with a Sorbothane pad may prove to be more conforming and to provide excellent protection (see figure 7.5).

Self-Adherence

Self-adherence refers to the strength with which the material bonds to itself. This factor determines the integrity and durability of a splint. A splint would be of little value if it uncoupled or separated as the athlete

Figure 7.5 Conformability is the ease with which material forms to fit the body part.

performed the sport. One product frequently used to ensure self-adherence is Velcro. One surface of this material sticks to almost nothing except its own other surface. This type of material is very useful in binding nonadherent materials together around a limb or joint. A brace or splint with internal padding glued inside might be an example of a device with poor self-adherence. The glue is often the point of failure for this type of brace. The heat and moisture inside the brace often destroy the bonds of the glue so that the padding pulls away.

Durability

Durability is the material's ability to withstand repeated stress during the sport activity. This simply means it will last longer if it is more durable. Although the desirability of this characteristic seems obvious, it becomes even more so when one is working within the limited budget of a club or school team where supplies and equipment are not plentiful. Materials that can be used only once or twice are not cost-effective if the same protection is required at every practice session over a prolonged period of time.

It is common for athletic equipment to wear out or break down; materials eventually stop doing their job if used repetitively. You would want to consider this, for example, if you needed arch support. You might have three main options: tape the arch, use a fabricated orthotic of soft neoprene or felt support with special pads to support the arch, or use a custom-made

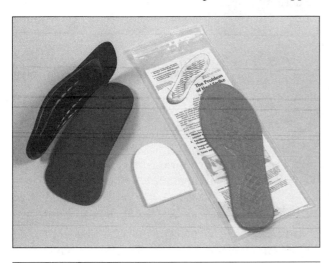

Figure 7.6   The prefabricated orthotic (left) and the custom-formed orthotic (right).

orthotic device constructed of special materials shaped and reinforced to support the arch (see figure 7.6). The tape is a one-time-use solution. Once wet, it will no longer work. The neoprene or felt can be used over and over again but needs to be replaced from time to time. The most durable of the options is the more expensive custom-made support. This device could serve the purpose well for several years.

Ease of Fabrication

Ease of fabrication relates to the time, equipment, and skill needed to shape the material into a form suitable for both protection and comfort. Forming some materials requires heat and thus access to an oven or other heating unit. These materials may be superior for the specific use you intend but are obviously unsatisfactory if you do not have the heating element. In this situation you are left to improvise with other off-the-shelf products that may not fit as well. Take the protective mouthpiece as an example. Many football players wear mouthpieces because of safety requirements. You may have seen or even used a "boil-and-bite" mouthpiece, a protective device that is designed to be molded by the athlete (see figure 7.7). Molding is quite easy if you have a hot pot, a **hydrocollator,** or another way to make very hot or boiling water. If you were traveling, you might not have access to water this hot. Unfortunately, athletes have sometimes played while wearing the unformed mouthpiece because of the problem of finding a heat source.

Fabrication of other types of protective devices can be difficult for various reasons; the special soft cast is an example. The equipment and supplies as well as the special skills needed to fabricate the rubber soft cast may lessen its attractiveness for daily use. If as an athletic trainer you become interested in such products, it will be important to learn the skills needed to fabricate the devices if the supplies are within your budget and you choose to have them on hand. If you don't have the necessary materials or skills, you may need to send athletes to another health care provider to obtain a particular device or find an alternative method of protection.

Availability and Cost

Availability and cost are the two factors that pose the greatest obstacles for many athletic programs. Sometimes you know of a material that would work well in a particular situation,

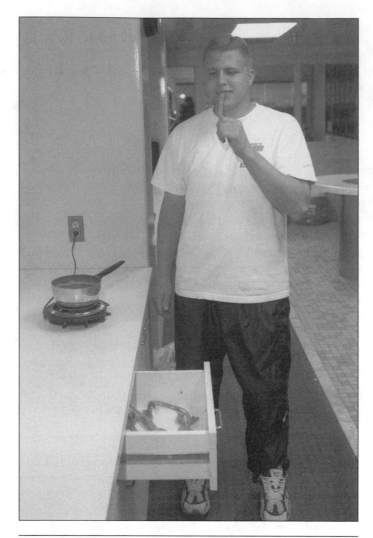

Figure 7.7 Boil-and-bite mouthpieces are designed to give a custom fit.

but it is not available; in this case you will need to devise an alternate solution using another material. In other cases a material that would be appropriate is expensive, and you would probably not expect to use that material at a school where the budget is limited. Some programs have sufficient capital resources to purchase all the materials one might want to use to fabricate various types of protective devices. It is more realistic, however, to understand the limitations imposed by the particular facility's budget and to plan to work within those limitations. If it is not possible to provide adequate protection of an injured part, it may be that the only sound decision is to withhold the athlete from participation until the condition resolves enough to make protection unnecessary.

Classification of Materials

There are four classes of protective splinting materials, categorized on the basis of the intensity of heat required to mold the material:

- No heat (layered)
- Low heat
- Moderate heat
- High temperature

Most materials used to make protective devices for sport fall into the two lowest-heat categories: no heat (layered) and low temperature.

No-Heat (Layered) Materials

No-heat or layered materials that are frequently used in athletics include athletic tape, self-adherent wraps, fiberglass casting materials, silicone rubber used in the fabrication of soft casts for the wrist and hand, and the somewhat outdated casting material plaster of paris. No heat is required to form these products into the appropriate splint, cast, or other type of padding. Although some products in the no-heat category are actually exothermic (giving off heat as they solidify), no heat is required to make the curing process occur. Perhaps the least desirable choice for a playing splint is the plaster of paris cast because of its poor strength-to-weight ratio as well as its poor resistance to moisture.

Low-Heat Products

The other class of materials most often used in fabrication of protective splints for athletes, the low-heat class, includes a variety of products (see figure 7.8). Low-heat materials include rubber, plastic, and other elastics that become very flexible when heated. The low-heat classification includes the rubber-based product Orthoplast, rubber and plastic material such as Polyflex II, plastic-based materials such as Polyform and Orthoplast II, and elastic-based materials such as Aquaplast and Orfit Soft, to name just a few. Forming all these materials requires a low temperature from a source such as hot water or a hot oven. The heat actually breaks the bonds that keep the material rigid, and while the material is warm it remains very malleable and easy to form. Once the material cools back down to normal temperature, the bonds reform and the material retains the shape that it was held in as the cooling took place.

One point you might consider when working with these low-temperature materials is that in some instances the temperatures that the splint is subjected to after fabrication are actually high enough to break the bond and reform the material (temperatures between 69° and 77°

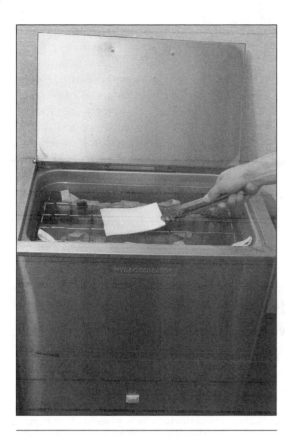

Figure 7.8   Some low-heat materials.

C). Think of a molded piece of plastic left on the dashboard of a car during June in a hot climate. Many plastic materials run the risk of meltdown in such conditions. But since heat is required to form the plastics in the low-temperature category, heat will also allow a change in the material after it has been shaped and molded.

Moderate- and High-Temperature Materials

Moderate- and high-temperature materials are not frequently used by the clinician to fabricate protective devices but are often used by manufacturers of athletic equipment. The temperature required to mold these materials could be dangerous for use in the athletic training room. One exception is manufactured splints or braces that must be custom formed when they are needed. Small adjustments in these moderate- and high-temperature braces can usually be made with the aid of a heating device such as a heat gun. The temperatures of the heat gun can reach 800° F, and care must be taken to avoid burning the athlete's skin, the clinician's skin, and any synthetic products near the heat outflow.

The Art of Fabricating Splints and Braces

Although not actually considered an art, making splints and braces seems to be a natural talent for some people whereas others struggle to get the device to fit and function properly. The ability to fabricate a protective device can be compared with the ability to tape. In athletic training, taping has long been the standard way of protecting a joint from injury. Some athletic trainers' process of applying athletic tape to support the anatomy is truly artistic. This talent in building support of an injured area can be directly applied to the fabrication of a brace or splint. One must take care to support the tissues that have been injured, to avoid areas of pressure, and to allow freedom of movement while providing sufficient restriction of the abnormal movement (see figure 7.9).

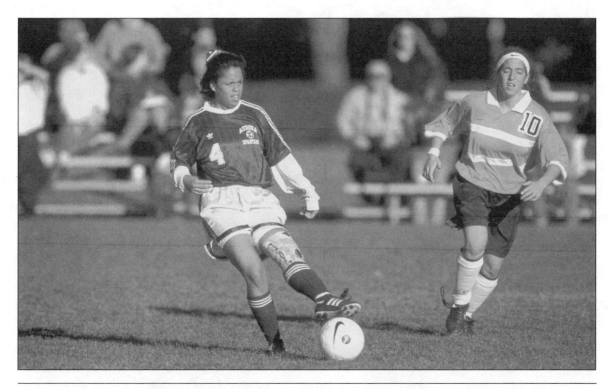

Figure 7.9   Fabricating effective braces and splints is a skill that takes practice and persistence.

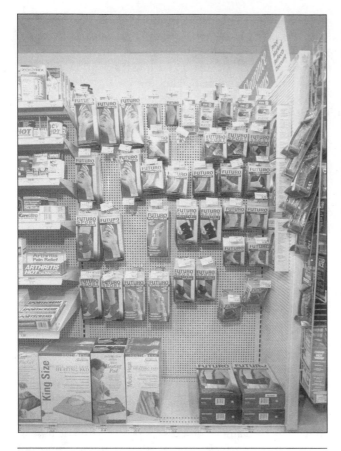

Figure 7.10   A variety of off-the-shelf products.

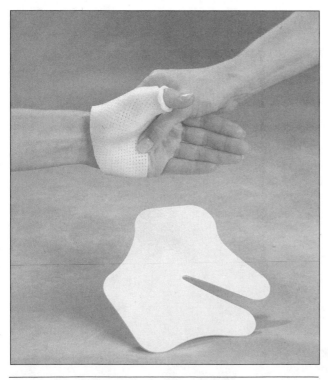

Figure 7.11   "Pre-cuts" come in a variety of sizes and splinting materials.

Photo courtesy of Sammons, Preston, Rolyan.

Fabricating a splint can be a simple or a complex process. When one is making a splint to protect an area from contact or from moving beyond a comfortable range of motion, the task is somewhat easier than when the purpose of the splint is to supplement the action of tendons in the hand (such splints are usually made by a trained hand therapist). Observing a skilled professional make a protective device should be the first step in your learning process. Watch closely and notice the care with which the person constructs the support. After you have seen a particular product such as foam rubber formed into a functioning device, you may want to try working with the material yourself. Ask a classmate to serve as your subject, and build a pad or brace using the material. Ask your friend to fully evaluate the feel and function of your product, and learn from any mistakes you may have made. Practice will help you improve your skills in this area.

Premade or Off-the-Shelf Products for Prevention and Protection

Many times you can find products that provide the exact support or protection that you need. Rather than devoting time and resources to fabricating a pad or support, you may want to look for a premade product (see figure 7.10). In addition to saving time, a purchased device often offers better fit and function than one you could fabricate. The major drawbacks to premade protective devices are that the use of such items is typically limited to one individual and that the fit may not be perfect for everyone. Among the premade items in common use in sport health care are insoles for the reduction of shock, and sleeves and braces for nearly every body part or area to provide support and sometimes relief of symptoms.

Shock-Absorbing Insoles

Often the athlete needs some type of protection that will reduce the shock transmitted through the soft tissue and into the bone or skeleton. Products such as neoprene, Sorbothane, and Viscolis are excellent materials for reducing shock through the feet or just about any bony area, and these materials are available in various sizes and designs to serve almost every need.

Sleeves and Braces

Manufacturers like Pro Orthopedics specialize in the fabrication of neoprene rubber sleeves, braces, and supports. Neoprene can be used for its shock-absorbing properties or for compression, support, and heat retention. Sleeves and braces made of neoprene offer support but are less apt to provide protection from external contact. A very thin neoprene sleeve may be used as a cushion under a brace, reducing the friction and pressure from the hard material of the brace.

Smith and Nephew offers a product line called Roylan pre-cuts that includes a number of splint forms precut in a variety of sizes and thermoplastic splinting materials (see figure 7.11). Products like these allow you to customize the splint by making simple changes in position of the joint or extremity, yet they offer convenience in that you do not have to design and cut a pattern in the material.

Many companies offer splints and braces for the patient in the healing stage of recovery; still others offer functional braces for the patient who is returning to activities and needs extra protection.

STANDARDS FOR EQUIPMENT DESIGN AND RECONDITIONING

Collision sports (American football, ice hockey) and some contact sports (rugby, soccer, lacrosse) use specialized equipment that is considered part of the player's uniform (see figure 7.12). The materials used in the manufacture of equipment for sport are governed by various standards, as you will learn in the following sections.

Occasionally athletes find equipment that is optional in another sport to be quite useful in protecting against injury or reinjury in their sport. For example, you may see a basketball player wearing volleyball knee pads to protect a bruised knee. A critical evaluation of equipment that has been purchased for all sport teams may allow management of some injuries without special fabrication of protective devices. Not only is manufactured protective equipment easy from a fabrication or modification standpoint; it is often more durable than something you would fabricate in the athletic training room.

REGULATING AGENCIES

Regulation of sport equipment manufacturers is necessary to prevent companies from producing inexpensive equipment that will not stand up to the stress of athletic competition. To ensure that equipment is of the requisite quality, governing bodies have been established to set the necessary standards. Additionally, every piece of athletic equipment must be reconditioned if it

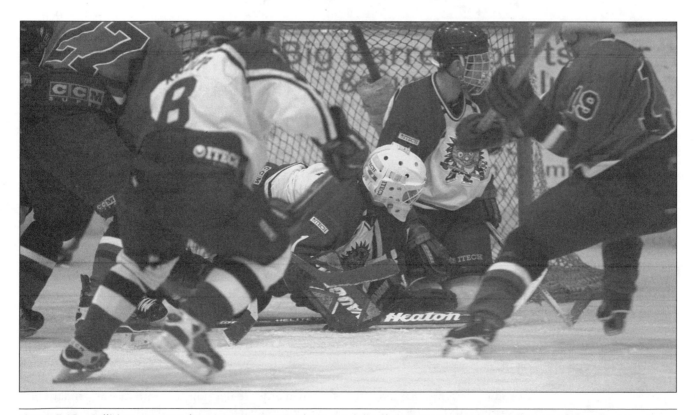

Figure 7.12 Collision sports and some contact sports have specialized equipment that is actually part of the player's uniform.

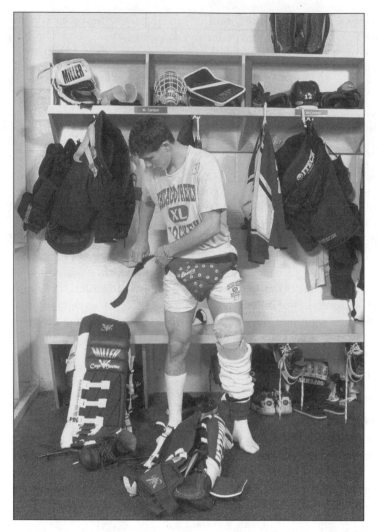

Figure 7.13 Agencies exist to standardize the protective qualities of athletic equipment, as well as the protective devices used by other active members of the community.

is to be used for more than one season of competitive play (see figure 7.13). Both the manufacturer and the reconditioner must comply with a set of standards.

Protective equipment has long been a concern of both the athletic community and the population in general. Agencies exist to standardize the protective qualities of athletic equipment, as well as of the protective devices used by other active members of the community. For instance, the motorcycle helmet is a piece of safety equipment, as is the bicycle helmet. Both helmets, just like sport helmets, are quality controlled by specific governing agencies. Familiarity with the governing agencies and some of the standards they are empowered with developing is helpful for understanding the criteria and conditions that protective sport equipment must meet.

Several organizations have specific roles in the issuance of standards. These include the International Organization for Standardization, the American National Standards Institute, the Consumer Products Safety Commission, the American Society for Testing and Materials, and the National Operating Committee on Standards for Athletic Equipment (NOCSAE). Many of these organizations are voluntary standards development organizations, which means that manufacturers meet the established standards voluntarily. From time to time, a governing body for a particular sport mandates that a piece of equipment must be "NOCSAE approved." This is a rule or mandate imposed by the sport organization rather than by the organization that established the standards.

International Organization for Standardization

On the global scale, there is the International Organization for Standardization (ISO: "ISO" is not an acronym, but means "equal"). This is a worldwide voluntary standards committee made up of representatives from most countries. The organization as a whole develops international standards for specific products ranging from microprocessors to swing sets. The mission of ISO is "to promote the development of standardization and related activities in the world with a view to facilitating the international exchange of goods and services, and to developing cooperation in the spheres of intellectual, scientific, technological and economic activity" (International Organization for Standardization 1999). For example, the format of credit cards, phone cards, and "smart" cards used all over the world is derived from an ISO standard. By adhering to the standard, which defines such features as an optimal thickness (0.76 mm), the manufacturer of the card assures the consumer that the card can be used worldwide.

American National Standards Institute

Within the United States, the governing agency for standards is the American National Standards Institute (ANSI). This is another voluntary standards development organization, serving as the international connection to the ISO standards network. Organizations wishing to submit a product design, system, or other service in order to develop an international standard may do so. The ANSI screens the product design, evaluates it, and eventually presents (if deemed acceptable) the developed standard to the ISO. The ANSI is the American representative to the ISO and also America's liaison from the ISO. Additionally, ANSI works on a more local basis in giving recommendations to many groups, including the Occupational Safety and Health Administration and the American Society for Testing and Materials.

Consumer Products Safety Commission

The Consumer Products Safety Commission (CPSC) is a governmental regulatory agency that deals with the safety of all products (not just athletic goods). Its mission is to protect the public from unreasonable risks of injury and death associated with consumer products. The commission's objective is to reduce the estimated 28.6 million injuries and 21,700 deaths that have been associated with the 15,000 different types of consumer products under its jurisdiction since the start of the commission in 1972. Since 1973, the epidemiological research group at the CPSC has operated the National Electronic Injury Surveillance System.

American Society for Testing and Materials

The American Society for Testing and Materials (ASTM) has a number of subcommittees that focus on testing materials and products used throughout industry, recreation, and leisure, among other areas. The ASTM is one of the largest voluntary standards development systems in the world. A not-for-profit organization, ASTM provides a forum in which producers, users, ultimate consumers, and those having a general interest (representatives of government and academia) can meet to write standards for materials, products, systems, and services. The ASTM is composed of 132 standards-writing committees that publish standard test methods, specifications, practices, guides, classifications, and terminology. The ASTM deals with all aspects of materials, products, and procedures. Many ASTM committees focus on the highway and construction industries, but some are concerned with sport products—the most prominent of these being the F8 committee.

The ASTM F8 committee, Sports Equipment and Facilities, is the ASTM committee most involved with sport equipment. Organized in 1898, it includes more than 30 subcommittees. All subcommittees have an interest in some aspect of the materials used in sport. Among the subcommittees are those listed in table 7.2.

Table 7.2

American Society for Testing and Materials F8 Subcommittees Involved With Sporting Equipment

Subcommittee no.	Subcommittee title	Sport equipment
12	Gymnastics and Wrestling Equipment	Mats and equipment
18	Golf Club Shafts	Club shafts
26	Baseball and Softball Equipment and Facilities	Protective gear, bats
52	Miscellaneous Playing Surfaces	Indoor and outdoor playing surfaces and other facility structures
53	Headgear and Helmets	Helmets worn in football, baseball, equestrian sports, etc.
55	Padding (Body)	Protective padding for all sports
57	Eye Safety for Sports	Protective eyewear

To learn more about the ASTM and their various activities and regulations, visit the ASTM home page at www.astm.org.

National Operating Committee on Standards for Athletic Equipment

In the United States, athletic equipment standards are issued by the NOCSAE. After being organized in 1969 at Wayne State University, NOCSAE began testing football helmets. Using a replica of a human skull, committee members tested various helmet designs to determine the safety of the model relative to concussion criteria in a severe football impact simulation. They established testing standards, and subsequently their test criteria were accepted as the "gold standard" for most sport helmets. Each sport has its own set of NOCSAE standards, which include standards for batting helmets, baseballs, softballs, lacrosse helmets and face masks, and football helmets and face masks. Those interested may obtain copies of all NOCSAE standards free of charge by contacting the executive director of the organization.

The NOCSAE has only two paid employees (a director of research and an attorney). Manufacturers, medical groups, school organizations, and equipment manager groups are invited to take part in NOCSAE developments. These individuals work to evaluate the standards and make any changes in any sport equipment that they deem necessary. Decisions to change the standards for the manufacture of a type of helmet, for example, would be based on evidence either that the current design is flawed or that some additional step could be taken to make the product safer. Each organization is offered two seats on the NOCSAE board. Some of the organizations represented on the board include the following:

- American College Health Association
- Sporting Goods Manufacturers Association
- National Athletic Trainers' Association
- National Collegiate Athletic Association (NCAA)
- National Federation of State High School Associations
- National Junior College Athletic Association
- The Sports Foundation
- National Athletic Equipment Reconditioners Association (NAERA)
- National Association of Intercollegiate Athletics
- National Association of Secondary School Principals
- National Equipment Managers Association

The NOCSAE symbol indicates that a product design meets NOCSAE standards. The committee also sets the standards for equipment reconditioners to use in evaluating and reevaluating helmets. The NOCSAE itself does not evaluate helmets after they have been manufactured; it only affirms that the design of a helmet meets NOCSAE standards and that the reconditioner's tests meet NOCSAE standards for testing. The organization also does not enforce the standard—it merely approves the use of the NOCSAE seal to be embossed on the helmet. If a helmet later fails to pass NOCSAE testing standards, the evaluating agency has the authority to revoke NOCSAE approval. The NOCSAE is just one of the many voluntary standards organizations for sporting equipment, and its standard in athletic **helmetry** is the one most widely accepted.

Some of the efforts of NOCSAE include the development of test standards for football helmets, baseball/softball batting helmets, baseballs/softballs, lacrosse helmets/face masks, and football face masks. For more about NOCSAE, visit www.nocsae.org.

Other Regulatory Agencies

There are other agencies that govern the manufacturing of sport equipment. Among these are regional associations such as the European Standards Association, the Canadian Standards Association, and the Swedish Standards Institute, just to name a few. Another agency crosses country borders and governs the testing and certification of equipment used in all forms of the sport of hockey—the Hockey Equipment Certification Council. Realize that these agencies all have one goal: to make equipment safer. If the agency is voluntary, that means that the manufacturer is not required to follow the standards the agency sets. But it is certainly positive for a company to advertise that its product meets standards of several of the pertinent agencies rather than only one or perhaps none.

RECONDITIONING AND MAINTENANCE OF ATHLETIC HEADGEAR

Several different standards exist for athletic headgear. The NOCSAE standard is the most recognized certification standard, although ANSI and ASTM still control some of the certification procedures.

A yearly inspection of all equipment should be performed by all groups distributing protective gear to athletes. Some school equipment supervisors elect to inspect their helmets themselves and to send only certain identified helmets to the reconditioner. Other schools or teams may find it necessary to send all helmets used during the season to the reconditioner.

The National Athletic Equipment Reconditioners Association (NAERA) suggests guidelines for reconditioning helmets as well as other sport equipment. Each area of the country typically has at least one equipment reconditioner. Some companies solicit business nationwide. These companies compete with the local company for the school's helmet-reconditioning business. The reconditioner, usually a member of the NAERA, inspects each helmet for defects and deficiencies. Loss of integrity of the helmet shell means an automatic rejection; other problems can be rectified in order to meet the helmet manufacturer's standards. Upon completion of the reconditioning, the reconditioner places a sticker on the helmet signifying that the reconditioning process has been completed and specifying the date it was completed.

Any helmet worn during practices or games should be evaluated periodically. Naturally, the higher the level of competition, the more abuse the helmet is likely to take. The athletic trainer or equipment manager, or both, should inspect each helmet for structural safety on a weekly basis at minimum. Fit should be inspected daily. Recent data from the NAERA indicate that over 1 million helmets were reconditioned in 1995, representing approximately 85% of all helmets in use. The average cost of reconditioning is $20; the cost varies if the face mask is damaged, as is typical with college and professional athletes' helmets.

The NOCSAE helmet test involves mounting the football helmet on a synthetic head and dropping it a total of 16 times onto a firm rubber pad. Six different contact points are used in dropping the helmet from a 60-in. (152-cm) height. Shock measurements are recorded and compared to an established severity index in order to determine acceptance or rejection of the helmet. Those helmets that pass the test get a NOCSAE recertification sticker; those failing are clearly marked "unfit for use" or "reject."

AGENCIES FOR DEVELOPMENT OF SPORT SAFETY RULES

The American Medical Association's Committee on the Medical Aspects of Sports and the NCAA Committee on Competitive Safeguards of Sports have both worked diligently in establishing policies and recommendations on safe sport participation. Among the many issues these guidelines cover are prohibition of athletic participation for an athlete with only one of a set of paired organs, weight loss due to hypohydration, and the procedure for medically disqualifying a student-athlete during an NCAA championship. These policies and recommendations are followed by the majority of schools and athletic clubs, yet individual allowances can be made by teams after careful consideration of the medical problem and the risks of athletic participation.

Many organizations play a leadership role in establishing rules for youth, high school, college, and professional sports. These organizations often include a committee to establish and evaluate rules of the sport with the aim of minimizing the potential hazards of participation. Many organizations such as the National Federation of State High School Associations and the NCAA establish guidelines for member institutions yet allow individual states or conferences to amend or add to the recommendations. Generally, all such organizations solicit the recommendations of medical and coaching personnel in changing the rules of games in order to reduce injuries (see figure 7.14). Careful evaluation of injury statistics is essential in establishing a relationship between a performance technique, a rule of play, or a piece of equipment and the occurrence of injury.

Rules and Regulations for the Use of Protective Equipment

To even begin to understand the rules and regulations concerning the use of protective equipment, we must first be consistent in differentiating between equipment that is required or recommended and equipment that is forbidden from use in a particular sport, which we will term illegal equipment. It is essential for people to be familiar with both the required equipment and the illegal equipment for any sport with which they might be associated.

Certainly there are similarities in the rules for equipment use in a particular sport across the various levels of competition, yet differences also exist. In general, the regulations governing younger players are more strict than those governing the professional athlete. The intent of the rule difference is to further protect the young, skeletally immature athlete.

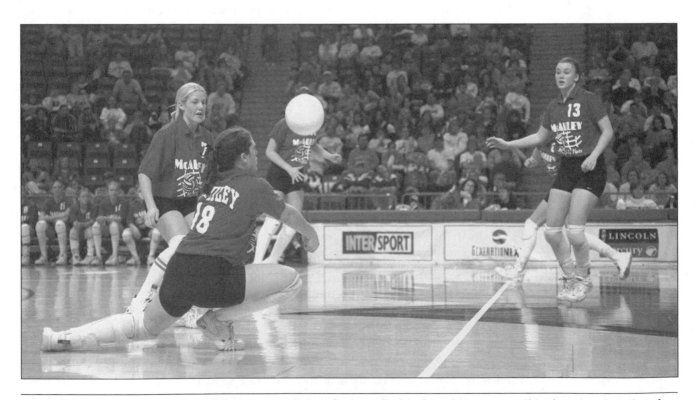

Figure 7.14 Regulatory agencies solicit recommendations from medical and coaching personnel in changing the rules of games to reduce injuries.

Visit the NCAA's website at www.ncaa.org for the *Sports Medicine Handbook* and sport liaison.

In order to understand some of the many equipment rules in athletics, it is wise to concentrate on one level of competition. Here we consider the regulations applicable to intercollegiate athletes. Guidelines for equipment use and regulations are published each year by the NCAA in the *Sports Medicine Handbook*. This handbook is distributed free of charge to all NCAA member institutions, and any nonmember institution may purchase a copy through the NCAA. Each NCAA-governed sport has a committee designated to review the sport rules on a yearly basis. This means that any sport classified as an NCAA sport, regardless of the division of play, undergoes rule review and potential revision each year. When working with an athletic team, to obtain the latest and most accurate information one would first review the published rule book for the sport; second, review the most current issue of the *Sports Medicine Handbook;* and lastly, contact the NCAA liaison for that sport (obtain the person's name and number from the NCAA).

In the following discussion of the rules regarding equipment use we consider equipment according to the various classes (headgear, face protection, etc.), as well as the rules that pertain to each sport using that class of equipment.

Required and Recommended Protective Equipment

For participation in athletics, some equipment is required prior to the start of the competition (is mandatory). In addition, some equipment, thought to provide some level of protection from injury, is referred to as recommended. When a player is seen to be without some part of the mandatory equipment, the referee will stop play and require the athlete to leave the playing area to obtain the appropriate protective equipment.

Headgear

Equipment considered headgear includes anything that is worn to protect the cranium or the scalp (see figure 7.15). Most often such an item is called a helmet, and it may be of the hard-shell variety or may be a soft covering of the scalp, ears, or both. Baseball, football, ice hockey, lacrosse, and softball require that all participants wear hard-shell helmets, while wrestling and water polo require protection over the ears by a soft padded material (table 7.3).

Face, Throat, and Mouth Protection

Sports with a risk of laceration of the face often involve use of a face mask to prevent fingers or other objects from coming too close to the participant's face. Many collision sports with a potential of concussion and oral trauma utilize an intraoral mouthpiece. Physically active persons who wear orthodontic devices may also use these mouthpieces to protect both the inside of the mouth and the somewhat fragile wires used in orthodontic bracing. Athletes who incur a risk of contusion to the throat area, such as baseball catchers,

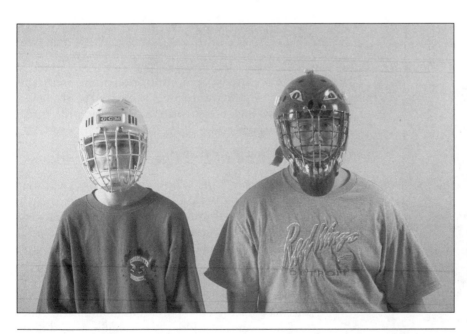

Figure 7.15   Protective headgear protects the cranium and scalp.

Table 7.3
Sports Specifying the Use of Helmets for Participants

Sport	Position(s)	Type of helmet	Comments
Baseball	Batting and base running	Hard-shell helmet with double earflaps	Helmets must carry the National Operating Committee on Standards for Athletic Equipment (NOCSAE) mark.
	Catchers	Hard-shell helmet for fielding the position	Helmet is made to allow face mask to be worn. Helmet must carry NOCSAE mark.
Football	All players	Hard-shell helmet secured with a four-point chin strap	Must carry a warning label regarding the risk of injury and manufacturer's or reconditioner's certification indicating satisfaction of NOCSAE test standards.
Ice hockey	All players	Hard-shell helmet with chin straps securely fastened	It is recommended, but not required, that the helmet meet Hockey Equipment Certification Committee standards.
Lacrosse	Women goalkeepers	Hard-shell helmet (either with face mask or without)	No standards exist.
	All men players	Hard-shell helmet secured with a cupped four-point chin strap (high-point hookup)	Helmets must carry the NOCSAE mark.
Softball	Batting and base running	Hard-shell helmet with double earflap	Helmets must carry the NOCSAE mark.
Water polo	All players	Soft-shell cap with protective ear guards	Cap also differentiates between teams.
Wrestling	All wrestlers	Protective ear guard	Any guard to prevent abrasion of ear on mat (cause of "cauliflower ear").

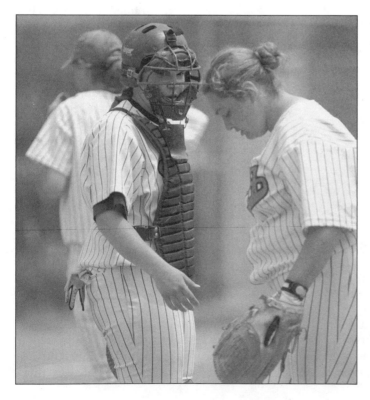

may be required to wear protection of this area (table 7.4). These athletes are usually required to wear a face mask to which an extension for covering the throat can be attached (see figure 7.16).

Protection of the Chest and Shoulders

Thick, open-cell padding material is utilized often in combination with a hard, plastic outer shell to distribute a local-impact shock onto the large surface area of the chest and shoulders. Various sports utilize shoulder pads, and other sports require simple chest protection of only some of the position players. Although both ice hockey players and football players must wear shoulder pads, the difference between the pads used for the two sports is quite dramatic. Since hockey players are seldom "fixed" but instead slide on the ice upon contact with another player, the need for heavy padding is reduced or eliminated in comparison to the situation in football. See table 7.5 for details on the chest protection needed for various sports.

Figure 7.16 Face, throat, and mouth protection.

Table 7.4
Face, Neck, and Mouth Protection Used in Sports

Sport	Position	Protection	Comment
Baseball	Catchers	Built-in or attachable throat guard on mask	No standard exists for the design.
Fencing	All participants	Mask with mesh face covering	Usually fits over the sides and front of the face but is open in the back.
Field hockey	All players	Intraoral mouthpiece	Can be colored or clear but must fit over upper teeth.
	Goalkeepers	Throat protectors, headgear, and face mask	Permitted, but not required.
Football	All players	Intraoral mouthpiece	Yellow or other color (not clear or white); must cover all upper teeth
	All players	Face mask	Must be attached to helmet.
Ice hockey	All players	Intraoral mouthpiece	Can be colored or clear but must fit over upper teeth.
	All players	Face mask	Must meet HECC-ASTM F 513-98 Eye and Face Protective Equipment for Hockey Players Standard.
Lacrosse	All players	Intraoral mouthpiece	Must cover upper teeth (women: any color or clear; men: yellow or other highly visible color).
	Goalies	Throat protector	Goalkeeper has the option of using face mask.
Softball	Catchers	Face mask with attached throat protector	Can be detachable but must be worn.
Wrestling	All participants	Protective mouth guard	Recommended.

Table 7.5
Protection of the Chest and Thorax in Sport Teams

Sport	Position	Protection	Comments
Baseball	Catchers	Chest protector	Shock-absorbing foam with plastic reinforcement in sternum area
Fencing	All participants	Vest of jacket and metallic lames and underarm protectors	Full coverage of chest with additional protection of vital points
Football	All players	Shoulder pads	Hard outer shell and open-cell foam padding inside
Ice hockey	All players	Shoulder pads	Lighter and thinner pads than for football
Lacrosse	Goalkeepers	Chest protector	Combination of hard and soft outer shell
Softball	Catchers	Chest protector	Similar to protection for baseball

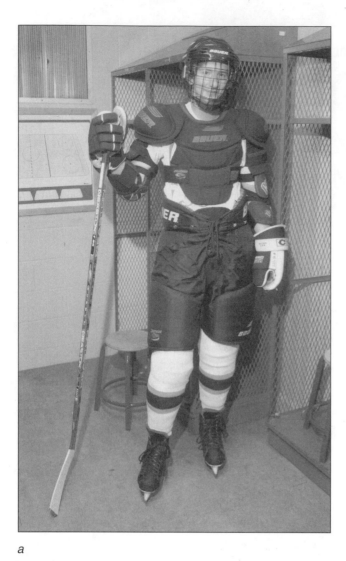

a

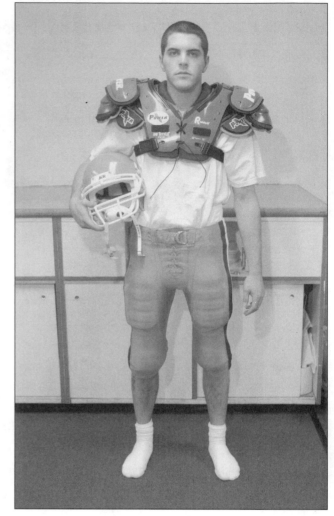

b

Figure 7.17   Protective wear in *(a)* hockey is not as heavy as the padding used in *(b)* football.

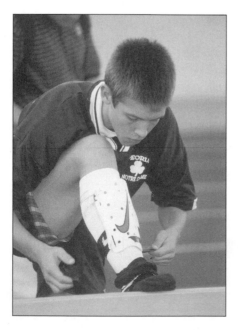

Lower Extremities

The joints of the lower extremity are often in contact with the ground or with other players. The superficial location of bony prominences makes protective padding valuable. Baseball catchers, hockey goalkeepers, and football and soccer players incur the risk of contact and are provided special protection (see figures 7.17 and 7.18). See table 7.6 for the details of sports requiring lower-extremity padding.

Illegal Equipment

In an effort to limit unintentional injury to other players, use of some equipment has been made illegal. In general, contact sports attempt to eliminate the potential for contusions or abrasions from casts or braces. Table 7.7 identifies illegal equipment by sport. In all cases, if a referee or other judge of the sport feels that a piece of equipment or another item (e.g., jewelry) worn by an athlete may be dangerous to another player, the player may be required to remove it or be disqualified from participation.

Figure 7.18   Shin guards and thigh pads are used in soccer.

Table 7.6
Lower-Extremity Protective Equipment by Sport

Sport	Position	Protection	Comments
Baseball	Catchers	Leg guards covering knees, shins, and top of feet	Should be easily removable for batting and base running.
Field hockey	Goalkeepers	Kickers (pads from top of feet to groin area)	Optional equipment.
Football	All players	Soft knee pads 1/2 in. thick	Must be covered by pants.
	All players	Hip pads, tailbone protector, and thigh pads	Pad must fit into uniform, covered by pants.
Soccer	All players	Shin guards	Thin, molded plastic.
Softball	Catchers	Protective leg coverings	Similar to baseball gear.

Table 7.7
Illegal or Restricted Equipment and Materials

Sport	Equipment	Specifications
Basketball	Braces or casts below the elbow	Must be pliable (no plaster, metal).
	Casts or braces of other body parts	May be used but must be padded.
Football	Protective braces between elbows and hands (to be used only to protect recent fracture/dislocation)	Must be covered on all sides with closed-cell, slow-recovery foam padding at least 1/2 in. thick.
	Hard thigh pads	Pads must be covered front and back with soft padding material.
	Knee braces unless entirely covered	No padding is necessary.
	Projection of metal or other hard substance	Any functional braces used for protection must be covered if made of hard material.
Ice hockey	No equipment that could endanger other players	Use "noninjurious" protective equipment.
Women's lacrosse	Any special equipment	Must be approved by umpires.
Men's lacrosse	Any "dangerous" equipment	As evaluated by official.
Soccer	Hard or dangerous equipment on the head, face, or body (braces, casts, etc.)	No hard materials can be used for protection if they may be harmful to an opponent.
	Knee braces	Must be covered, no metal exposed.
	Casts	Permitted if covered and not considered dangerous.
Softball	Plaster or other hard substances	Any hard material that could cause harm to another player.
	Exposed metal	Must be covered by soft material and taped.
Track	Taping of any part of the hands or fingers of hammer, discus, javelin, and 35-lb weight throwers	Not permitted unless an injury, cut, or wound requires protection by tape.
Wrestling	Anything that prohibits normal movement of the joints	Equipment cannot prevent the opponent from applying normal holds.
	Hard and abrasive materials	Must be padded and covered.
	Loose pads	May allow an opponent an unfair hold.

Fabricating Custom Protective Equipment

Training personnel certainly fabricate custom protective equipment in a typical athletic training room, yet the clinician must first evaluate several important variables. First and foremost it is critical to carefully evaluate legal liability issues. If the equipment could cause an injury or worsen an existing condition, it should not be fabricated. If there is no potential of increased harm, the design of the equipment must adhere to the rules and guidelines for the sport. Fabric selection should take into account the factors mentioned at the outset of this chapter, and those factors should be considered in relation to the sport and playing style of the athlete. When fabricating protective devices, always consider all the factors we have discussed before spending time, money, and energy in a misguided effort.

LEGAL CONCERNS ABOUT EQUIPMENT USE IN SPORT

Since the purpose of protective equipment is to safeguard the athlete from harm, it should be easy to understand why the consumer (or the family of the consumer in some cases) might think there has been a legal wrong when an athlete suffers an injury due to failure of the protective equipment. Carry this thought just a bit further and realize that spectators or workers in the athletic facility also expect proper protection from injury. Spectators attending a practice or game certainly do not attend with the thought that they may be injured by a flying bat, ball, stick, puck, or any other piece of equipment.

The majority of legal cases brought against an athletic department or its staff entail tort. **Tort** cases usually involve an athlete's seeking to blame someone other than himself or herself for an injury or resulting condition. A tort must be classified into one of seven areas, meaning that the person filing the suit (the **plaintiff**) must show one of the following seven reasons for issuing the legal action:

1. Intentional harm to the person
2. Intentional harm to tangible property
3. Negligence
4. Strict liability
5. Nuisance
6. Harm to tangible personal interests
7. Harm to tangible property interests

In a tort case in sport, the injured person would probably attempt to show **negligence.** This means that the plaintiff will attempt to show that the responsible person (the **defendant**) failed to take the action that another person of equal abilities and training would have taken in the same circumstances. For example, if an athletic trainer stops to help the victim of an accident, the care the athletic trainer provides should be the same as what any person of the same level of knowledge would provide. If the care failed to meet that standard of care, the athletic trainer could be held negligent. Each case involving an attempt to show negligence is considered by the court on the basis of its particular set of circumstances; if the circumstances indicate some negligence, a liability issue will result. Specifically, liability results from five factors:

1. Ignorance of the law
2. Ignoring the law
3. Failure to act
4. Failure to warn
5. Expense

These five factors would all be considered when an injured person tried to establish a tort liability case with a charge of negligence. First, let's define the factors. Later in the chapter we'll look at liability, or *who* is responsible.

Ignorance of the Law

You may have heard your parents say something like "Ignorance is no excuse," and this is never more true than in cases of sport liability. Consider, for example, a situation in which a diving coach decides to have the athletes work on the trampoline to perfect some of their diving skills. Let's suppose that the coach fails to supervise the athletes on the trampoline, that two of the divers get on the apparatus at the same time, and that during their trials at doing simultaneous flips they collide. Assume also that the collision results in some permanent disability of one of the divers.

Now, realize that in 1977 the American Academy of Pediatrics issued a statement opposing the use of the trampoline in physical education, recreation, and sport programs. This statement was issued not because the number of injuries resulting from trampoline use was great, but rather because of the number of injuries that were serious and debilitating. Safety guidelines have since been established through the combined effort of several organizations; and all supervisors, as well as all participants using the trampoline, must follow these guidelines. Now, this is not to say that the statement of opposition to the use of the trampoline is a law; but the court would expect the coach to be aware of this decision by the national association. The fact that neither the coach nor the athletes were aware of the recommendations against the use of the trampoline does not make those individuals less responsible or less liable.

It is certainly expected that coaches know the regulations and laws that pertain to their sport and to the equipment used in training for their sport. When you look at a piece of equipment, do so with a very critical eye regarding the potential for injury. If you are unaware of rules and regulations associated with equipment, check with the manufacturer, attorneys, or other coaches or administrators in order to gain knowledge of any and all potential ramifications associated with the use of that equipment.

Ignoring the Law

Since everyone is expected to know the law, the next step is to obey the law. Unfortunately, some people still believe that "rules are made to be broken" and consequently ignore rules, regulations, and laws until they are forced to pay attention. Some people may suggest that a school or coach will continue to get away with disobeying a rule or regulation until something serious happens. Examples of ignoring the law or ignoring the rules can be found in every sport and probably in every school or team. It is not difficult to think of injuries that could have been avoided if an athlete had been wearing the proper protective equipment. People who decide to ride a bike without a helmet can hardly complain of the concussion that occurs when their tire catches a pothole and they are thrown to the ground. The same concept applies in a high-contact sport like football when athletes fail to wear protective thigh pads that are provided and required. A contusion to the quadriceps muscle can incapacitate the athlete for several days or even weeks. Although quite minor as compared to a life-threatening injury, a quadriceps contusion resulting from inappropriate athletic equipment could be the start of a negligence case citing "ignorance of the law" as the grounds.

Failure to Act

A person who is aware of a rule or regulation and consciously elects to ignore it is guilty of "failure to act." This typically applies when adherence to a rule or regulation is intended (stated in writing or in some other manner) but for some reason the intention has not been carried out. It is expected that regulations will be followed regardless of financial concerns or other issues that may delay the intended action. You may have heard stories about athletes or spectators who were injured when a flying object hit them in the head. If the incident occurred because the injured person was permitted to come too close to the practice or competition area, there may be negligence on the part of the athletic department.

As an example, if regulations specify that protective barriers must be placed between the hockey rink and the spectator area but the athletic department—failing to act on the regulations—allows visitors to watch practices and attend games in that facility, liability is assumed by the athletic department. A flying puck that strikes an inattentive fan in the head, causing a fractured skull, would become a much different case if it became known that the request for funds to erect a protective barrier in front of the spectator area had been denied. Failure to act can take many forms, but the bottom line is that the proper procedures were not carried out. In contrast to the issue of ignoring the law, this failure to act is a failure to provide or prevent rather than a failure to comply (as when a rule or law is ignored).

Failure to Warn

Some sports have unique associated dangers, regardless of how safe the participants might attempt to be. The actor Christopher Reeve was an accomplished horseman, yet all his training and skill could not prevent the spinal cord injury that rendered him quadriplegic when he was thrown from his horse. Accidents can and do happen; and the coach, trainer, or other person responsible must fully warn the athlete of the potential dangers. It is not only important to provide printed information regarding the risks of participation; in addition, those risks must be conveyed verbally and must be well understood by all participants (see figure 7.19).

A widely publicized case involving the failure to warn occurred in Seattle in 1982—*Thompson v. Seattle Public School District* (Appenzeller 1985). The athlete, Thompson, was awarded $6.3 million when the court found the coach and the school district liable for failure to warn of the dangers inherent in football. Thompson had been injured in 1975 as a sophomore football player. He suffered a fracture of the spine when he lowered his head to ward off a tackle.

Prior to this landmark case in the early 1980s, warning athletes of potential dangers was not considered very important. Today, not only must the coach explain the dangers of football

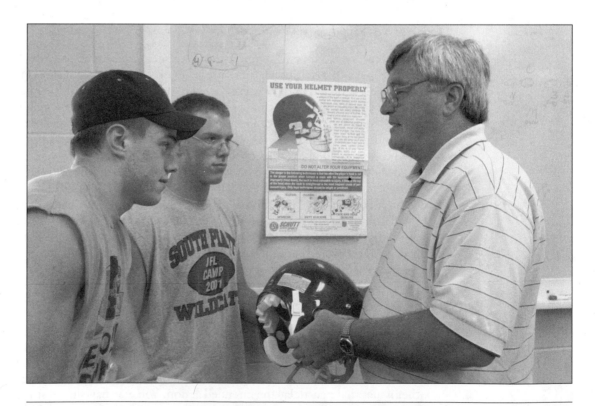

Figure 7.19   Coaches should explain the dangers of athletic participation or risk a lawsuit if someone is injured.

participation; the athlete will see a warning sticker inside his helmet, and he may be asked to sign a statement saying that he has been informed of, and that he understands, the risks of permanent injury associated with football participation.

Expense

Although expense is not as easy as the other issues to immediately relate to liability in sport injury, you might recognize the element of expense in other situations. For example, let's say that you wanted to learn to skydive. You are a starving college student and don't have much money. You save and save and finally have enough money to take the lessons. You love it. You want to go again and again, but you can't afford the parachute rental. Would you accept a "deal" offered in the classified ads if the parachute was substandard? Budget concerns may cause teams or individuals to use old equipment that they have repaired and refurbished. As discussed earlier, if the equipment must be used over and over again, it is critical that it be reconditioned and its safety recertified. There are agencies that provide the reconditioning service for athletic equipment; and when budgets are limited, the expense of reconditioning must be allowed even when funds are insufficient for new equipment.

Other forms of expense issues could look the same as those discussed in connection with failure to act. When a proposal for providing some protective equipment or improving the safety of a facility is declined for budget reasons, the issue of expense comes into play. One lost life or one serious injury may be far more expensive than the preventive measure would have been.

LIABILITY NEGLIGENCE

When a healthy, athletic person leaves home to go to school in the morning, the parents naturally expect that their son or daughter will return home that evening healthy and happy. When a catastrophic injury occurs, changing that young person's life forever, it may appear to the community only as a tragic consequence of participation in sport. To the family and the injured individual it is obviously much more than a consequence of sport; neither the athlete nor the parents will want to admit that they did in fact accept the risk of athletic participation. Too often, the injured person and the family are overwhelmed with grief and feel the need to shift blame to some other person in order to explain the tragedy.

In the attempt to shift the focus of responsibility onto someone else's shoulders, the injured party may name any number of athletic department employees as defendants or codefendants: the administrators, athletic trainers, equipment managers, coaches, and even teammates.

DETERMINATION OF LIABILITY

First and foremost, the courts will want to see the degree to which the injured person was responsible (liable) for the actions that resulted in an injury. When an individual chooses to play a sport, the knowledge of potential risk is in most cases clearly understood. This knowledge is termed "assumption of risk" because every person must take responsibility for his or her own safety. In the unusual case in which the athlete is not warned of the dangers of participation, he or she assumes none of the risk. On the other hand, in the situation in which athletes have no knowledge of the dangers but make no effort to determine the hazards, there may be "contributory negligence."

In a 1979 case (*Brahatcek v. Millard School District*), the plaintiff (Brahatcek) brought a wrongful death action against the defendant school district after her son David died following an accident in a physical education class. David, a ninth-grade student, was fatally injured when he was struck in the head by a golf club swung by a fellow student. The class was being conducted in the gym because of inclement weather. David's class consisted of 58 students supervised by two teachers. David had missed the first day of indoor instruction but had returned to school the next day and participated without the benefit of the first day's safety instructions. The trial court found the school negligent and therefore ruled in favor of the plaintiff. The school board appealed, asserting that both David and the classmate who struck him were in some way responsible for the mishap. This attempt to diminish the level of negligence of the teacher would shift some of the responsibility for preventing the injury onto the injured person (contributory negligence).

Contributory negligence may prevent the injured person from recovering damages (collecting on a legal liability suit) because it means that the person was in some way responsible for his or her own injury. It is up to the court to decide the level of responsibility and what action is appropriate. Factors that help the court determine the amount of negligence the injured person is responsible for include the person's age, physical capabilities, level of training, and other factors. In *Brahatcek v. Millard*, the state supreme court upheld the trial court's decision that the 14-year-old was insufficiently prepared to anticipate the dangers of the situation, rejecting the school district's contention that David was guilty of contributory negligence.

In some states, a level of negligence is determined, and that percentage is used to calculate the award. This prorating of damages reflects "comparative" negligence and may mean that both the plaintiff and the defendant are partially responsible. A person who lives in a contributory negligence state would receive nothing if he or she were found to be partially at fault, while the same circumstances might yield a partial award in a state that observes comparative negligence.

An injured athlete may try to point a finger toward the person or persons who issued protective equipment, those who provided medical care, or those who did coaching on particular techniques. Usually, if the equipment person or the coach is named in a lawsuit, the employer is also named. Two reasons for naming two or more persons in a lawsuit are the "deep-pocket" concept and the doctrine of "respondent superior."

The deep-pocket concept seems self-explanatory: When the plaintiff is seeking to recover a large amount of money (damages) for a serious injury, the effort is of little use if the defendant cannot afford to pay the full amount of damages. Thus, more people may be named in the suit, or the school system may be named, to ensure that it will be possible to recover the total damages awarded by the courts.

The respondent superior doctrine allows the plaintiff to name additional defendants due to the established covenant that the employer may be held responsible for actions committed by its employees if they are acting within the scope of their employment. When the employer is named in the lawsuit the employee may, and usually is, still named as a codefendant. An employee named in a lawsuit in which negligence is claimed often suffers a great deal emotionally and perhaps financially. If the employee is considered negligent for his or her actions, there may be reason to question that employee's abilities. The employer may discontinue the service of the employee, and other potential employers evaluating this person for the same position in which negligence was found may not want to take the risk of employing the person. When the court finds the employee guilty of negligence and damages are awarded, insurance may offset some of the costs of the lawsuit, but if insurance does not fully cover the damages awarded, the employee must come up with the money out of pocket (or out of future wages), and this debt cannot be alleviated by declaring bankruptcy. Overall, negligence and liability are devastating to the individual and, with proper care and attention, should be totally avoidable.

As we realize, the coach, athletic trainer, and equipment person work directly with the athletes, and their actions or lack of actions may have a direct relationship to an athlete's injury. The person who hires or supervises these employees can be held equally responsible for the employees' actions. The courts expect supervisors to have control of the actions of their staffs; the athletic director is expected to have control of the actions of the coaches, trainers, and equipment people. We see this in an example from New York in which a young athlete with a heart condition died during participation in the school football program. It was found that the school district had a preparticipation physical examination policy but that the school, and other schools in the district, failed to follow the policy. The administrator responsible for the school district athletic programs was sued and subsequently removed from his position as a supervisor of the athletic programs because he had failed to make sure that his member schools followed the policy *(Monaco v. Raymond)*. Administrators must take an active role in the selection, hiring, and supervision of the coaches, volunteers, and all department employees associated with the health and welfare of the athlete. If a person is hired and it were found that the individual committed negligence but was insufficiently qualified for the position, the person responsible for the hiring would be guilty of vicarious liability.

PRODUCT AND MANUFACTURER LIABILITY

If a product is found to be defective for the purpose for which it was intended, the manufacturer is held liable. The "product" need not be a piece of equipment like a football helmet or shin guards; it could be a diving board, a pool, or even the land upon which an athletic field is constructed. If there is some defect in the product—that is, some reason that the product was not adequate for the purpose intended—the manufacturer (or seller in the case of the land) is liable.

Facility or Playing Surface Problems

In a major Pacific-Ten Conference school, a baseball player's death was alleged to be due to faulty artificial grass surface on the athletic playing field. This case, *Halbrook v. Oregon State University*, was a $2.5 million liability suit that named the artificial turf manufacturer, the installer, the subsurface manufacturer and its installer, and the university as responsible for the faulty surface and thus liable for the athlete's death. Manufacturers are held responsible for the design, manufacture, and consumer support related to the playing surface. The manufacturer must ensure that the consumer uses the product in the manner in which it was intended and also must issue warnings to the consumer if the product has any chance of being dangerous. This case should illustrate how far the plaintiff may reach to find the party responsible in the case of a catastrophic injury.

Sporting Equipment

As we have noted, products are expected to be safe for the purpose for which they were designed. Litigation has been a great financial burden in American football over the past 20 years. Lawsuits between manufacturers and athletes have attempted to show that equipment was improperly designed or perhaps defective in some way. One of many examples of this type of suit is *Austria v. Bike Athletic Co.* Austria, a junior on the high school football team, was hit on the front of the helmet by another player's knee during football practice. The plaintiff was initially dazed but seemed to be fine. Two weeks later, Austria was complaining of severe headaches, and one day at practice he collapsed on the field. He underwent a special radiograph evaluation and subsequent surgery to relieve a **subdural hematoma** (blood clot on the brain), and although his life was saved he was left with permanent disability.

The court found no reason to think that the blow to the helmet was unusual for the sport and therefore concluded that the injury was due to a defective helmet. The court ruled in favor of the plaintiff. Cases such as this were quite frequent especially in the early 1980s, when suits against helmet manufacturers cost various companies over $20 million. After these cases were settled, usually at great expense to the defendant's insurance company, the cost of premiums to insure the manufacturers of football helmets averaged $2.5 million a year (Appenzeller 1985). The higher cost of insurance had to be offset in the price of the helmet, which jumped from $40 per helmet in the 1980s to over $100 today. The fact that legal action against a manufacturer will ultimately affect the consumer is unfortunate but is a part of athletics that is well recognized and reasonably well accepted.

Improper Care or Modification of Manufactured Products

It is not uncommon for an athlete to attempt to alter a piece of protective equipment to make it lighter, less bulky, or generally more comfortable to wear. It is important to realize that any modification of equipment will void any legal liability the manufacturer would have due to failure of the product. In *Bonoconti v. The Citadel*, the athletic trainer was held liable for a spinal cord injury suffered during a football contest. The athletic trainer had modified the athlete's helmet to prevent him from excessive neck extension in an attempt to preclude "stingers" from occurring. The modification included a strap, attached from the shoulder pads to the face mask of the helmet, that would tighten as the athlete's neck was forced into extension and hypertension. The plaintiff held the athletic trainer liable because the strap seemed to actually cause the athlete's neck to be held in a flexed position—a vulnerable position for the cervical spine that increases the potential for vertebral injury in the event of impact with the top of the helmet. This modification of the helmet negated any responsibility of the helmet manufacturer, shifting the blame to the athletic department employee.

Manufacturer's Liability

Only equipment that is unaltered and regularly inspected and reconditioned can be considered within the scope of the manufacturer's responsibility. In *Rawlings Sporting Goods Co., Inc. v. Daniels*, Rawlings attempted to convince the court that a defect in the helmet worn by the injured plaintiff (Daniels) could be due to the failure of the school to inspect and recondition the football helmets. Unfortunately for the sporting goods company, the helmet did not have warning labels to inform the wearer of the potential for injury while playing football. The defendants tried to demonstrate that the school was partially negligent for not reconditioning all of the helmets and not keeping proper records on each helmet in its inventory. The court found no fault on the part of the school but found the defendants guilty of gross negligence influenced in part by the company's attitude toward the matter.

PROTECTING ONESELF FROM LEGAL MISFORTUNE

The best protection people have from legal misfortune is prevention, yet it is virtually impossible to avoid injuries in athletics. In an effort to protect themselves from the financial drain of attorney fees and court costs, all professionals should consider liability insurance coverage. Often the employer provides health care employees with liability coverage. In addition to the protection offered by the employer, an athletic trainer may wish to obtain professional liability insurance from a private insurance company, which may cost around $50 to $100 per year for persons employed by an organization or about $100 to $200 per year for persons who are self-employed.

SUMMARY

1. *Identify the eight factors to consider in fabricating a protective splint for a physically active individual, and present examples of times when each of those factors would become critical.*

    (1) **Density:** Weight (or mass) per unit of volume. When the splint needs to be of a particular size, the density of the material will affect the total weight. Thus density becomes important when a large splint is needed and you wish to keep it as lightweight as possible.

    (2) **Strength:** How much force the material can withstand. This becomes important when the splint is being made for a high-impact, high-collision sport. Strength of a material would not be as important for a synchronized swimmer as for a diver.

    (3) **Rigidity or stiffness:** A characteristic of a material that is measured by the modulus of elasticity. Although elasticity brings recoil to mind, elasticity in this sense means the ability to resist deformation. The higher the modulus of elasticity, the more difficult it will be to deform (bend) the material. This factor is of great importance when one is fabricating a brace to protect an injured bone, for example. If you used a low-modulus material, the brace might bend and thus fail to fully stabilize the broken bone.

(4) **Conformability:** The degree to which a material can be shaped into various forms. Some materials used to fabricate splints and braces are very conformable when heated, but once cooled they cannot be manipulated so freely. Other materials, like foams, may be very conformable if they are very thinly cut but become less manageable when thicker. Although a material that can conform to the body part is usually preferable, if you needed to fabricate a splint to bring a part back into its normal position you would not want to use a material that will conform.

(5) **Self-adherence:** The ability of a material to stick to itself. This feature is convenient when you are trying to attach a pad or splint to the body part, but a disadvantage is that the material usually cannot be reused. Velcro is a self-adherent material that is very reusable, in contrast to self-adherent stretch bandages, which once removed cannot be reapplied.

(6) **Durability:** The ability of a material to withstand repeated use. One factor to remember in working with the physically active is that "repeated use" carries a slightly different meaning than it would for a sedentary individual. Durability is important whenever you fabricate a protective device for someone who will be physically active.

(7) **Ease of fabrication:** The ease with which a person without special training can work with a material to fabricate a device. A level of knowledge or training is required to fabricate some protective devices, but often the difficulty relates to the material itself rather than the device. A material that conforms well is typically easy to fabricate. This factor is important when one is selecting a material that many different people will be using.

(8) **Availability and cost:** Two of the greatest obstacles for an athletic program. When a material is low in cost and abundant, these factors will not be important. However, many items advertised in magazines or demonstrated by sales representatives seem to have wonderful uses for fabrication purposes until you discover the high cost. On the other hand, when a material that is perfect for the job is not available, you will need to devise an alternate solution using another material.

2. *Explain the various types of materials according to their requirement for heat in the molding process.*

Materials are classified according to the degree of heat required to make them into useful shapes and products. The four classifications are high, moderate, low, and no heat (layered). Most high- and moderate-heat materials used in sport require such high temperatures that they are formed by the manufacturer rather than on-site. Yet some moderate-heat products can be adjusted to achieve a perfect fit with the aid of an industrial heat gun. Low-heat items are firm when cool but become malleable when heated in an oven or with hot water. Most of these materials come with excellent instructions about the process and the intensity of heat required to bring the product to the workable stage. No-heat products include wraps that are layered, as well as products that are exothermic (that give off heat) in the curing process. Such exothermic no-heat materials include casting materials like fiberglass and even plaster of paris.

3. *Explain the function of a voluntary standards organization and describe how such an organization might impact sport equipment.*

Many standards organizations exist, each with the common goal of establishing consistency in the manufacture of specific items. The voluntary nature of these organizations means that manufacturers voluntarily follow the standards; if the product does not follow the standards, the manufacturer cannot display the symbol of that standards organization. Certain standards have been adopted in sport and recreation, and equipment not meeting those standards is not accepted for use. Often a product bears the symbols of various standards organizations, signifying that the product is of specified size, shape, and quality.

4. *Explain the significance of the NOCSAE seal on protective headgear and discuss ways in which that seal would serve to protect the wearer.*

The NOCSAE sets standards for various pieces of athletic equipment, and the seal indicates that the particular product (headgear) design meets the NOCSAE standards. This organization also sets the standards for equipment reconditioners to follow in evaluating helmets. When a used helmet passes the recertification process it again meets the NOCSAE standards—this time the standards for a reconditioned helmet.

5. *Identify the factors considered in determining legal liability for an injury that occurred after alteration of protective equipment.*

If the alteration of the protective equipment is found to have been a causative factor in the injury, the person who altered the equipment may be found liable. This assignment of responsibility for the injury is moved away from the manufacturer as soon as the product design or structure is altered; the person making the adjustments then becomes responsible. The five factors that help to establish this liability include ignorance of the law, ignoring the law, failure to act, failure to warn, and expense.

CRITICAL THINKING QUESTIONS

1. One of your basketball players has received repeated contusions to the iliac crest, specifically, the anterior superior iliac spine. You decide to pad the area using some kind of padding that you will tape to the affected area. Describe three types of materials you might use and give the pros and cons of each. Use the Internet, ask the school athletic trainer, or do both in order to obtain names of different materials.

2. You have been asked to make recommendations on the types of material to purchase for the local soccer club. There are 20 athletes on the team, and last year the team was plagued with shin contusions, quad contusions, and a few upper-extremity contusions that limited participation solely because of the pain associated with getting the bruised area hit again. You are informed that the budget for padding material is $500. Research the items you will suggest and provide the cost and rationale for each suggested purchase. Include the quantity of the materials you choose.

3. You have been charged with the job of evaluating all headgear before the next school season. This includes baseball and softball batting helmets and football helmets. Explain how you would progress in this task. Explain the rationale for any suggestions you make.

4. Your athletic director called you to his office after reading your recommendations (from question 3). He asks you to explain the significance of NOCSAE and why this is of any importance in evaluating the helmets. Please do so.

5. You have witnessed situations that you feel may be putting the athlete at risk of injury, but the situation is not within your power to change. You decide to approach the athletic director to discuss the situation and what you think should be done about it. What legal concerns are involved in this discussion? What legal issues are in play if the athletic director suggests that you just "ignore" the situation? Discuss what you would do if you were asked to "ignore" the problem.

CITED SOURCES

Appenzeller, H. 1985. *Sports and law: Contemporary issues.* Charlottesville, VA: Michie.

Austria v. Bike Athletic Co. 810 P. 2d 1312 (1991).

Brahatcek v. Millard School District. 273 N.W. 2d 680, 202 Neb. 86 (1979).

International Organization for Standardization. 1999. www.iso.org/iso/en/ISOOnline.frontpage (accessed September 15, 2004).

Rawlings Sporting Goods Co., Inc. v. Daniels. 619 S.W. 2d 435 (Tex. Civ. App. 1981).

ADDITIONAL READINGS

Appenzeller, H. 1980. *Sport and the court.* Charlottesville, VA: Michie.

Champion, W.T. 1990. *Fundamentals of sports law.* Rochester, NY: Clark Boardman Callaghan.

Garner, B.A., ed., H.C. Black, and H.L. Black. 1999. *Black's law dictionary,* 7th ed. Eagan, MN: West Group.

Jones, M.E. 1998. *Sports law.* Upper Saddle River, NJ: Prentice Hall Business.

Wade, S.C. 1988. *Sports law for educational institutions.* New York: Quorum Books.

CHAPTER 8

Emergency Care and Medical Management of Athletic Injury

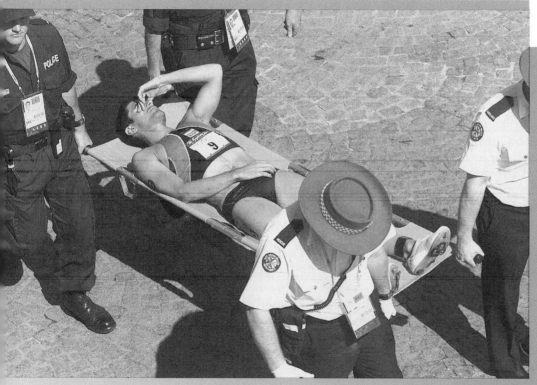

© Sport The Library

Objectives

After reading this chapter, the student should be able to do the following:

1. Identify the appropriate first aid procedures for a variety of injuries and illnesses.

2. Explain the "ABCs" of emergency care.

3. Identify the main features of an emergency care plan for an athletic team.

4. Explain methods for obtaining consent for various levels and situations of treatment.

5. Identify the members of the emergency medical services team and their roles in helping an injured athlete.

6. Discuss the importance of Universal Precautions.

Kathy, a junior student-trainer, was in the team van on the way to a volleyball meet. She and six other young women and an assistant coach were traveling between West Lafayette and Muncie on a rural highway when they came upon a man lying facedown on the road. Nancy, the assistant coach who was driving the van, stopped to see why the man was lying there. Quickly Nancy returned to the van and called for Kathy's help. Since they all knew that Kathy was the "medical" person on the van, everyone expected her to take charge of the scene. Kathy responded immediately.

"Sir! Sir! Are you all right?" Kathy shouted without touching the man.

She could see that he had already lost quite a bit of blood from an open wound about midthigh. More blood was slowly seeping from a small cut below his ear. The man was able to open his eyes but only muttered, "Please help me."

"Okay, sir, we can help. Just relax and keep talking if you can," Kathy said with a calm voice.

Kathy ordered the coach to go to a nearby house and alert someone to the problem. "You'll need to call 911. Tell them where we are and let them know we have a 60-year-old male with possible vascular problems and a potential head injury. Tell them to hurry!"

The coach took off toward the house to find help or a phone.

Kathy turned her attention back to the man and quickly realized that she needed to do something to stop the flow of blood from the leg. "Carol, would you get my training kit from the back of the van? And Jenny, see if the glove box has a first aid kit—if so, please bring it," Kathy ordered, calm but obviously in control of the situation.

Carol returned with the trainer's bag and placed it within Kathy's reach, and Jenny returned empty-handed. Kathy zipped open the trainer's bag and pulled out gloves, sterile gauze, a pair of scissors, and a stethoscope and blood pressure cuff. "Jenny, would you put these gloves on and put a sterile pad against the blood from his ear area? And Carol, you've had first aid class—do you remember how to take blood pressure?" Kathy asked as she put on her gloves and began cutting the man's pants to expose the cause of the pool of blood. As she suspected, the man had a compound (through the skin) fracture of the femur. Immediately she placed a wad of sterile gauze into the open wound to slow the bleeding.

Carol had seen the stethoscope, and before Kathy had gotten the whole thought expressed Carol had already put the cuff on the man's arm. "BP is 100 over 60," Carol said with a tone of doubt.

"Keep talking to him, Carol—make sure he's still with us," Kathy instructed. "He's lost a lot of blood and his pressure is dropping."

Nancy returned and informed Kathy and Carol that emergency medical services was on its way and that the police would also be sent. "His wife was in the house; she's in a wheelchair. She had already called the police when she saw the car hit her husband on his way back from the mailbox."

Kathy's gauze and gloves were becoming saturated with blood, so she instinctively began applying pressure with her other hand to an area on the front of the man's hip—an area over the main artery to the leg.

"Oh my gosh, that explains this fracture," Kathy muttered.

Just then they began to hear the sounds of approaching sirens. Within seconds the emergency medical services crew were at Kathy's side, saying, "What do you have?"

Kathy quickly summarized the situation: "BP is 100/60; he's lost a lot of blood from this compound fracture of the femur, but I've got it controlled with femoral artery pressure. I'm not sure what's going on with the blood by his ear; he's talking, but not too alert."

"Great job, we'll take him from here," said one of the paramedics while the other two were busy getting a splint and a box of medicines.

Relieved that the man was in good hands now, Kathy took off her gloves and began gathering her supplies. She could tell that her heart was still racing, and her mind was full of thoughts. "Hey coach, can we just run up to tell the wife he's looking okay?" Kathy asked as they all headed back to the van.

"Sure, she'll be glad to hear something. She was really scared," Nancy said. "I'll come with!"

Have you ever taken a first aid course? If so, do you remember why you should perform the skills you learned, or merely how to perform the skills? Don't feel bad if you remember only the how: The first step in learning skills of injury management is often what to do and how to do it. If you have not taken a first aid course yet, you certainly will in the near future. Just realize, we all begin our athletic training or coaching exposure by watching someone else do something. Soon we are allowed to take over, to lead the drill, exercise, or conditioning; but we're so intent on doing the job correctly that sometimes we fail to understand why we are doing what we're doing. As we become more and more comfortable with the process of performing the skill or the job, we can step back and question ourselves: why a particular technique was chosen, what other techniques could be used, and, perhaps most importantly, whether the technique works—and if it does, why it does.

Understanding the why, what, how, and when of injury management is our ultimate goal. This allows us to become thinkers rather than just robots. If you already know some of the injury-management skills from a previous first aid course, this chapter will assist you in the application of that knowledge. If you haven't had your first aid course yet, this chapter will expose you to some of the first aid skills used in athletics.

FIRST AID, EMERGENCY CARE, AND CARDIOPULMONARY RESUSCITATION

If someone asked you what to do for a patient needing CPR (cardiopulmonary resuscitation), you would probably respond, "ABCs!" To those who have been trained in the area of first aid, ABCs is a mnemonic that stands for

- A = airway: Is the victim's airway open so he or she can breathe?
- B = breathing: Is the breathing smooth, or does it sound obstructed or noisy in some way?
- C = circulation: Is the heart beating to provide circulation to the rest of the body?

We all know that many other questions are answered, almost subconsciously, prior to initiation of CPR. If we were not present when the person collapsed, we survey the scene. If you come upon a car wreck with gasoline spilled over the road, you might decide that the scene is unsafe for evaluation of the victim and that it is necessary to immediately relocate the victim. On the game field, if you see an athlete "go down" you might perform the evaluation of the scene subconsciously and already be at the next question—"What happened?" All of these steps are important in the overall care of an injured person.

Two major organizations instruct and credential people in the performance of CPR: the American Heart Association and the American Red Cross. The differences are minor; the important thing is to be trained and then to be retrained at regular intervals (see figure 8.1). We might think that once we know CPR we could perform it at any time. The fact is that when we first learn the skills we are concentrating on the tasks at hand, and the procedures are quite rehearsed. If we encounter an actual emergency, we may not have time to think—we have to react quickly and automatically.

If you have not yet been instructed in CPR, you may want to plan to attend a course. Often local agencies offer training, or you may have a first aid course on your campus that will include training, testing, and certification in CPR.

The emergency situation necessitates two evaluations, or surveys. Even though the athletic trainer is often present at athletic practices and events, they cannot see everything that occurs. Unless the entire injury is seen, the medical provider should perform both the primary and secondary survey. The primary survey, the ABCs, is the first step in the evaluation of the injured person. Obviously, if you come to the aid of an injured person who is alert and speaking to you, you will not need to render CPR, but taking the pulse and monitoring respiration rate are still important. Once the ABCs have been established, the spine and

Two major organizations instruct and credential people in the performance of CPR: American Heart Association (www.americanheart.org) and American Red Cross (www.redcross.org).

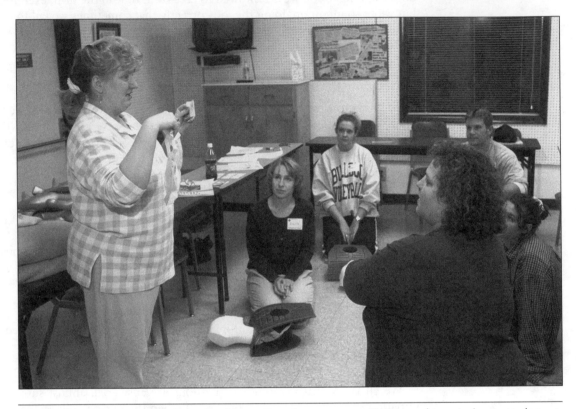

Figure 8.1   It is important to be trained in cardiopulmonary resuscitation and to retrain at regular intervals.

extremities must be evaluated. This second evaluation, of the spine and extremities, is called the "secondary survey."

Uncontrolled Bleeding

Bleeding is a problem if it is uncontrolled. A little bit of blood should warn the rescuer to take precautions. Remember to use Universal Precautions! In some accidents the victim is bleeding badly and may be in need of immediate help, like the man in the scenario on the roadway.

Remember that controlling bleeding is not your first concern; the biggest concern is to keep the patient breathing. Once the airway is established and breathing is spontaneous or assisted, bleeding can be managed. There are four ways to control bleeding. The first three are the most practical and useful; the last one can be used if necessary and if the rescuer has the equipment and training.

Direct Pressure

Applying pressure with a soft, sterile cloth or bandage will often slow the flow of blood enough to allow natural clot formation to occur (figure 8.2). Preventing contamination may be the first thought when one encounters a bleeding patient. This should be a concern, not just in relation to the safety of the wound itself but also in relation to the safety of the care providers as well as the patient.

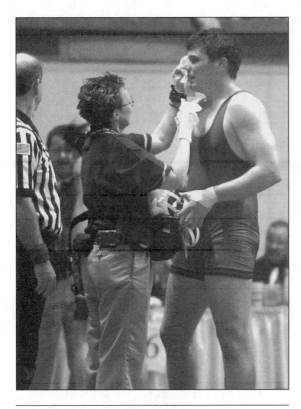

Figure 8.2 To control bleeding, apply pressure directly on the wound.

Anyone working with an individual who has an open wound should exercise Universal Precautions. Gloves are one means of preventing spread of bloodborne pathogens to or from the patient; but even if gloves are not immediately available, bleeding control can begin immediately. If the patient is conscious and able to place pressure on the wound, you may give the person a sterile cloth or gauze while you find and apply your gloves (figure 8.3). People who are severely injured may be unable to apply pressure to their own wound. In this case, if you are ungloved, you must use sufficient cloth to prevent saturation and penetration through the barrier.

Splinting

The rationale for using a splint to control bleeding is that in the case of broken bones, the bleeding occurs because the ends of the bones are injuring adjacent tissues. As long as the bones are free to move, they can continue to damage vessels and dislodge clots that are beginning to form. Immobilization of the fracture may, by itself, be sufficient to stop bleeding. Think about an individual with a severely broken leg as in the opening scenario. We know it is a compound fracture, meaning that the end of the bone has pierced through the skin. The leg should be held in the position in which it was found, and one or more objects made of firm material, like a board, should be used to stabilize the bones. The wound should be padded with sterile cloth if possible—clean cloth if not—and bandaged to the immobilization device.

Sterile cloths are often not readily available at the scene of a traffic accident. Profuse bleeding needs to be controlled. If it is not, the patient may die. It is less likely that a person will die because you applied a clean, but not sterile, cloth to the wound to control the flow of blood. The cloth should be clean and free of any known bacteria, dirt, grease, or other soil.

Figure 8.3 An injured athlete who is conscious may apply pressure to his wound while the athletic trainer pulls on his gloves.

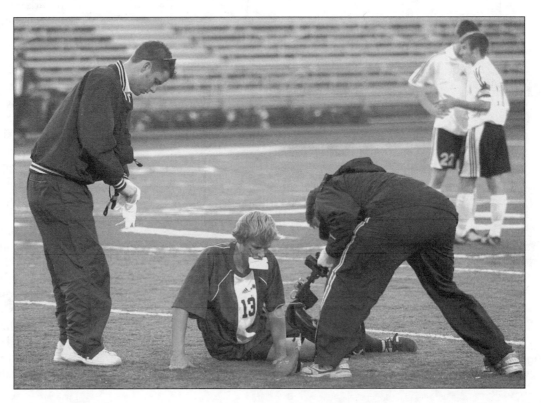

Pressure Over the Major Artery

In the case of the man on the highway, the major artery supplying the limb is the femoral artery, which is in the area of the groin. Pressure on the artery will slow the flow of blood to all areas below the point of artery compression. Application of this technique may be necessary if direct pressure and splinting prove ineffective or too difficult to provide. Pressure over the femoral artery could be provided even after the splint has been applied.

Tourniquet

A tourniquet is the last thing to try in order to control bleeding and should be avoided unless you are also a trained paramedical professional. A tourniquet should not be applied unless bleeding is copious and cannot be controlled by direct pressure. Vigorous attempts to control with direct pressure should be continued. Once a tourniquet is placed, it should not be removed or loosened by anyone but a doctor. A tourniquet should be used only when a decision has been made to save the patient's life by sacrificing the limb. It is a decision that only the trained emergency care provider should make.

Obvious Orthopedic Deformity

In addition to checking for bleeding, we will need to know whether there is something torn or broken that may be causing bleeding we can't see. If patients are alert, you must tell them you are going to check for broken bones. As you feel along the contours of each of the limbs, the hips and pelvis, and the trunk, you should continue to talk to the patient. Ask questions like "Can you feel me touching you?" "Do you have any pain here?" "Can you wiggle your toes? Your fingers?" Questions such as these will apprise you of the patient's level of consciousness as well as tell you more about where the injury may be. This scenario is more like the typical situation one might encounter on the athletic field—the athlete is injured, but we may not know the exact nature of the injury. Bleeding is suspected whenever there is significant trauma. Internal structures may be bleeding if torn, and this bleeding must be controlled just as the bleeding from an open wound must be controlled. Remember the flowchart shown in figure 8.4 as you progress through your evaluation of the injured person, and you will be able to prioritize these steps much more quickly.

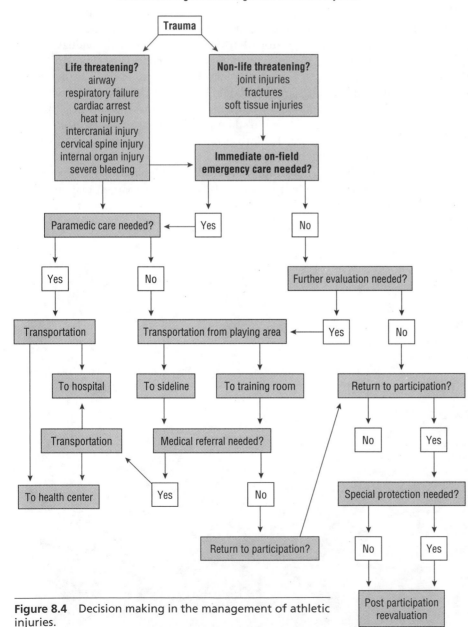

Decision making in the management of athletic injuries

Figure 8.4 Decision making in the management of athletic injuries.

FIRST AID PROCEDURES FOR SUDDEN ILLNESSES

Athletes are not often overcome with sudden illness, but that emergency certainly may occur. When people become ill suddenly, they often exhibit some warning signs before an emergency situation develops. Signs that there may be some problem include changes in skin color (the skin becomes pale or flushed); unusually heavy perspiration; complaints of feeling dizzy, light-headed, or weak; and vomiting or diarrhea. The problem has become much worse if the athlete exhibits changes in level of consciousness or an inability to move, demonstrates slurred speech, complains of severe headache, or has difficulty breathing.

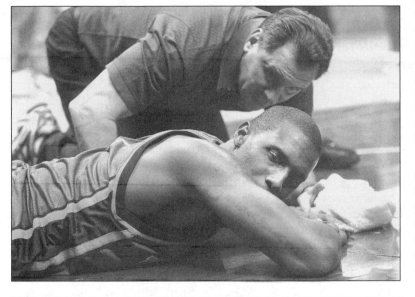

Figure 8.5 An athlete who is suddenly ill should be monitored until medical assistance arrives.
© Icon SMI

Sometimes the athlete or the situation can give you a good idea of what is wrong. For example, if the temperature and humidity are quite high, the person may be experiencing heat illness; or, if you know someone has diabetes, you may reason that the problem is a diabetic coma or an insulin reaction. When you know the cause of the problem, you can provide better care.

When there is no clue to the reason for a sudden illness, the best measures are to care for any life-threatening conditions first and then, if the person's life is not in danger, to treat the symptoms (see figure 8.5). Help get the individual comfortable, prevent overchilling or overheating, watch for signs of decreased level of consciousness, and seek medical assistance or call emergency medical services (EMS). Always remain with the athlete to monitor his or her condition and to provide any emergency care needed. Don't leave the scene until the ambulance personnel or the physician has taken over the athlete's care and you have provided all the vital information you have gained.

Athletes With Diabetes

If the athlete is experiencing a diabetic emergency but can continue to communicate with you, ask about the person's last dosage of insulin and last meal. Other illnesses that result in vomiting or diarrhea can cause an athlete who has diabetes to go into acute distress. Usually the patient with diabetes knows what is wrong and what needs to be done to help. If the athlete has not been diagnosed with diabetes, you may be able to recognize some of the warning signs of diabetes as listed here. You should not be the one to make the diagnosis of diabetes, but be aware of the common signs and know when the athlete should be referred to a doctor for further evaluation.

For athletes thought to be having a sudden illness related to diabetes, the best thing to do (if they are conscious) is to offer them something to eat or drink that contains sugar (candy,

Warning Signs of Diabetes

- Increased frequency of urination
- Excessive thirst or hunger
- Sweet or fruity (acetone) breath odor
- Intoxicated appearance
- Irritability; aggressive or unusual behavior
- Weakness and fatigue, faintness, seizure, or coma

fruit juice, non-diet soft drink). Athletes with known diabetes may keep candy with them to use in such an emergency. If the problem is excessive sugar, additional sugar will not harm them, but it will not make the situation any better. If after about 5 min of ingesting sugar the athlete does not improve or continues to worsen, call for medical care immediately. Be sure to stay with the athlete until help arrives, because what you know about the strenuousness of the athletic activity will allow a better understanding of the exact needs of the patient.

Athletes With Bronchospasm

Usually, athletes who have been diagnosed with asthma or a form of exercise-induced bronchospasm identify themselves to the coach, athletic trainer, and team physician. They may ask you to carry an inhaler for use shortly after the start of the exercise warm-up. When athletes who have this condition (or even those with no previous diagnosis of airway problems) begin to experience difficulty catching their breath, have coughing episodes that last several minutes, or otherwise manifest airway obstruction, medical assistance may be necessary. If an individual experiences extreme difficulties in oxygen exchange, one must observe closely for signs of tissue hypoxia. If the person's breathing continues to be labored, transportation to a medical facility may be necessary. Usually an ambulance is not required if there is any other way the individual can be safely transported.

Sickle Cell Crisis

Episodes of severe pain that can be triggered by infection, low oxygen, or stress, or that can occur spontaneously, are the result of a sickle cell crisis. Virtually any body part can be involved during a crisis. Sickle cells are fragile and tend to break apart. These cell fragments and misshapen cells clog blood vessels and disrupt the supply of oxygen and other vital nutrients to tissues and organs. If this occurs, the health care provider needs to quickly recognize the symptoms (often the individual complains of pain in the chest or abdomen or painful joints) and transport the individual to a medical facility.

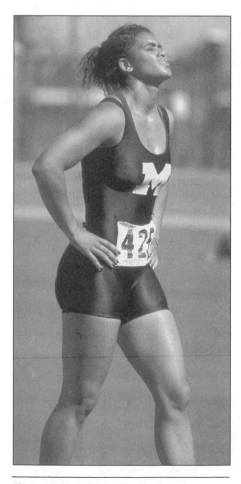

Once identified as having sickle cell disease, individuals need to learn about the ill effects of overexertion. Since people carrying the sickle cell trait are more prone than others to **rhabdomyolysis,** which may occur after excessive muscular activity, they must be cautious about engaging in such activity (see figure 8.6). When someone with known sickle cell trait complains of muscle pain, weakness, or unusual fatigue, it may be that the activity is causing damage to or death **(necrosis)** of some of the muscles. If the muscle damage continues, it may cause damage to the kidney as the kidney attempts to filter the myoglobin produced by the muscle damage. After any exercise, hydration should be provided to dilute the urine and flush the myoglobin out of the kidney. It may be necessary to provide intravenous (IV) fluids, and an ambulance service should be called if this cannot be done by the on-site medical staff. The sickle crisis can develop into an emergency situation if not properly managed.

Epilepsy

Management of the individual with epilepsy during a seizure consists of ensuring a safe area for the person. After the seizure is over, transportation to a medical facility should be provided so that the person can be evaluated and treated. There is little to no need for immediate medical care during the episode.

Heart Conditions

When a person is diagnosed with a heart condition, all team personnel who understand the condition and can render care should be involved in the emer-

Figure 8.6 Sickle cell anemia can cause rhabdomyolysis, which may occur after excessive muscular activity.

gency plan. If a participant suddenly develops cardiac difficulties, the health care provider should seek medical assistance while monitoring the pulse and blood pressure (BP). Cardiopulmonary resuscitation is necessary for individuals in cardiac arrest. In all instances of heart disease, first aid must be provided if the person is unable to sustain his or her own heartbeat.

THE EMERGENCY CARE PLAN

One can never be too prepared for an emergency situation. Just as in the case of doing CPR, if and when we need to use the emergency procedures, our minds will be flooded with information—and the more automatic the response can be, the better. It is wise to practice the steps of the emergency plan several times throughout the school year or sport season. Having every member of the coaching and medical staff familiar with the emergency care plan will be a great asset if an emergency ever arises. As an example, consider a situation that actually occurred during a football practice. During tackling drills in the early phase of the practice, a linebacker made a hit, lowering his head and striking the ball carrier. The linebacker collapsed suddenly and then lay motionless on the field. Since this was a practice day, the only staff on the field were three athletic trainers, several coaches, and one equipment person. The athlete could not move; his level of consciousness was diminished, and he was calling people by the wrong name and making strange requests.

This player had a concussion, and in view of the type of drill that had led to the concussion, one could suspect that his neck may also have been injured. The athletic trainer, coaches, and equipment man safely and quickly immobilized the athlete's spine on a **spine board** as one of the players ran to the phone to call an ambulance. Preplanning with the entire staff allowed smooth teamwork in helping this athlete.

Every member of the sport staff has a responsibility in the total athletic injury emergency care plan. In an emergency situation, anyone may be called upon, and everyone must be knowledgeable and ready to help. Every team should develop an emergency care plan that outlines game and practice coverage, emergency procedure steps, and other elements of emergency care such as communication, transportation, and record keeping. For a sample emergency plan from the National Youth Sports Safety Foundation, Inc., see page 266.

Game and Practice Coverage

Regardless of the setting, sports with a high potential of serious injury should have medical coverage during practices and games. The list of sports with a high potential of serious injury may vary from school to school. If the staff are trained and the emergency guidelines allow the staff to place an injured athlete on a spine board, the necessary equipment should be at hand. Each individual athletic trainer responsible for a sport team should know which athletes have conditions that might predispose them to sudden illness. Knowledge of athletes with diabetes, sickle cell anemia, epilepsy, or heart conditions allows the sports medicine specialist to prepare for any potential problems. This emergency plan should be discussed and practiced with all members of the support and coaching staffs so that any person available at the time of an emergency can be of significant assistance.

As discussed in the Athletic Training Education Series text *Management Strategies in Athletic Training, Third Edition*, emergency care to be provided for game coverage should be established each year. Sometimes schools contract with local emergency providers. Ambulance staff on hand for the game should be dedicated to emergencies on the playing field or court, and a separate ambulance should be available for emergencies in the stands. In the event one ambulance is taken from the site, a replacement ambulance should be sent for immediately. These services should be formulated before the season begins, and members of the ambulance company should meet with the team coaches, medical staff, or both, prior to the first game.

Emergency Procedure Steps

When an emergency situation arises we want to be prepared. The best way to prepare for an emergency is to plan. If you were not very familiar with the team, facility, or community, it

National Youth Sports Safety Foundation, Inc.
EMERGENCY PLAN

Designated Personnel

1. Person designated to stay with injured athlete: _____

2. Person designated to phone for medical assistance: _____

3. Person designated to meet emergency medical assistance at gate and accompany them to injured athlete: _____
_____

4. Person designated to immediately call parents and inform them of circumstances: _____
_____

5. Person designated to accompany injured athlete to the hospital: _____

6. Person responsible for documenting all information relating to injury and emergency response: _____
_____

Emergency Information

1. Location of closest phone: _____

2. Keys to access phone are located at: _____

3. Change for pay phone is kept in: _____

4. Address of the athletic facility is: _____

5. Entry location for the closest emergency vehicle is: _____

6. To access the athletic facility, emergency medical personnel must pass through _____ gates and _____ doors
   Keys to unlock these areas are available from: _____

7. Phone number of emergency facility if 911 is not available: _____

8. The closest emergency care facility is _____, which is located at _____
   and is _____ miles from the athletic facility. Average travel time is _____

9. The closest trauma facility is _____, which is located at _____ and is _____ miles
   from the athletic facility. Average travel time is _____

Emergency Call Instructions

When you call an emergency medical service (911) you should:

- Identify yourself and your exact location
- Explain what happened and the type of injury (head/neck/spine, fracture, loss of consciouness, etc.)
- Give address of athletic facility and exact instructions on how the ambulance is to reach the injured athlete. This would include street address, gate information, building location, and entry information.
- Stay on the line until the operator disconnects the call.
- Return to the injury scene.

Additional Phone Numbers

Team Physician: _____

Ambulance Service: _____

Fire Department: _____

Police Department: _____

School Nurse: _____

Athletic Director: _____

Principal: _____

Emergency Care Plan

- Game and practice coverage: Outline the duties of those regularly in attendance. Anticipate the personnel who might be available, delineate duties, and discuss contingency plans.
- Procedure steps: Know what will be done. Outline the steps to be taken in various emergency situations.
- Communication systems: Know how to contact emergency medical services. Ensure that there is a working telephone near all practice and game facilities. On or next to each telephone, have appropriate emergency numbers and directions for calling for an ambulance.
- Equipment: Appropriate emergency care equipment and supplies must be available and in proper condition for use. Include emergency equipment in annual inventory and ordering.
- Emergency care facilities: Contact local emergency care facilities to establish protocol for registration of injured athlete. Preregister entire team if possible. Discuss procedures to be followed when emergency medical needs arise.
- Transportation: Arrange for ambulance crew to be in attendance during events, or notify local ambulance company of event location, time, and preferred access routes.
- Personnel training: Training and retraining of all personnel need to be accomplished periodically.
- Record keeping: Review commonly used and accepted abbreviations for medical terms as well as metods of recording medical information. Always make a record of injuries and treatment provided.

---

would be wise to involve the athlete administrator, coach, team physician, and community EMS personnel in formulating your plan for emergency care at specific events as well as issues concerning team and crowd control, immobilization, and transportation preferences and communication protocols. All questions should be addressed prior to the start of the sport season. The following steps should be taken in any emergency situation:

- First responder assesses the situation for severity and nature of the injury and calls for help if needed.
- Begin providing needed injury management.
- Second responder assists in managing injury, directing functions of various personnel available to help, or both.
- Team (first responder, second responder, and other personnel) stabilizes the injury to allow for transportation.

The activation of the EMS system depends on the nature and severity of the injury and the level of knowledge and skill of the responders. Further discussion of these concepts is presented here and in the *Management Strategies* textbook of this series.

Communication Systems

Telephone communication has become much more convenient than it was 10 years ago. Today, with the low cost of cellular phones, immediate access to EMS is possible. If the practice or game area is indoors and cellular phone reception is hampered by the architecture of the building, it is essential to have a regular phone with a dedicated line. This phone access must be very convenient—not through dark hallways and locked doors. Immediate access to EMS may make all the difference in the well-being of an athlete.

At some schools where athletic fields are spread out over the campus, communication occurs through a central dispatcher, often through walkie-talkie radio transmission. Although this system involves an additional step for contacting EMS, it can function quite well in some situations. It is very important that the line stay clear of idle chitchat so that the response to an emergency call can occur without delay.

Wherever the telephone is located, written instructions for contacting EMS should be on or near it. This information should include the telephone number to call, the words to say, and the exact directions to the location of the injured player. As soon as EMS has been contacted, someone should be sent to whatever entrance or other specific location the ambulance has been instructed to go to. This person should direct the ambulance to the appropriate building or field.

In addition to the communication that might occur prior to the telephone call (internal communication) and the call to the emergency care service (external communication), on-site communication is critical in the total care of the athlete. The first responder (the first medical person to render attention to the victim) is often the athletic trainer. It becomes that first responder's duty to give the EMT or paramedic (or both) any medical information known about this patient. By passing on bits of information pertaining to etiology (cause) and any pathology (physical problems) relating to the athlete, one gives the emergency personnel a better understanding of what is occurring.

Once the ambulance crew determine that the athlete needs to be taken to the hospital, they will notify the emergency care facility. If the condition of the athlete is not a threat to life or limb, it is permissible to call upon a parent or other authorized person for transportation. In this case it is necessary to call the hospital or health care provider to alert the medical staff of the athlete's problem, the method of transportation, and the estimated time of arrival. When possible, it is best to speak directly to the person who will be caring for the athlete upon arrival.

One final form of communication, which may be among the most important, is notification of the athlete's parents and the school administrators. Certainly the parents need to know what has happened, and in general it is best to have the team athletic trainer or team physician make this notification. If the athlete is under the age of consent, or a minor, the hospital will want to contact the parent or guardian for permission to treat. Of course there are situations, such as a true emergency, in which consent to treat the minor is implied, allowing care to be rendered immediately. Notification of the school administrators may be thought of as a courtesy, yet these are usually the people who receive requests from parents and the press for information about the incident. The administrator need only have sufficient information to understand what happened (e.g., Joe Black collided with the goalpost and was unconscious) and where the athlete is being taken for further care (e.g., he is being taken by ambulance to St. Vincent's Hospital). Other information may be helpful for the administrator (including the coach) and, with the exception of confidential medical information, may be provided.

Sample of Emergency Procedures for Posting at Telephone

EMERGENCY PROCEDURES, McKALE BASKETBALL FLOOR

1. Call 9-911 from this phone.

2. Identify yourself: name, position. "This is Joe White, head athletic trainer at State University."

3. Explain the emergency: "A forward on the men's basketball team fell and is unconscious."

4. Be ready to answer any questions: Is there a pulse, is he breathing?

5. Explain how to enter McKale: "Enter from McKale Drive, going west off Campbell. Turn right at the entrance to the loading dock (just before the parking garage). Come down the ramp. The rolling door will be open."

6. Stay connected until THE OTHER PERSON HANGS UP.

7. Go open the rolling door (use the #91 key in the desk drawer). Meet the ambulance at McKale Drive and Campbell; direct them toward McKale. Get someone to stand at the top of the ramp to signal the ambulance and direct them down the ramp.

Equipment

Emergency equipment is important to have at hand when it is needed (see figure 8.7). Many companies manufacture storage bags that can be used to organize storage and to transport stretchers, spine boards (see figure 8.8), cervical immobilization devices, and other equipment that may be needed on the athletic field or court. This equipment should be the same equipment that is used in emergency situation practice sessions. It is important that EMTs and paramedics (EMT-P) who are responsible for the ambulance coverage at the particular athletic event(s) check all materials. Emergency care providers are usually more familiar with equipment standards and are also often able to repair damaged supplies.

Some schools may not have sufficient personnel to provide emergency care to an injured athlete, relying instead on local emergency services. There are no known regulations that

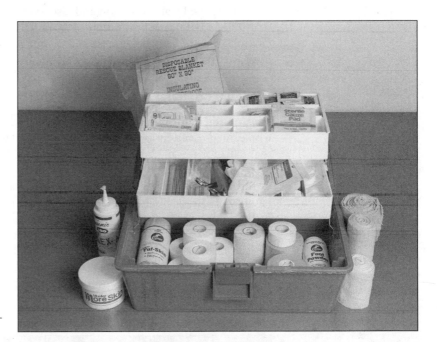

Figure 8.7   Contents of a first aid kit.

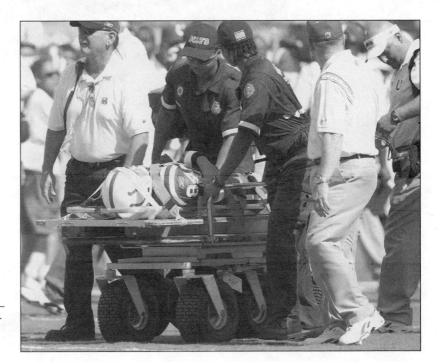

Figure 8.8   A spine board is used to immobilize an injured individual.

© G. Newman Lowrence

require schools to have emergency equipment on hand, yet it may be very wise to be sure that life support could be provided in the case of an emergency.

Emergency Care Facilities

Most communities have an emergency care facility nearby. In some small, rural towns, the only emergency service may be through the volunteer fire department. Most firefighters are trained as EMTs, and this care is certainly helpful during an athletic crisis or other emergency.

In large metropolitan areas, where emergency care facilities are available locally, there may be many hospitals within a short distance of the athletic facility. Knowing the locations of the hospitals and the best routes to get to them is important if you ever plan to transport ill or injured athletes yourself or to have a family member transport them. Additionally, it is helpful to know where the closest fire station is in the event an ambulance is needed.

Visiting the local fire station and discussing the potential emergency needs of the team or school may be of help in the future. Familiarizing fire station personnel with your practice facilities may be beneficial if an ambulance is needed at a practice site. Information about how to enter the restricted grounds of some schools can be especially critical.

Transportation

The injured or ill athlete must be transported with extreme care. If the problem could become worse, medical attention during transport could be required (see figure 8.9). This is a situation that calls for use of an ambulance. There may be situations in athletics in which the injury is significant but life or limb would not be at risk during transport to the emergency room or physician's office via a school or personal car. However, you should be familiar with the liability involved should you elect to use your personal car for such purposes.

If one decides that transportation of the athlete is safe, it is prudent to document as much of the case as possible. Aspects such as peripheral circulation (distal to the injury) and neurological status should be noted and recorded. Additionally, before the person is moved, proper immobilization of injured joints or bones must be provided. If there is any doubt about the safety of personal transportation of the individual, professional services (EMS) should be employed for that purpose.

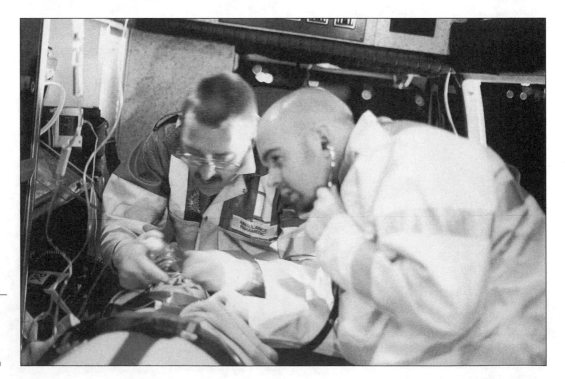

Figure 8.9 Emergency medical services transport of an injured player.

© Digitalvisiononline.com

Obviously if the injury necessitates CPR, EMS should be activated immediately. Whether summoned for life support or for transportation of a spinal injury or other orthopedic or medical reasons, once EMS personnel arrive, care of the athlete becomes the job of the ambulance personnel, and transportation as well as medical care will be provided by the EMS team. The responsibilities of the on-site medical team are transferred to the EMS personnel at that time.

Personnel Training

Whenever a number of people will be on hand for an athletic event, everyone associated with medical services should be familiar with the emergency procedures to be conducted. When only a few medical and athletic training personnel are present, coaches and sometimes other support staff may be called upon to provide help.

Yearly completion of CPR training should be a requirement for all students and staff members expected to help in a cardiac emergency (see figure 8.10). Training of all teachers and administrators in CPR is beneficial, not only for the sake of the athletes and students, but also to better prepare each person to handle an emergency at school or home.

If the emergency policy includes preparing injured athletes for transport by ambulance, those who will be involved should receive instruction and should also have practice—before the season begins—in the preferred techniques for lifting and turning the victim. The physicians responsible at the games should play an active role in establishing the procedure the emergency team is to follow. Involving the ambulance staff with the medical staff is critical to assure good understanding and open communication between the groups. Schedule a meeting in which all members of the emergency response team will plan, review, and rehearse the procedures to follow in the event of an emergency on the playing field. Be sure to discuss the specific duties of each individual who will be present at each type of event.

Record Keeping

Just as with any injury, emergency care rendered must be documented for the athlete's medical records. The record should include all treatments performed by the school personnel, as well

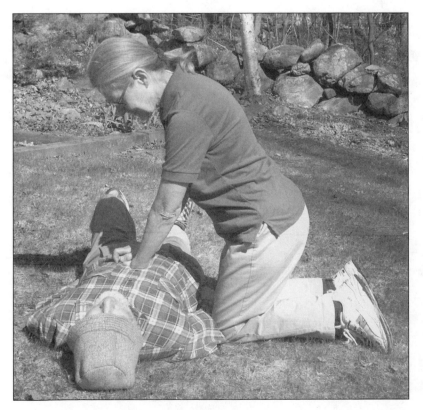

as the times of the EMS call and ambulance arrival. The ambulance crew, according to regulations set forth by their governing parties, will monitor the condition of the athlete. The ambulance crew may be required to perform particular tests regardless of what information the first responders have provided. This should not pose a problem, especially if lines of communication are well developed and active.

Careful documentation of the emergency situation is very important in the event that the athlete or family later files a lawsuit against the medical care providers. This is likely to happen in the situation in which an athlete suffers loss of limb or life. Naturally, the family will want to know exactly what happened and what was done, and the court may call for this information. Relying on memory is not good enough; you must have carefully written records. See "Sample Emergency Report Form" on page 272.

Figure 8.10 Cardiopulmonary resuscitation.
© Schwartz

Sample Emergency Report Form

Name of injured person: _____

Time of injury: _____ Date of injury: _____

Place injury occurred: _____

Nature of emergency: _____

Immediate steps taken: _____

Primary survey

    Vital signs: _____

    Pulse: _____ Blood pressure: _____ Respiration rate: _____

Secondary survey:

    Bone or joint injury: _____

    Soft tissue injury: _____

First respondent _____

    Secondary respondent(s): _____

Immediate management: _____

    EMS notification time: _____ EMS arrival time: _____

Emergency care facility: _____

Attending physician: _____

Notification of parent/guardian: _____

    Time and date of notification: _____

    Person contacted: _____

Name of person completing report: _____ Date: _____

LEGAL AND ETHICAL ISSUES IN TREATMENT

In athletics, the individual athlete is a potential patient. As a health care provider or coach, you must give the patient the best health care you can, each day, every day. Your emergency care skills may not be expected to be as good as those of a paramedic or physician, yet knowledge of CPR and first aid procedures might be within the scope of your particular position. If you face an injury situation, your reaction and your management of the injury will always be subject to scrutiny. If the injury is serious and the patient suffers loss of life or limb, or is rendered physically limited in some other way, all medical care given the patient will be scrutinized. There is but one thing to do: Stay current with your skills and techniques and perform your best in all situations.

Consent

Consent for treatment, by law, is required for any medical treatment to a patient. Consent is often assumed because of the relationship of the athlete to the coach or athletic trainer. Usually that assumption is correct because of prior planning and documentation by the school administration. Legally, consent should be obtained from every athlete prior to the first day of practice. If the athlete is under the legal age of consent, the parents or guardian should sign consent-for-treatment forms that will allow medical aid should it ever be necessary during athletic participation on the team(s) with which you are working. Some states have laws that permit minors to give their own binding consent for medical attention. In terms of consent for medical care, your state may have a law that permits minors to be treated as adults if they are self-supporting, married, or pregnant. As the person in charge of medical care of the athletes, you may want to contact the legal department (your athletic director can refer you to the appropriate person) to obtain help in designing medical consent-for-care forms. See the form "Emergency Medical Authorization" on page 274.

Negligence

Negligence involves four key elements: duty, breach of that duty, physical or psychological injury, and cause. These are defined as follows:

- Duty: something you are assigned or expected to do
- Breach of duty: failure to fulfill the duty
- Physical or psychological injury: bodily injury or some psychological trauma caused by the incident
- Cause: a causal relationship between the lack of care and the injury (the fact that an injury happened and that care was not provided is not enough)

To examine negligence, let's imagine a situation in which you are the only adult responsible for the team. You are at soccer practice when two players collide. Neither appears to be moving, so you run onto the field. You see that one of the players is alert and responsive; the other tries to look at you (opens her eyes), but then seems to become unconscious. What would you do?

You have a duty to help the athlete (patient). If you fail to perform that duty, you commit a breach of duty. That duty is what anyone with similar training and responsibility would do in the same circumstance. If doing something or the failure to do something causes physical or psychological harm, you will be acting in a negligent manner. Thus, if you fail to provide care and this failure results in some physical injury or psychological trauma, you could be found negligent if it can be proven that the injury would not have happened had you provided appropriate (and reasonable) care. Thus, as with liability, you have certain responsibilities—and if harm comes to someone because you failed to fulfill your responsibilities, you could be found negligent (or liable when the error did not involve your service or care but involved

Emergency Medical Authorization

I/we, the undersigned, am/are the parent(s) of _____, minor(s).

Consent

I/we hereby give consent, in the event I/we cannot be contacted within a reasonable time, for (1) the administration of any treatment deemed necessary for my/our children by Dr. _____, or any of his/her associates, the preferred physician, or Dr. _____, or any of his/her associates, the preferred dentist, or in the event the appropriate preferred practitioner is not available, by another licensed, qualified physician or dentist; and (2) the transfer of any of my/our children to _____ Hospital, the preferred hospital, or any hospital reasonably accessible.

Major surgery

This authorization does not cover nonemergency major surgery unless the medical opinions of two other licensed physicians or dentists concurring in the necessity for such surgery are obtained prior to the performance of such surgery and unless all reasonable attempts to contact me/us have been unsuccessful, defining such period for nonemergency surgery as 24 hours.

Medical data

The following is needed by any hospital or practitioner not having access to my/our children's medical history:

Allergies: _____

Medication being taken: _____

Physical impairments: _____

Other pertinent facts to which physician should be alerted: _____

_____

Medical insurance coverage: _____

I/we, the undersigned parent(s), also do by these premises appoint and constitute _____ and _____ _____ and/or _____ as temporary custodians of my/our children above mentioned, for the period of _____, 20____, through and including _____, 20____, and do hereby authorize them to obtain any x-ray examination, anesthesia, medical or surgical diagnosis or treatment, and hospital care to be rendered to my/our children in my/our absence, under the general or special supervision, and on the advice of a licensed physician, surgeon, anesthesiologist, dentist, or other qualified personnel acting under their supervision.

Witnesses

_____

_____

State of _____

SS:

_____ County

Note. The law varies from state to state. No form should be adopted or used by any program without individualized legal advice.

Adapted by permission from Herbert 1994.

materials, facilities, equipment, etc.). In the soccer example, the respondent is expected to act (perform a duty) in a way that others with the same level of training would act.

In addition to the responsibility to give care in emergency situations, you have the responsibility to give care in the same manner when life is not threatened. Daily attention to athletes during activities is critical and sometimes cannot be accomplished by one person alone. Often, coaches are so intent on stressing the need to get in shape that they fail to recognize signs and symptoms of trouble in a player. As an example, consider a situation that actually occurred in a hot, desert climate.

A young athlete, Tommy, had just returned to the high school football team, which had been practicing for the past two days. Tommy had spent the summer with relatives in a cooler coastal city and was coming back just for football. He went through the entire practice and then began the postpractice conditioning with the team. Other players got sips of water from their personal water bottles, but Tommy hadn't known to bring one and was too shy to ask another player for a drink of his water. After a couple of the sprints at the end of practice, Tommy just couldn't go any more. He sat down under a goalpost to rest. The coach yelled at Tommy to "get up," and Tommy struggled to his feet and ran another sprint. At the end of the running, he collapsed—tired, actually exhausted, boiling hot, and thirsty.

Unfortunately, Tommy had collapsed with heat exhaustion, and that exhaustion developed into heatstroke; Tommy died before help could arrive. The situation went to court, and the court determined negligence. The coach had a duty to take care of the student-athletes. He had failed to provide the care expected. The injury (heatstroke) could have been prevented if the coach had given proper care. Thus the court ruled in favor of the plaintiff and against the coach and the school.

It shouldn't take an athlete's death to get us to think about ways to prevent medical problems in athletics. Certainly we never want an athlete under our supervision to be seriously injured, much less die. Proper training and knowledge of first aid will not keep athletes safe if we fail to exercise good judgment and do not learn to understand the warning signs of serious medical problems.

COMMUNITY-BASED EMERGENCY MEDICAL SERVICES

Anyone working in athletics will have occasion to call on or work with the community-based EMS. A visit to the nearby fire station to introduce yourself will go a long way in establishing lines of communication between your athletic team or school and the ambulance and paramedic team. Often, if you devote the time and energy to meeting those responsible for emergency transport, they will work with you in establishing preferred methods of transport, open lines for communication, and other details of your emergency care needs. To learn more about establishing lines of communication with EMS agencies, refer to Richard Ray's text in this series, *Management Strategies in Athletic Training, Third Edition.*

Brief History of the Emergency Medical Services

Emergency medical services, as it is now known, began in 1966. Several agencies investigated aspects of accidental death and disability and found that pre-hospital care was inadequate in many areas of the United States. This information triggered Congress to direct two federal agencies to address the issue. Those agencies, the National Highway Traffic Safety Administration (NHTSA) and the Department of Health and Human Services, created funding sources to develop and improve systems of emergency, pre-hospital care.

After the development of EMS systems in the '60s and '70s, the focus changed in the '80s toward standardizing training programs for those people most closely involved in pre-hospital care: the EMT and the EMT-P (emergency medical technician-paramedic).

Table 8.1
Members of the Emergency Medical Services Network

Personnel	Individuals involved and job duty relating to EMS network
Dispatchers	Triage 911 calls to appropriate DPS (Department of Public Safety) team.
Emergency medical technicians, emergency medical technicians-paramedic	Emergency care on the scene, transportation to medical facility.
Hospital personnel	Admissions, nurses, and technicians prepare the patient for medical care.
Poison control centers	When needed, provide antidote for ingested poisons.
Physicians	Hospital- or community-based physicians care for the injured.
Other allied health personnel	Radiologists, anesthesiologists, medical specialists provide special care.

In the '90s, demand for EMS became greater than the supply of EMTs, so the U.S. Department of Transportation developed an EMT-Basic National Standard Curriculum. Addition of the EMT-B to the EMS team increased the number of trained individuals available for pre-hospital emergency services.

Today, EMS involves a number of professionals who all work to provide emergency care in the shortest time possible. The members of the EMS network are listed in table 8.1.

Community-Based Emergency Health Care Delivery Plans

When the community has an established emergency system, there is usually a central location from which appropriate teams are dispatched to the caller, depending on the type of emergency. When a call is received, decisions are made regarding the type of help needed, and a call goes out to the agency from which help is required (fire, police, ambulance). In large cities this system becomes much more involved than in the rural towns of America, yet most communities have some system to expedite the response to calls for help.

Accessing the Emergency Network

In the United States, the emergency network is usually activated by dialing 911 on any telephone. Although many think of this number merely as a way to call police, fire, and ambulance, it has other important functions. A 911 call coming in to the dispatch desk automatically generates certain information (see figure 8.11). Even if someone were only to dial 911 and hang up, the dispatcher would know the telephone number from which the call had originated. This system is the same as the systems people purchase for their homes that let them call a special number to find out where missed calls originated. The same system is operating in caller-ID devices. Knowledge of the caller's telephone number enables the dispatcher to return an interrupted 911 call to attempt to find out whether there actually is some kind of trouble.

You should not assume that 911 for emergency is the number to dial when visiting another country. Whenever you are traveling outside the United States, especially with sport teams, it is important to know the local emergency access numbers. For example, in the United Kingdom, the number for emergencies is 999, and in Australia it is 000. Take the time to check with local health care providers to establish the protocol for obtaining emergency medical assistance.

As mentioned earlier, a visit to the local provider of ambulance service is extremely valuable. Usually this is the nearest fire department; most firefighters are also trained as EMTs. When you contact or visit the EMTs, it is helpful to discuss all aspects of your emergency plan—from the preferred gate for entering the practice or game area to the techniques for placing an athlete on a spine board for immobilization and transport.

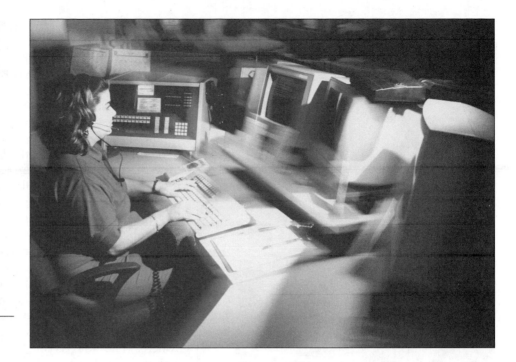

Figure 8.11   A 911 dispatcher.
© Getty Images

In addition to establishing the lines of communication and discussing the emergency care plan, it is advisable to schedule a training session. During this session, all members of the medical/emergency care team work together to perform actual techniques to be used in the event of head injury, spinal injury, or cardiac emergency. This cooperation between the athletic training staff, the ambulance crew, and the attending physicians will allow all members of the emergency response team to understand the concerns and skills of the others.

Transportation Systems

Because of the cross-training of many public safety personnel, transportation may be provided by groups other than ambulance crews. Depending on the local policies and the level of trauma, police or fire departments may dispatch officers to provide assistance in transporting the injured subject to the emergency facility or to the hospital.

Regardless of the means by which your athlete arrives at the hospital, if a DPS (Department of Public Safety) agency provides the transportation from your location to an area hospital, agency protocols and orders must be followed. When working with a medical/emergency care team that has its own physician, you must realize that your physician's orders will become secondary to the orders given by the medical director responsible for that team. Be sure to discuss this issue with your team physician to avoid misunderstandings that can arise in emergency situations when the EMS chain of command is not understood in advance.

COMMUNITY-BASED EMERGENCY CARE FACILITIES

Whether you live in a large city or small town or on a college campus, the local community often has some emergency care facilities or some type of network. Understanding the local system is essential to providing the best medical care for an injured person.

Availability and Capabilities

With regard to pre-hospital care, response times for the EMS team in busy cities may be longer than in small, quiet towns. This availability may also be affected by the capabilities of the responding team. Many items needed in the care of home and road trauma victims are carried on all emergency vehicles, but special equipment that is sometimes needed in

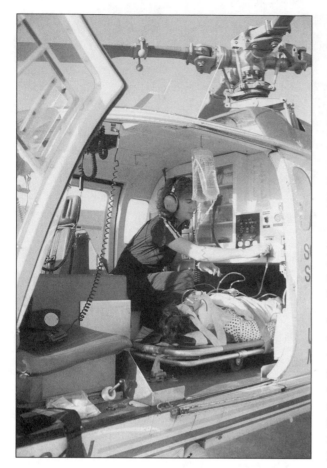

Figure 8.12 Special equipment sometimes needed in the care of athletic trauma may not be available on all vehicles. Tell the dispatcher that you have an athletic injury; that information can be relayed to the emergency medical services, hospital, or both.

the care of athletic trauma may not be available on all vehicles (see figure 8.12). When you have information that would be helpful for understanding the special needs of an athlete, you should give that information to the dispatcher during the initial call to 911.

For example, suppose that during a fast break at basketball practice, the athlete with the ball is in the air for a layup and another player undercuts her, causing the ball handler's feet to be knocked out from under her. The player who is hurt, a forward, lands on the floor on the back of her flexed neck. She is lying motionless on the floor, obviously dazed. When you reach her, you recognize the decreased level of consciousness, but are relieved to see that she is breathing without difficulty. She is obviously in pain but cannot say much other than "my neck" in response to your questions about where the pain is located. You determine there is a possibility of spine injury in addition to a probable head injury, and you decide to call for an ambulance for transport to the hospital.

What information would you want to give the dispatcher? This information should include "who," "what," "when," and "where." The "who" is you. State your name and your position with the school or team. The "what" is the situation you are reporting: the injured basketball player, alert but complaining of neck pain. The "when" relates to the time (circumstances) of injury. The basketball player was injured on a layup when someone ran under her and she fell on her head. The "where" is your exact location, including directions to the nearest access point to pick up the injured person.

From time to time when using the EMS system for sport injuries, you may wonder why an athlete is not taken to a hospital just a couple of blocks away from the school but instead to one that is farther away. Depending on the type of injury or trauma suspected, the ambulance crew may be directed to one hospital over another. For example, an athlete with apparent neurological trauma may be taken to a level-one trauma center that is farther from the site than the non-trauma hospital two blocks away. Remember that when you ask EMS for transport and care, they are responsible to their medical director, not to the school medical staff.

Admission and Treatment Policies

Most hospitals will admit patients who are brought in for an emergency, regardless of their insurance coverage. This is not always the case when the emergency is not a threat to life or limb. It can happen that an injured individual is taken to one hospital but transferred to another one after the insurance information has been obtained. Analogously, patients are occasionally transferred from one physician to another. Be assured that the transfer to another hospital would not occur if the medical condition were serious and the patient's health would be jeopardized by the transport.

Roles and Responsibilities

The EMS system is made up of several professionals working together to provide the best and fastest emergency care (see figure 8.13). Each member of the emergency team has specific roles and responsibilities set forth by federal, state, and local agencies. Each state may have some rules of its own; if interested, you could check with the local professionals to obtain complete information about the roles and restrictions for each of the emergency response team members.

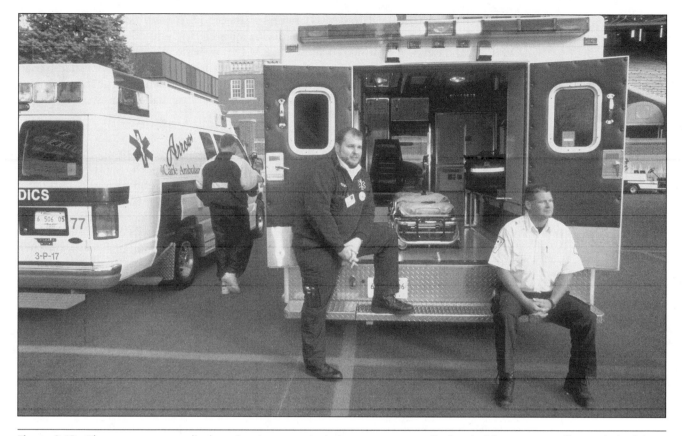

Figure 8.13   The emergency medical services team can include emergency medical technicians, paramedics, and physicians.

First Responders

Although not a specifically trained person in all states, the first responder is the first medically trained individual to arrive at the scene of an injury or sudden illness. This person may be a firefighter, police officer, school nurse, coach, athletic trainer, lifeguard, teacher, or one among many other professionals with some level of emergency training. The first responder, at the least, has successfully completed a first aid course. This person's duty is to provide the specific care that he or she has been trained to provide. If the first responder is a lifeguard and the injury is a diabetic coma, the lifeguard may only treat for shock or may call 911 and monitor the vital signs. If you are the first person on the scene of an injury, you are the first responder. You are obligated to provide whatever care a person with your training and experience level would afford the injured person; this is your duty.

Emergency Medical Technician

The EMT is the allied health professional most commonly associated with ambulance calls. One should realize, however, that there are two levels of EMTs: basic (EMT-B) and intermediate (EMT-I). There are greater differences than one might think between the "B" and the "I," in that the EMT-I is nearer to the level of the paramedic. The EMT-B (commonly called the EMT) is often the first member of the EMS team to arrive at the scene of an accident or to respond to an emergency call. The EMT typically attempts to care for the patient after having learned what preliminary care was given by the first responder, the first non-EMS person on the scene.

Working with the first responder, the EMT will attempt to stabilize the patient and prepare for transport. The limitations on the EMT are continually changing because of advances in technology and levels of training. Some techniques previously reserved for paramedics, such as defibrillation of the patient's heart, can now be performed by the EMT with the aid of an automated external defibrillator (AED). In most states, the EMT is trained in the **pneumatic antishock garment (PASG)**, AED, epinephrine autoinjector, and inhaler bronchodilators. Other technology will continue to allow the EMT to provide increasingly advanced health and cardiac care. The EMT-I has additional hours of training in the areas of cardiac care and additional areas of expertise including, but not limited to, endotracheal intubation, advanced life support (ALS) such as IV therapy, and interpretation of cardiac rhythms.

Paramedic

The paramedic (EMT-P), as well as the EMT-I, has had advanced training in pre-hospital care. The paramedic is the team member who has the most advanced training in ALS care, including skills in IV therapy, advanced pharmacology, cardiac monitoring, defibrillation, advanced airway maintenance, and intubation as well as other advanced assessment and treatment skills. This person can provide further immediate treatment before the patient is transported to the hospital.

The number of attendants and the range of qualifications on an ambulance can vary from one district to another and from one ambulance company to another. There are times when a dispatcher would like to send an EMT-P to a 911 call but, because of availability, sends a less highly trained EMS crew instead. There may seem to be an overlap of duties when the fire truck (with EMTs) that you see responding to an accident scene is followed within a few minutes by an ambulance (with paramedics). In emergency medicine, the goal is to provide the most skilled professional available to every person in need. If you had an emergency and all the paramedics were on other calls, would you want to wait for the response until they finished? Or would you feel better knowing that some help for the immediate emergency would be arriving shortly? Perhaps you wouldn't even need the paramedics but only transportation to the hospital. Sometimes the patient is too unstable to move by ambulance, so the EMT crew must attempt to stabilize the person while calling for paramedic support. Although the EMS system may be redundant, the intent is to get some help to the patient as soon as possible; if nothing else, that help can get the patient to the hospital.

Emergency Room Physician

The physician on duty in the emergency room is often the medical director of the EMS team. Through an understanding of the situation that has caused the injury (etiology of the injury), the physician can continue the care initiated by the EMTs and EMT-P. Physicians often assist the EMTs and paramedics in developing skills of assessment and treatment, allowing the physicians to "extend their arms" through the EMS team. This is done through continued training in various situations. Just like athletic trainers who come to know the team physician so well that they can predict with high confidence what the doctor will do, the EMS personnel out in the field often have to act on behalf of the doctor. They need to know the tests the doctor is going to want and what treatment he or she would want to try first, second, and third. The paramedics and EMTs working closely with the emergency physician often build a trusting relationship that allows the physician additional insight into the patient's exact condition at the remote location.

Ambulance Crew Guidelines

Persons in the ambulance responding to the scene are responsible to the medical director of their "home" hospital. The protocols established by the medical director and hospital must be carried out and should not interfere with the expedient health care of the injured athlete. Tempers may flare when the sport team physician fails to understand that the ambulance

For more information about emergency medicine, visit the American Academy of Emergency Medicine Web site at www.aaem.org.

attendants' responsibility is first to the patient and secondly to the hospital/medical director, and not to the team physician.

From time to time, an observer may be riding along in an ambulance. This arrangement, if available in your area, is an excellent way to learn more about the skills, roles, and responsibilities of those you may come to depend upon. When we understand the duties of the EMTs and paramedics, we learn to appreciate the care and treatment they can provide when called to an athletic emergency.

EMERGENCY CARE EQUIPMENT AND SUPPLIES

Not only is it wise to understand what to do in the case of a broken leg or "blown-out" knee; it is critical to understand what to do in the case of a life-threatening emergency. It is the life-threatening injury that will remain in your memory for years to come. Let's try to make that memory a pleasant one! Having the proper equipment available in the event of an injury is not the only step in being prepared; having the proper training to allow use of that equipment is essential. It is not wise to purchase equipment that you are not trained or skilled enough to use. Purchase and provide only equipment that will be useful to the majority of the staff members providing medical coverage for the contest or event.

Airway Management

Management of airway conditions, although infrequently required in sport, is essential; and all medical, allied medical, and coaching staff members should possess the skills involved. Every athletic trainer should possess certain supplies for managing airways, and some can provide supplemental oxygen. Various airway-management devices and supplies for delivery of supplemental oxygen are available on the ambulance.

Oropharyngeal Airway

Emergency care providers, physicians, and ambulance personnel quite frequently use a measured device called an **oropharyngeal** airway (see figure 8.14). The airway is graded from 00 to 6, and fit is determined by the distance from the center of the patient's mouth to the angle of his or her jaw. Analogous to ranges in clothing size, the range from 00 (for an infant) to 6 (for a large adult) indicates a relative size scale. Use of this device requires that the patient be unconscious and not have a gag reflex. The airway is inverted from its final direction and inserted into the patient's mouth. Once in the mouth, the airway is rotated 180°. Insertion into the unconscious patient's mouth allows the airway to be established and held open and permits secretions to be aspirated without compromise of the airway. This is not an absolute airway, yet it is often used in emergency situations by the team physician, the paramedic, or ambulance personnel.

Positive Pressure Ventilation

Positive pressure **ventilation** is used to force air into patients' lungs when breathing is inadequate. Ventilations can be given without the aid of any equipment or supplies, but it is always best to use some barrier between you and the victim.

Pocket Mask

The pocket mask is a personal item often carried by the athletic trainer. The mask is used to deliver mouth-to-mask ventilation and minimizes contact between rescuer and victim. Use of the mask may be supplemented by applying oxygen, which a trained emergency care technician would do.

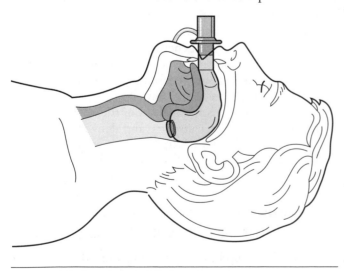

Figure 8.14   Oropharyngeal airway.

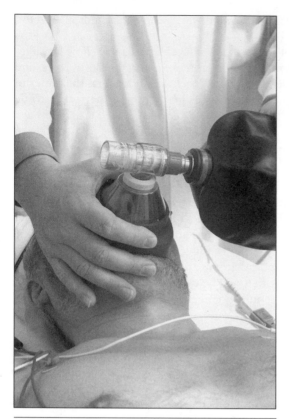

Figure 8.15   Bag-valve mask resuscitator for ventilation that minimizes contact between the rescuer and victim.

© Photo Researchers

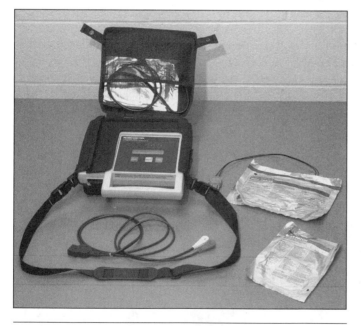

Figure 8.16   Automated external defibrillator.

Bag-Valve Mask Resuscitators

The bag-valve mask resuscitator can be used on any patient, conscious or unconscious, who requires ventilation (see figure 8.15). Use of the bag-valve mask can be supplemented with oxygen, but this is a procedure that requires considerable practice and training and must be performed by a trained technician.

Supplemental Oxygen

If the patient is ventilating but not perfusing the tissues, supplemental oxygen may be needed. All ambulance and emergency care vehicles have oxygen cylinders; some athletic departments (especially in schools at high altitudes) may have an oxygen cylinder at the sideline at events. Most often the athlete is able to perfuse sufficiently with normal respiration, yet an athlete suffering from a head injury—or sometimes a cervical spine injury—may not be able to gain sufficient oxygen with normal breathing. Simple oxygen masks are the masks often provided along with the oxygen canister at the sideline at high-altitude contests. Injured patients do not always tolerate these masks well; but when in full control of their faculties, most athletes tolerate them very well.

Cardiac Equipment

In the 1980s and early 1990s, the public became aware of athletes who had suffered life-ending cardiac emergencies during participation. Because of these incidents, sports medicine teams, coaches, and administrators became more concerned with providing the training and equipment necessary for preventing cardiac emergencies during sport activity.

Most of the cardiac emergencies that occurred involved ventricular fibrillation or cardiac arrest. In the case of cardiac fibrillation, shock is required to reestablish normal heart rhythms. Similarly, if the heart stops as in cardiac arrest, a shock may be sufficient to restart the heart, but should not be employed until manual methods of resuscitation are attempted.

Some years ago, cardiac care was provided only by paramedics or hospital personnel. Today, many athletic trainers, coaches, and others who may be involved in a potential cardiac emergency (such as airline attendants) are able to provide cardiac monitoring and defibrillation using the AED, a portable monitor and defibrillator (see figure 8.16). These devices have verbal and visual step-by-step instructions for analysis of the heart's rhythm, application of the electrodes, and delivery of cardiac conversion techniques. Large companies are beginning to train employees in AED use and CPR and to provide AEDs throughout the workplace.

Availability of Equipment and Supplies in Athletic Facilities

Not all athletic facilities have sufficient funds to purchase all the equipment that would be needed for all sorts of medical emergencies. And not only is some of the equipment quite expensive; use of some items, such as the oropharyngeal airway, requires considerable skill.

Most emergency ambulance services provide a complete array of emergency care devices, as well as the personnel to operate them.

In communicating with the local providers of emergency services, you need to discuss the topic of equipment. If the ambulance crew wish your staff to provide initial management of the injured athlete, they may also suggest a vendor or even provide the equipment and training necessary to allow you to complete this level of care. Many times the EMS team will want to modify your equipment, such as a spine board, for easier application and handling to allow better care of athletes.

Maintenance of Equipment

All equipment used for emergency care of the injured athlete must be available and in proper condition for use when the need arises. Checking the equipment on a regular basis is essential to ensure its working order. Any time a piece of equipment is used, a designated staff member should check all supplies associated with it and make sure that all items are returned to their proper locations.

It is wise to inspect all emergency care equipment prior to each season, regardless of how often it was used during the previous season. Electrical equipment, such as semiautomatic defibrillators, should be professionally checked for power output, circuitry, and other functions. Equipment that is expendable (single use) should be discarded once it has been used and should be replaced immediately. Products such as vacuum splints should be tested to ensure against leaks or malfunctions of the pump apparatus.

Athletic Trainer's Kit

Depending on the sport, the emergencies will vary to some degree. In addition to the type of injury you are likely to encounter, you need to keep in mind any known preexisting conditions in any of the participants. In general, one must prepare for all types of emergencies; the following discussion may help you decide what equipment and supplies you will want to have available at an athletic practice or contest (see figure 8.17).

Certain equipment and supplies are needed just for head and neck trauma in collision sports. In collision sports, the risk of head and neck injury is fairly high. When a player hits their head hard enough to cause a concussion, it is wise to carefully examine the neck to make sure there is no significant damage there as well. Caring for a head or neck injury may require a spine board. It is not prudent to provide a spine board unless at least one person is present who is well trained in the transport of an injured patient. If staff are unfamiliar with the precautions needed to safely move a patient with a potential spinal cord injury, it is advisable to keep the athlete calm and protected in the same position in which he or she was found on the field. You need to care for the athlete until the ambulance arrives—keeping the person calm and quiet, making sure no other injuries exist (secondary survey), and protecting the person from shock. If other conditions exist, medical care should be given to minimize the pain and control any bleeding (see "Four Methods of Controlling Bleeding" on p. 284).

Full evaluation of the risks versus benefits of moving the athlete should be discussed with the local provider of ambulance care and the team physician. If the risks are numerous, it is best to rely on the EMT and paramedic crew to move the athlete and transport him or her to the medical facility.

Airway and cardiac emergencies pose an additional concern because they require immediate attention. All

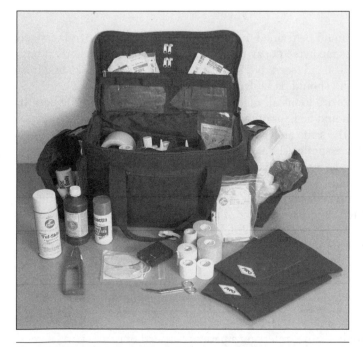

Figure 8.17 Athletic trainer's kit.

Four Methods of Controlling Bleeding

- Direct pressure on the wound
- Splinting/Bandaging and elevation of the extremity

- Pressure over the major supplying artery
- Tourniquet

Table 8.2

Emergency Care Equipment and Supplies to Be Available at All Athletic Sites

Emergency care equipment	Typical application purpose
Spine board	Immobilization of spine while on the field
Nonstretch straps	To secure athlete to the spine board
Stretcher	Spine board placed on stretcher for transport
Immobilization device	Head and neck stabilization padding and/or straps
Pocket mask	For rescue breathing
Airways	For team physician use in obtaining airway
Automated external defibrillator	For cardiac conversion
Sterile gauze, cotton, and bandages	For lacerations, abrasions, and other wounds
Rubber gloves	Universal Precautions for the treatment of open wounds
Splints and slings	For the treatment of fractures, dislocations, and sprains
Tape or elastic wrap	For securing bandages or splints

members of the coaching staff should be trained in CPR, as should all athletic trainers and assistants working with the sports medicine department. Pocket masks, airways, and, if possible, an AED are items to have at hand (see table 8.2). At least one pocket mask should be located in every emergency kit and should be replaced if it is ever used.

First aid and splinting supplies are items all medical kits should contain. Sterile cotton, gauze, and bandaging supplies should be kept on hand in case of lacerations. Several sets of rubber gloves should be kept in the same area as the bandaging supplies. Splints to be used to immobilize fractures and severe sprains should also be available and should be kept near the practice and contest sites. And, in the event of an injury to the upper extremity, a sling should be kept in the medical bag.

Other special emergency equipment may be selected according to the sport, the athletes (e.g., an athlete who has diabetes), and the location of medical assistance. Unless there is a functioning telephone on the sideline, a cellular phone should be kept in the medical bag. Emergency numbers and instructions for calling 911 should be posted or located near each telephone.

REFERRING THE ATHLETE FOR FURTHER CARE

As any health care provider should realize, referring a patient for further care is part of good practice. One of the most important aspects of athletic training is understanding the limits to our skills and knowing other medical professionals who could continue the primary care we have been able to provide. Establishing the protocol for referring the athlete is covered in the book in this series titled *Management Strategies in Athletic Training, Third Edition.* Two aspects of referring athletes for further care are the most important for everyone to understand: documenting your observations and care and communicating those thoughts and procedures to the medical professional.

Standard Nomenclature for Athletic Injuries

Communication is the keystone of a well-conducted sports medicine program. The fact that little can be accomplished by one individual is what makes a team approach critical. When personnel are added to the medical care team, communication among team members, as well as from the sports medicine department to outside providers or consumers, becomes increasingly important.

Each member of the medical services team should give full attention to the accurate and timely reporting of medical findings and also should supply clear and complete medical information when communicating with other health care providers.

Medical Terminology

There is no greater frustration than to read a medical note on a patient only to find unfamiliar medical terminology. Readers in this situation may wonder whether the problem is their own lack of knowledge or the writer's use of nonstandard expressions. Whatever the case, the final outcome is a failure in communication. It is wise to become familiar with the names of special tests that are used to establish clinical signs; yet if one refers to a test that others do not know about, the significance may be lost.

In communicating about clinical signs and symptoms it is perhaps most important to first understand the difference between a sign and a symptom. In general, a sign is a concrete finding that could be quantified and objectively evaluated. A symptom, on the other hand, is a more subjective finding that the patient would report.

Clinical signs of a problem would include measurable findings such as a temperature, the range of motion of a joint, the amount of blood, the size or angle of a deformity, or even the amount or separation between bones as determined in a stress test of a joint. Regardless of the location or nature of the problem, findings that can be quantified are considered "signs" indicating a particular condition or pathology.

Symptoms are things the patient reports to the clinician or physician. An athlete may report a feeling of instability by saying "my knee gives out." Feelings of fullness upon bending a joint may be indicative of edema or swelling. The word "symptom" is defined in *Stedman's Concise Medical Dictionary* (1997) as "any . . . departure from the normal in function, appearance or sensation, experienced by the patient and indicative of disease."

Medical terminology is often quite different from "ordinary" language. Students of sports medicine typically build their vocabulary of medical terms slowly unless they make a concerted effort to memorize a textbook of terms.

Clarity and Accuracy in Reporting

Often students learn "shorthand" for common terms during their classroom work in athletic training. Sometimes instructors present the shortened version or abbreviation along with the whole word or phrase in order to help students learn. But written alone and without sufficient context, the shortened version may be meaningless.

When recording information on a patient's chart or in any other type of document, it is best to remember: "If in doubt, write it out." If you are not sure a particular abbreviation has one well-known interpretation, avoid abbreviating. When writing a medical report or notes, you may be able to take the time to refer to a medical dictionary that lists commonly accepted abbreviations; these you can assume others will understand easily.

To see how abbreviations stand in the way of comprehension, read the following and try to decipher the meaning: Rbt. c/o acute pain in the L. knee following practice on 4/3/99. He reports previous ACL injury in high school FB. ROM and MMT are WNL. No swelling

Commonly Accepted Abbreviations

activities of daily living: ADL

anteroposterior: AP or A/P

approximately: approx

bis in die (Latin: twice daily): bid

blood pressure: BP

cum (Latin: with): w/ or c

cervical vertebrae (level): C1, C2, . . . C7

complains of: c/o

continue: cont

discontinue: dc

diagnosis: Dx

examination: ex

gastrointestinal: GI

intravenous: IV

left: L or Ⓛ

lumbar vertebrae (level): L1, L2, . . . L5

left lower quadrant (abdomen): LLQ

last menstrual period: LMP

level of consciousness: LOC

left upper quadrant (abdomen): LUQ

negative: neg

nothing by mouth: NPO

operating room: OR

posteroanterior: PA or P/A

Physician's Desk Reference: PDR

pro re nata (Latin: as needed or desired): prn

four times a day: qid

right (direction or side): R orⓇ

red blood cell count: RBC

right lower quadrant (abdomen): RLQ

rule out: r/o

right upper quadrant (abdomen): RUQ

without: w/o or s

immediately: stat

symptoms: Sx

thoracic vertebrae (level): T1, T2, . . . T12

temperature: T

tablets: tab(s)

three times a day: tid

ointment (unguents): ung

white blood cell count: WBC

negative: −

female: F

male: M

pound or number: #

increase: ↑

decrease: ↓

greater than: >

less than: <

equal to: =

or discoloration are present. +1 Lachman, + Pivot Shift. MCL/LCL & PCL are normal as compared to R. knee.

In other words, Robert complains of acute pain in the left knee following practice on 4/3/99. He reports previous anterior cruciate ligament injury in high school football. Range of motion and manual muscle testing are within normal limits. No swelling or discoloration is present. Grade One Lachman (test) is found (is positive); there is (+) a pivot shift. The medial collateral ligament, lateral collateral ligament, and posterior cruciate ligament are all equal to the ligaments of the right knee.

Remember that words are how we communicate. If the words and terms you choose are unclear because of lack of precision, or incorrect spelling, or because an abbreviation is not "standard," communication may suffer. In all cases of medical record keeping, writers need to keep in mind the possibility that some day their words will be used in court. Be sure you write clearly and accurately in reporting your clinical findings.

TRANSMISSION OF BLOODBORNE PATHOGENS

As an athletic trainer, you always have to guard against disease transmission in athletics. In chapter 2, we discussed bloodborne pathogens in general, but here we'll take a closer look.

Any infectious agent found in human blood is considered a bloodborne pathogen. With use of Universal Precautions, the risk of exposure to all bloodborne pathogens is controlled. **Hepatitis B** (Hep B) is a bloodborne pathogen virus said to be more tenacious and more highly contagious than human immunodeficiency virus (HIV). The fear of hepatitis B transmission is not nearly as great as that associated with HIV. Precautions taken to prevent hepatitis B virus (HBV) infection vary according to the concerns of hospital staff. Most, however, feel that the low morbidity associated with hepatitis B is the major reason this pathogen does not elicit the fears that HIV does.

In all organizations in the United States, bloodborne pathogen training is required for all employees who have the potential of coming into contact with human blood. The team, school, clinic, or other facility must offer the hepatitis B vaccine to all persons with exposure potential. In addition to the inoculation, any worker who reports an incident with the potential of infection will receive immediate hepatitis B **prophylaxis** as further prevention against contracting the disease.

Considering the mere potential of exposure to bloodborne pathogens, one might feel a bit apprehensive in treating open wounds even with close attention to proper precautions. Every individual working in an environment (figure 8.18, for example) where there is potential for contact with another person's blood or body products can obtain, free of personal charge, the full series of HBV vaccinations. This program, established by the U.S. government, requires all employers to provide this opportunity to all employees who have this contact potential. The series of vaccination injections is well worth the time and minor discomfort when one considers the high potential for accidental exposure and the lifelong consequences of liver damage if hepatitis B is contracted through incidental exposure on the athletic field.

In addition to transmission of common bacteria or spores of an airborne virus, transmission of bloodborne pathogens has become an increasing concern. With the media coverage of **acquired** immunodeficiency syndrome (AIDS) and HIV, the general population has become increasingly aware of health practices to avoid disease transmission. People not falling into

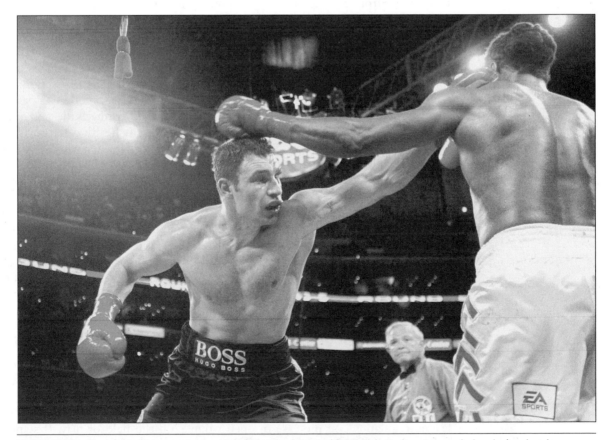

Figure 8.18 The risk of human immunodeficiency virus and hepatitis B virus transmission in boxing is greater than in other sports because there is often significant bleeding on both sides. Boxing is currently the only sport in which testing for human immunodeficiency virus is mandatory.

Further information on the Centers for Disease Control and Prevention, Universal Precautions, infectious diseases, and bloodborne pathogens can be found at Web site www.cdc.gov.

"high-risk" groups once thought themselves immune to the disease; many coaches and athletic trainers felt that they were in this "safe" category. However, when the flamboyant, ever personable National Basketball Association star Earvin "Magic" Johnson announced to the public that he was HIV positive, sport health care views changed. The announcement, and Johnson's subsequent retirement from the Los Angeles Lakers, served as a wake-up call to the entire athletic population. Young, strong athletes realized they were not "bulletproof"; they could contract diseases just like any other person. Concerns of teammates, coaches, and the sport health care providers soon surfaced. All persons working with athletes and any of those who come into bodily contact with others must be aware of the methods of transmission of HIV and other bloodborne pathogens and take all precautionary measures to avoid inadvertent transmission.

Potential Causes of Increased Risk

In an attempt to limit the risks of infection with a bloodborne pathogen, the Centers for Disease Control and Prevention recommends that blood and certain body fluids of all patients be considered potentially infectious. This assumption encourages individuals to take Universal Precautions, meaning that care should be routinely taken to prevent skin and mucous membranes from coming into contact with the patient's blood or with the body fluids listed in this section.

Blood and body fluids containing visible blood, semen, vaginal secretions, tissues, and bodily fluids such as **synovial fluid** are potentially infectious. Tears, nasal secretions, saliva, sputum, sweat, urine, feces, or vomit are not unless such bodily products contain visible blood.

Appropriate barriers include gloves, a mask, a gown, and eye protection. However, the Centers for Disease Control and Prevention also recognizes something as simple as a thick gauze pad, which may be used to cover a small spot of blood as long as the gauze is thick enough to prevent blood from soaking through and contacting the health care provider's skin.

Other precautions include frequent, regular hand washing when working with patients and disposal of any used sharp instruments into impervious ("sharps") containers. Those working with needles must remember that a needle should not be recapped by hand, but immediately disposed of into the sharps container. Sharps containers should be located throughout the health care facility to allow immediate access wherever wounds are treated. Additionally, soiled cloth or gauze should be disposed of into clearly marked biohazard bags. Gloves worn during the care of a patient must also be disposed of into the biohazard bag, and those bags must be closed and disposed of according to strict guidelines (see figure 8.19). The Occupational Safety and Health Association (**OSHA**) publishes guidelines for preventing occupational hazards as well as the National Athletic Trainers' Association guidelines for preventing transmission of bloodborne pathogens.

Increased Risk of Disease Transmission Due to Behaviors

In watching a televised game, viewers sometimes see the team physician or athletic trainer cleaning the bloody turf wound of a football player. Does the trainer wear gloves? Does the viewer see what happens to the soiled cloth or gauze?

The public attention to Universal Precautions serves to reinforce school, university, and league regulations on the care of open wounds on the field of play. If standards are not enforced, will they be practiced? All individuals owe it to themselves to practice the safest possible precautions in treating the broken skin of any patient. Without "Big Brother" watching, you and the patient may be the only ones to know if you did or did not practice Universal Precautions. You owe it to yourself and to your athlete to do so.

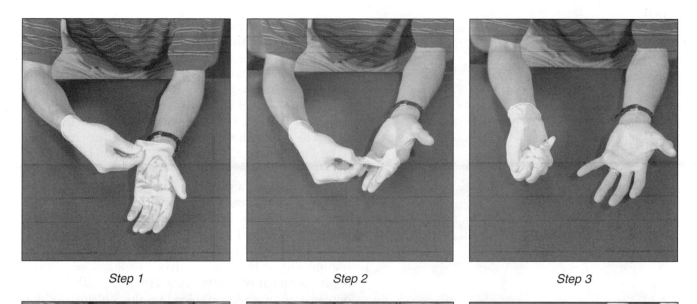

Step 1   Step 2   Step 3

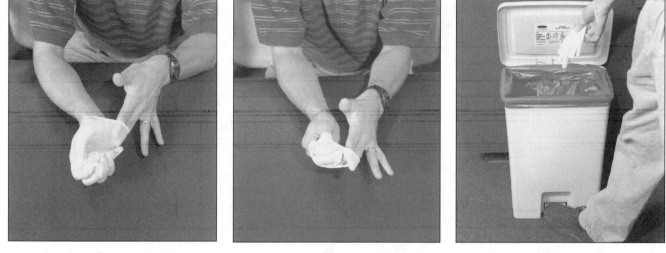

Step 4   Step 5   Step 6

Figure 8.19   Contaminated disposable gloves should be removed in the following systematic manner so that they do not contaminate the skin. Step 1: Use your dominant hand to grasp your nondominant hand at the palm. Step 2: Carefully pull off the glove of the nondominant hand. Step 3: Hold it in your dominant hand. Step 4: Work your nondominant hand under the palm side of the glove on the dominant hand. Step 5: Once the fingers of your nondominant hand are to the glove finger holes, slowly push the glove over the fingers of your dominant hand. Carefully pull the glove off. Step 6: Dispose of gloves in proper container.

Copies of any OSHA documents can be obtained online at www.OSHA.gov.

Transmission by Direct Physical Contact

Skin-to-skin contact with a person infected with HIV or HBV does not mean you will be automatically infected. In most cases, if the skin of the health care provider is closed and free of sores, the virus will have difficulty entering. If, however, you have an open sore on your finger, you must protect yourself and put on gloves before treating the wound.

In the case of a player coming off the court or field with a bleeding wound, you as the health care provider must think before you react. Even if the wound is bleeding heavily, you must take the time to get the proper supplies (see figure 8.20) and to glove before touching

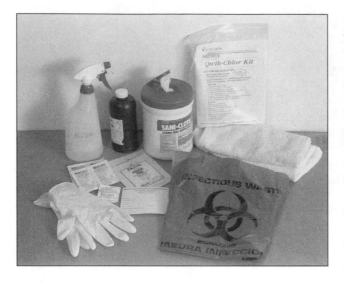

Figure 8.20 A biohazard kit contains disposable paper towels, a squirt bottle filled with a 1:10 bleach-to-water solution, hydrogen peroxide (to clean blood off of clothing), assorted sizes of disposable gloves, disposable gauze, two small cloth towels (for larger spills or wounds), and a red biohazard bag.

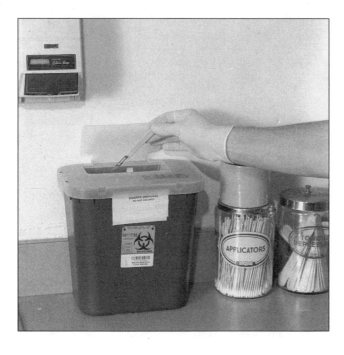

Figure 8.21 The risk of human immunodeficiency virus transmission can be greatly reduced by careful handling of contaminated needles and blades. Dispose of sharps in a puncture-resistant container.

the wound. As the athletic trainer for the team, you may want to hand the athlete a gauze pad—the athlete can use the pad as a compress while you prepare your supplies and don your gloves. During the time it takes you to prepare, the bleeding may be under control.

Too often we find a bloody towel at the sideline of a football game. Who used the towel to stop the bleeding? What should be done with the towel? Use the proper supplies, or if the wound is so large that a gauze pad would not control the bleeding, be sure to dispose of whatever cloth you used in the same way you would if you had used a gauze pad.

Players who fall and suffer a laceration or abrasion to the skin may not realize that the injury has occurred until the uniform is soiled with blood. Contact between the soiled clothing and another person's skin may not normally cause transmission of HIV, yet this type of contact has a much higher potential of transmitting HBV. Regardless of the potential of transmission, blood on the athlete's clothing should be washed off or the clothing changed prior to return to play. Products are currently on the market that will effectively kill both HIV and HBV to prevent transmission. These products also change the color of the blood from the bright red associated with fresh blood, thus decreasing the apprehension of other team members and opponents.

Transmission by Direct Contact With Blood or Body Fluids

Contact between the health care provider and blood or at-risk body fluids is as high a risk factor as is currently known. Typically, these exposures occur when a health care worker is attempting to recap a needle used on an infected patient. In athletic health care, the needle may have been used to drain a bloody blister on the athlete's foot. The needle-stick penetrates the skin of the athletic trainer, producing blood. The chance of transmitting either HIV or HBV is quite high in this situation if the patient happens to be positive for either of these two bloodborne pathogens. The best defense against this type of transmission is to avoid recapping any needle used in the care of an athlete's wound. You do not need to recap, because the procedure is typically over—the needle-stick occurs after the job is done. Dispose of the needle, without recapping, into the sharps container (see figure 8.21).

Since direct contact with blood or body fluids is a potential risk, any incident must be reported. A very simple form that may be helpful if your employer does not have one is the "Report of Exposure to Human Blood or Other Potentially Infectious Materials" on pages 291–292. It is much better to make the report and follow up with proper testing and observation than to let the fear of the unknown hang over your head.

Report of Exposure to Human Blood or Other Potentially Infectious Materials

Exposed Employee

1. Wash the exposed area thoroughly. Use soap for skin; use only water if eyes, nose, or mouth.

2. Notify your supervisor of this exposure.

3. Please complete this section. If you have any questions, please ask your supervisor.

Name: _____ Title: _____

Home Address: _____ Home Phone: _____

City: _____ State: ____ Zip: _____ Work Phone: _____

On _____ at _____ AM/PM, at _____ ,
   (date)   (location)

I received an exposure to: [ ] blood [ ] other potentially infectious body fluid (specify, if possible):

_____

This material came into contact with my:

❑ right/left/both eye(s) ❑ nose ❑ mouth ❑ cut/scratched/damaged/punctured skin

This exposure occurred while I _____

_____

_____

I was wearing: ❑ gloves ❑ protective clothing ❑ face protection ❑ protective eyewear

Immediately after I received the exposure, I:

❑ washed the exposed area thoroughly ❑ reported the exposure to my supervisor

I ❑ have ❑ have not been vaccinated against the hepatitis B virus.

I ❑ can ❑ cannot identify the individual to whose blood or body fluid I was exposed:

Name: _____

Address: _____ Phone: _____

4. When you are finished, sign and date this section and give this report to your supervisor.

5. Promptly report to the health care professional to whom your supervisor refers you.

Signature of Exposed Employee _____ Date _____

(continued)

Report of Exposure to Human Blood
or Other Potentially Infectious Materials *(continued)*

Exposed Employee _____ Exposure Date _____

Supervisor

1. Confirm that the exposed employee has washed the exposed area and has completed the form as completely as possible.

2. Complete the following information. If you have any questions, please ask your unit head.

Your name: _____ Title: _____ Phone: _____

On _____ at _____ AM/PM, the above-named employee reported this exposure to me:
    (date)

❑ as described above

❑ as follows: _____

_____

According to unit records, the exposed employee:

❑ has received ❑ 1   ❑ 2   ❑ 3 hepatitis B vaccinations

❑ has not received hepatitis B vaccination

❑ has   ❑ has not received training in Occupational Exposure to Bloodborne Pathogens

Source individual identification ❑ cannot ❑ can be confirmed. Complete a Source Individual Identification form.

I referred the exposed employee to the following health care professional:

❑ _____
    (list local health care professional here)

❑ _____
    (list local health care professional here)

Signature of Supervisor _____ Date _____

3. Photocopy this form for your unit's records.

4. Send the original form and a copy of the employee's task description with the employee to the health care professional.

Reprinted from Zeigler 1997.

Transmission by Indirect Contact

Indirect contact with an HIV- or HBV-positive patient is not likely to cause transmission of the disease. Indirect contact includes such actions as drinking from the same cup as the infected individual or using the same towel to dry your hands. Although it is possible, even HBV is unlikely to survive the time between contacts; and even if it did, the virus would have to be present in the form of blood or other specific bodily fluids, and this in and of itself would be an unlikely circumstance for indirect contact.

Changes in The Perception of Risk

Suppose that you, a health care provider, are asked to debride the wound of an athlete. You don gloves and a mask, and through your attention and care, the task is completed very safely. Now suppose that you are performing the same procedure on an athlete known to be positive for HIV. Do the precautions change? Does your anxiety? Now reverse the two positions and imagine you are the athlete. You observe as the Universal Precautions are performed; your wound is covered, and you feel comfortable. But if you knew that the health care provider was HIV positive, would you request that someone else work on your open wound? Often perception is the reason people wish to keep the knowledge of their medical condition private. The stigma associated with HIV and AIDS is so firmly established in our society that people have fears about how others will treat them should the diagnosis be known. As health care providers we must remember that every patient, every athlete, deserves the best medical care you can provide. Exercising the proper precautions enables the health care practitioner to provide the quality of care the patient deserves while protecting both the provider and the patient.

Although OSHA has issued recommendations for preventing transmission of bloodborne pathogens (HIV and hepatitis B) from health care workers to patients, no federal policy or legislation is currently in force to restrict HIV-positive health care workers from practicing. The feeling that HIV-positive health care providers must reveal their HIV-**seropositive** status continues to be heavily burdened by legal and ethical issues.

SUMMARY

1. *Identify the appropriate first aid procedures for a variety of injuries and illnesses.*

   In general, first aid procedures are intended to supplement normal physiology until the individual's system takes over (as in CPR) or to stop or control the progression of injurious conditions (such as bleeding). When the individual's heart, lungs, and circulatory system are not affected, first aid provides care for the particular pathology presented such as immobilizing fractures, splinting, sprained joints, padding contusions, etc.

2. *Explain the ABCs of emergency care.*

   A is for airway and means that the air passage is open and clear so that the victim should be able to breathe. B is for breathing and means that the air is moving in and out of the lungs without resistance or compromise. C, for circulation, means that the heart is beating and the blood is assumed to be moving throughout the body. Once these ABCs are identified as satisfactory, evaluation and care can be directed to other areas.

3. *Identify the main features of an emergency care plan for an athletic team.*

   Game and practice coverage: Outline the duties of those regularly in attendance. Anticipate the personnel who might be available, delineate duties, and discuss contingency plans. Emergency procedure steps: Know what will be done. Outline the steps to be taken in various emergency situations. Communication systems: Know how to contact EMS. Ensure that there is a working telephone near all practice and game facilities. Have posted, on or next to each telephone, appropriate emergency numbers and directions for calling for an ambulance. Equipment: Appropriate emergency care equipment and supplies must be available and in proper condition for use. Include emergency equipment on the annual inventory and in the ordering process. Emergency care facilities: Establish open lines of communication with the nearby emergency care facilities to allow more expedient care of individuals if needed. Transportation: Establish the methods available for transportation of an ill or injured individual. Contact local ambulance companies to establish on-site ambulance service if desired. Personnel training: Training and retraining of all personnel need to occur periodically. Record keeping: Establish a system of recording all injuries and the treatment provided for each participant.

4. *Explain methods for obtaining consent for various levels and situations of treatment.*

   Although in an emergency, consent is not required before one provides life-saving treatment, all non-emergency treatment requires the patient's consent. If the patient is under the legal age of consent, a parent or guardian must sign on the patient's behalf. There must be proper written documentation indicating the problem, the nature of treatment, the location and provider of the treatment, and any foreseeable complications to that treatment; and the signature on the consent form is the indication that approval for treatment has been given.

5. *Identify the members of the EMS team and their roles in helping an injured athlete.*

   The EMS team comprises four levels of providers. The first is the "first responder." This individual is usually a person who was in the immediate vicinity when the accident occurred. Although the first responder is not a recognized member of the EMS staff, this individual serves as the gateway into the emergency care system. The EMT (or EMT-B) is the basic level of emergency care technician. This EMS crew member can provide immediate care including CPR and advanced first aid. In most states, the EMT is trained in the PASG, AED, epinephrine autoinjector, and inhaler bronchodilators. The EMT-B will attempt to stabilize the patient sufficiently to allow safe transportation to a medical care facility. If the EMT-B cannot sufficiently stabilize the patient, this person will call for further EMS assistance. The EMT-I (intermediate) has additional hours of training in the areas of cardiac care and additional areas of expertise including, but not limited to, endotracheal intubation, ALS such as IV therapy, and interpretation of cardiac rhythms. This professional may be able to render treatment to allow a more involved patient to be stabilized enough for transportation to a medical facility. The final level of EMS provider is the EMT-P (paramedic); this person can provide IV therapy, advanced pharmacology, cardiac monitoring, defibrillation, and advanced airway maintenance.

6. *Discuss the importance of Universal Precautions.*

   Since the transmission of bloodborne pathogens has lifelong ramifications, and since it is virtually impossible to know the medical history and HIV status of every individual, it is best to take full precautions with every patient.

CRITICAL THINKING QUESTIONS

1. You have been asked to establish the emergency medical coverage for a 10K run that your school is sponsoring. The course is entirely contained on your campus. Using a campus map, draw a course (regardless if you know the actual distance around campus) for the race to follow. On that map, draw in any aid stations and the location of any emergency medical station(s), taking into consideration the climate you live in and the type of runners you will attract. Allow, at minimum, two stations. Suggest ways to obtain coverage of the aid stations you designate.

2. You recognize that you have very little help in the medical coverage of your sport teams and begin to think of options you would have if an emergency arose. Make suggestions for choosing individuals you could train for the potential emergency situation. Give your rationale for selecting those people for training.

3. You have been notified that one of your athletes has been diagnosed as HIV positive but are not told which athlete it is. You ask and are told that this information is confidential and that you should treat all athletes as if they are infected. Discuss the pros and cons of this situation from the perspective of infection control.

4. You are working in the situation described in question 3, with the softball team. The pitcher takes a line drive right in the face and is bleeding profusely. Explain the steps you would take in managing this situation. Include the steps taken to control the bleeding as well as any other evaluation you think should be conducted.

5. One of the girls on your college track team has diabetes. She has shared with you some of her fears and concerns. You ask her if you can share this information with the other team members and she gives you the permission to do so. Design a lecture for the team members that will help them recognize the signs, symptoms, and complications of diabetic problems.

6. Visit your local fire department and interview the EMT or EMT-P regarding emergency protocols they are required to follow in transporting an injured patient. Compare and contrast the EMT/EMT-P protocols with the procedures of injury management followed by your athletic training staff (interview a member of the staff if necessary).

7. Design an athletic trainer's kit for the coverage of a basketball tournament (do not include prophylactic taping). Compare and contrast the contents of that kit with the contents you would include in a kit for the coverage of a swim meet.

CITED SOURCE

Stedman's concise medical dictionary. 1997. Baltimore: Williams & Wilkins.

ADDITIONAL READINGS

Editorial. 1994. Establish communication with EMTs. *NATA News* 6: 4-9.
Kleinknecht v. Gettysburg College. 786 F. Supp. 449 (M.D. Pa. 1992).
Kleinknecht v. Gettysburg College. 989 F. 2d 1360 (3d Cir. 1993).

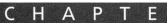
Nutritional Aspects of Health and Performance

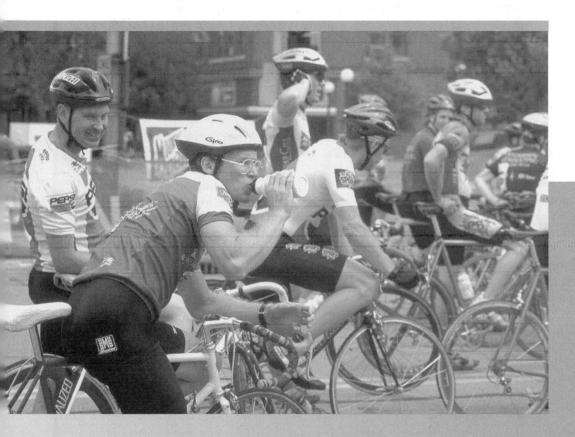

Objectives

After reading this chapter, the student should be able to do the following:

1. Discuss the recommended dietary intake of carbohydrates, fats, and proteins and explain how one would calculate the caloric content of a meal or diet.

2. Explain the role of carbohydrates as an energy source and list the types of carbohydrates found in foods.

3. Discuss the recommended amount of water that should be consumed daily and explain the suitable alternatives to plain drinking water for replenishing body fluids.

4. Explain the difference between "good" and "bad" cholesterol and suggest the method one might use to minimize the negative effects of cholesterol.

5. Discuss the concepts of a "pre-event meal" versus "pre-event nutrition" and explain why some people may feel they are able to eat anything they want prior to competition.

It was September, and Retesha was excited for the end of the month to come because that was the start of tryouts for the school's lacrosse team. This was Retesha's first year in college, and classes were going pretty well. Adjusting to life away from home was difficult at times, but it was lots of fun meeting new people and learning new things. But now, the tryouts.

After the first two days of drills and situation practice, Retesha was ready for it all to be over.

"These practices are wearing me out," she mentioned to another student who was trying out for the team too.

"You think this is bad? Just wait. If you make the team, it gets worse. I've heard other players say the practices last nearly three hours. We've just been going half that long!" her new friend responded.

Retesha was worried. Not only was she worried about making the team because she felt so drained of energy by the end of the practice, she worried about her grades. After the practice she hardly had the energy to do her assignments, much less open a book to read.

After talking with her roommate, Retesha decided to take advantage of the services offered by the student health center. During a break between classes she walked to the student health center and told the receptionist why she was there. The receptionist suggested she see the physician and scheduled her for an appointment right away.

After reviewing Retesha's medical history, physical exam, and blood test results, the doctor reported, "Everything appears fine. But," he said, "I'd really like you to see the people in the nutrition counseling center before we give up on this problem."

Retesha went down the hall to the nutrition counseling center and was immediately referred to one of the nutritionists. After a review of Retesha's eating habits, the nutritionist suggested that Retesha start looking carefully at her food choices. They discussed the food options around campus, and Retesha left the nutrition counseling center with some great ideas of ways to eat better and a little homework from the nutritionist: keeping a food diary and recording the types and duration of all activities throughout the day.

After the second meeting with the nutritionist, Retesha was convinced that the changes she had made in her diet gave her not only more energy during the tryouts, but also a renewed energy to do her reading and studying after practices. She made the team and found the three hours of practice a great break from homework!

At the end of the year, Retesha was given the team's Most Improved Player award. What an honor, and what a great feeling to have others see how much improvement there had been. In her speech at the awards dinner, Retesha thanked the coach for giving her the chance and the nutritionist for giving her the energy to play. Retesha was convinced that without those changes in her diet, she would never have made it through the year.

Nutrition has become a concern of almost every physically active individual. The concept that a diet is a program for losing weight is as far from fact as the generalization that athletes should not have to think about the foods that they eat. Good nutrition should be viewed as a method to provide the body with the best tools for growth and development as well as an aid to recovery when injury or illness strikes. When the physically active individual fails to consider the nutritional demands of increased activity levels, both performance and health suffer. Understanding the role that nutrition plays in keeping the body healthy is as important as understanding the need for a regular workout schedule. Nutrition should be viewed as an asset to performance. Every physically active person must attempt to understand the effect of nutrition on performance and health. Good nutrition can help the physically active person prevent injury and illness as well as help improve performance.

WHY STUDY NUTRITION?

It seems reasonable that a competitive athlete would want to employ as many techniques as possible in the quest for excellence. In this age of athletic competition, the skill levels of the participants are so closely matched that the athlete's nutritional practices make the difference between winning and losing. Not only will nutrition help the athlete with performance issues, it is imperative that the physically active individual understand the demands that athletic participation places on the body's fluid and fuel supplies. Trying to win at sports with poor nutrition is similar to a race car driver's trying to win a race using low-grade or limited fuel sources.

BASIC NUTRITIONAL NEEDS OF ATHLETES

The basic nutritional needs of the physically active person are quite similar to those of any other individual. A well-balanced diet with protein, fat, and carbohydrate at every meal is the key to both optimal performance and health (see table 9.1).

Table 9.1
Typical Sources of Carbohydrates, Proteins, and Fats

High-carbohydrate foods	Protein-rich foods	High-fat foods
Breads	Meat, fish, poultry, eggs	Fats and oils (used in cooking)
Fruit juices	Dairy products	Meat, fish, poultry
Dried fruits	Cereals	Dairy products
Fresh (or canned) fruits	Fruits, vegetables	Eggs
Grains, pastas, starches	Beans, peas, nuts	Beans

To determine if you are meeting the criteria of a well-balanced diet, first you must understand how to calculate the total calories (energy) consumed and determine the percentages of energy sources provided. Both carbohydrates and proteins provide about 4 calories (energy) per gram, while fats contribute 9 calories per gram. To calculate the total calories in a meal, you need to know how many grams of protein, fat, and carbohydrates are in each item. Multiply the number of grams of each energy source by its specific factor (4 or 9) and add the values of the three energy sources together. This total is the total caloric (Kcal) content of the item. Add all the items consumed in a meal and you

An Example of Calorie Calculations for a Meal

Description of food	Fat (g)	Carb (g)	Protein (g)
1 plain bagel	2	38	7
1 oz cream cheese	10	1	2
1 cup 2% milk	5	12	8
Total grams	17	51	17

Here are the calculations for a meal of one plain bagel with cream cheese and an 8-oz glass of 2% milk.

To calculate the calories for this meal, multiply the number of grams of fat by 9, the number of grams of carbohydrate by 4, and the number of grams of protein by 4:

$$17 \text{ g fat} \times 9 \text{ Kcal/g} = 153 \text{ Kcal}$$
$$51 \text{ g carb} \times 4 \text{ Kcal/g} = 204 \text{ Kcal}$$
$$17 \text{ g protein} \times 4 \text{ Kcal/g} = 68 \text{ Kcal}$$

This calculation gives you 425 Kcals total.

can calculate the calories consumed in that meal. Adding all foods consumed during a full day can provide the daily intake. If you average several days' intake, you should come close to the average daily caloric consumption.

Generally, for physically active individuals, 60% of total calories should be derived from carbohydrate foods, 30% or less from fat, and 10% to 15% from protein (see table 9.2). Athletes benefit from a fairly high consumption of carbohydrates because the storage for carbohydrates is glycogen, and glycogen is the source the muscle depends on for energy. Physically active and competing individuals need higher levels of carbohydrates to provide

Table 9.2
Example of Approximately 60/25/15 Meal (60% Carbohydrates, 25% Fats, 15% Protein)

Food item (size)	Calories	Protein	Fat	Carbohydrate
Breakfast				
English muffin with margarine (1 tsp)	190	6	5	30
Banana (1)	105	1	1	27
Yoplait yogurt, fruit flavored (1 serving)	190	8	3	32
Orange juice, frozen-reconstituted (1 cup)	112	2	0	27
Lunch				
Turkey breast (2 slices)	47	10	1	0
Butterhead lettuce (2 leaves)	2	0	0	0
Whole wheat bread (2 slices)	135	3	1	28
Mustard (1 tsp)	4	0	0	0
Romaine lettuce (1 cup)	10	<1	<1	1
Raw broccoli flowers (1/2 cup)	12	1	0	2
Raw cauliflower (1/2 cup)	12	1	0	2
French dressing (5 tbsp)	290	0	22	23
Peach (1)	37	1	0	10
Snack				
Grapes (1 cup)	116	1	1	31
Dinner				
Baked potato (1) with margarine (1 tbsp)	364	6	11	61
Beef round, broiled (3 oz)	162	25	6	0
Steamed broccoli (1 cup)	44	5	1	8
Snack				
Popcorn, popped plain with margarine (1 tsp)	103	2	5	14
Totals				
Grams		73g	58g	296g
Calories	1,935	292	522	1,184
Percent of total calories		15%	25%	60%

the fuel (glycogen) for workouts and competition. Additionally, physically active people do need slightly more protein (about 0.9 to 1.34 g of protein per pound of body weight per day) than the nonathletic individual (0.8 g of protein per pound of body weight per day). When the physically active person follows a well-balanced diet and consumes adequate calories to meet the energy demands of the sport, he or she can usually obtain the additional protein needed. Many of the foods that contain high amounts of necessary carbohydrates (e.g., breads, pasta, and cereals) also contribute to the protein goals.

FLUID NEEDS FOR ACTIVE INDIVIDUALS

In addition to a well-balanced food intake, physically active people must pay close attention to their fluid intake. Some people have the misconception that soft drinks contribute to the goal of providing the body with fluid. Actually, some soft drinks can contribute to fluid loss. The caffeine in many soft drinks acts as a diuretic and depletes your body of fluids. Drinking these beverages increases the need for water. The body's need for fluid is best satisfied by water unless specific electrolytes or carbohydrates are also needed. As a general rule, the average person should consume eight 8-oz glasses of water each day (64 oz). Active people require even more water to make up for the water lost in perspiration. Unfortunately, thirst cannot be used to indicate your need for water. By the time you feel thirsty, you are already slightly dehydrated.

Most people tend to drink more of a particular fluid if it tastes good. If the water from a drinking fountain has a bad odor or taste, you'll tend not to drink it. This comes into play in efforts to get physically active people to drink more fluids. Because of the taste factor, sport drinks are often preferred even if there is little or no need for the extra carbohydrates or electrolytes. Take care to ensure that the concentration of carbohydrates is low enough (less than 7%) to allow rapid intestinal absorption if people are using sport drinks for hydration

---

Sweat Rate Calculation

To calculate sweat rate, you'll need a few measurements. First subtract body weight (in grams) after exercise from the body weight before exercise. This gives you the difference in body weight (DBW). Next, measure total drink volume in milliliters (DV) consumed during exercise. Then measure the urine volume (UV) in milliliters.

$$\text{sweat loss (SL)} = DBW + DV - UV$$

$$\text{sweat rate (ml/hr)} = SL \div \text{duration of exercise (in hours)}$$

For example, Retesha weighed in before practice at 120 lb; following practice she weighed again and found she weighed only 118 lb. During practice she consumed the entire contents of two sport bottles, each containing 1 L water (total of 2 L or 2,000 ml). The practice lasted 2 hr, and after practice Retesha emptied her bladder into a special cup for measuring urine and found that she had eliminated 300 ml. The calculations would be as follows:

pre-practice weight (120 lb × 453.6)	54,432.0 g
postpractice weight (118 lb × 452.6)	− 53,524.8 g

DBW = 907.2 g

DV = 2,000 ml

UV = 300 ml

(Note that 1 ml of water is approximately 1 g.)

Thus sweat loss = 907.2 ml + 2,000 ml − 300 ml = 2,607.2 ml / practice session or sweat rate = 2,607.2 ml / 2 hr = 1,307.2 ml / hr or 1.3 L/hr during physical activity. Ideally, a flavored sport drink with 6% carbohydrates (60 g carbohydrate per liter of drink) is well tolerated and will aid in replenishing body fluids as well as providing an additional energy source.

Every physically active person should establish his or her own fluid replacement schedule based on that person's individual sweat rate (see p. 301), exercise parameters (availability of rest breaks and fluid; duration of exercise; and exercise intensity), environmental factors, and degree of acclimatization. People unaccustomed to exercise in certain environmental conditions usually require more frequent rest breaks and a greater intake of fluid than indicated by the sweat rate alone. Those who are acclimatized may be able to consume fluids at a rate equal to or slightly higher than the sweat rate without compromising performance. A general rule is that fluids should be consumed prior to the event as well as during the event, and also until about an hour or more following the event.

CALORIC DEMANDS OF ACTIVE INDIVIDUALS

The major nutritional need of the active individual is increased calories. The obvious reason for the increased need for calories is the increased use of calories as energy to perform. When the number of calories consumed in the diet is lower than the number of calories burned throughout the day, weight loss will result. On the other hand, if the number of calories consumed is greater than the number of calories burned, weight gain will result. Depending on the sport and the athlete's role on the team or in the sport, body weight may be important. A lineman on the football team may be able to gain weight and still perform very well in his position; the distance runner carrying extra pounds may suffer greatly from the added weight.

THE FOOD GUIDE PYRAMID

The Food Guide Pyramid is a system designed by the United States Department of Agriculture (USDA) to teach people to eat a balanced diet from a variety of food groups without counting calories or other nutrients (see figure 9.1). The USDA expanded the original four food groups to six and expanded the number of servings to meet the caloric needs of most persons. The current recommendations include

- 3 to 5 servings of vegetables (serving size: approximately 1/2 cup);
- 2 to 4 servings of fruits (serving size: one medium fruit or 1/2 cup);
- 2 to 3 servings of dairy products (serving size: 6 oz milk, 1 container yogurt, or 3 oz cheese);
- 6 to 11 servings of bread, cereal, rice, and pasta (serving size: 1 slice, 1/2 cup);
- 2 to 3 servings of meat, poultry, fish, tofu, meat substitutes, dried beans, eggs, and nuts (serving size: 3 oz); and
- sparing use of fats, oils, and sweets.

The size of a serving in this system is provided for each food group and is included on the labels of the products we buy in the grocery store. This pyramid is quite similar to the exchange list that people with diabetes use as a guide in food selection and nutrition.

The diabetic exchange list is available from your local chapter of the American Diabetes Association. You can also find the USDA Food Guide Pyramid and other nutrition information at www.nal.usda.gov/fnic.

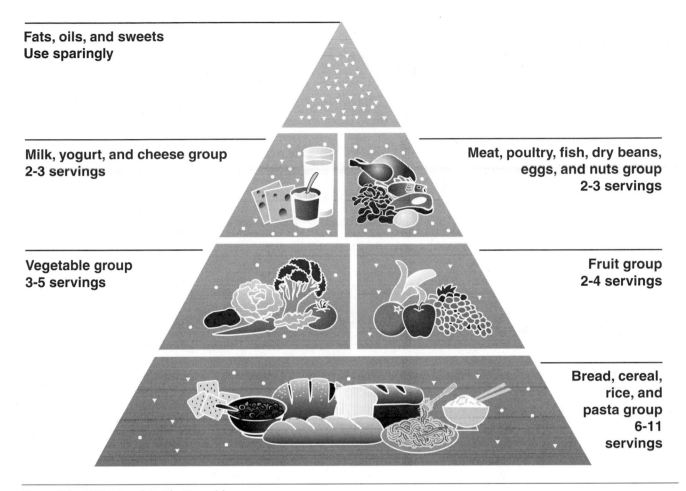

**Fats, oils, and sweets
Use sparingly**

**Milk, yogurt, and cheese group
2-3 servings**

**Meat, poultry, fish, dry beans,
eggs, and nuts group
2-3 servings**

**Vegetable group
3-5 servings**

**Fruit group
2-4 servings**

**Bread, cereal,
rice, and
pasta group
6-11
servings**

Figure 9.1 USDA Food Guide Pyramid.

Carbohydrates in the Diet

Since carbohydrates are such an important source of energy for working muscles, it should be easy to understand why at least 60% of the calories in an active individual's diet should come from carbohydrates. Some foods may be high in carbohydrates but also high in dietary fat. It is important for people to distinguish carbohydrate calories from fat calories when consuming a combined food. Menu items high in carbohydrates and low in fat include breads, grains (brown rice, oats, barley, etc.), pastas, vegetables, fruits, fruit juices, and juice drinks. Muscles replenish stored carbohydrates most efficiently within the first 2 hr following exercise. Therefore, the active person should begin to replenish his or her carbohydrate stores as soon as possible after exercise and then again a few hours later.

Because carbohydrates are such an important source of energy for short-duration or intense exercise, it is wise to understand the foods that supply the needed nutrients. Carbohydrates can be classified as monosaccharides (fructose, galactose, or glucose), disaccharides (in which two or more of the monosaccharides are chemically linked), or polysaccharides (hundreds or thousands of linked monosaccharides). Simple (monosaccharides and disaccharides) and

Table 9.3
Types of Carbohydrates

Carbohydrate class	Type	Source
Monosaccharides (simple carbohydrates)	Fructose	Fruit sugar
	Galactose	
	Glucose	Blood sugar
Disaccharides (simple carbohydrates)	Sucrose (glucose + fructose)	Table sugar
	Lactose (glucose + galactose)	Milk sugar
	Maltose (glucose + glucose)	
Polysaccharides (complex carbohydrates)	Amylose (straight chain of glucose)	Starchy foods like bread, potatoes, corn
	Amylopectins (branched chain of glucose)	

complex carbohydrates (polysaccharides) are also terms used to describe the types of carbohydrates. Both are outlined in table 9.3.

Different types of carbohydrates are composed of different combinations of monosaccharides. During digestion, carbohydrates are broken down into their component monosaccharides. This process occurs to a limited degree in the mouth and stomach, but most of the digestion happens in the small intestine. In the small intestine, enzymes from the pancreas (insulin) break the large carbohydrates into fructose, galactose, and, mainly, glucose. After the breakdown, galactose and glucose leave the mucosa of the intestine by a process called active transport, which requires energy. Fructose can pass through the mucosal membrane by diffusion (no energy required) as long as the concentration gradient is low on the opposite side of the membrane.

Once in the blood, the monosaccharides enter the bloodstream and progress to the liver. The liver converts the fructose and galactose to glucose or another product of glucose metabolism. Glucose is stored in the liver in the form of glycogen. Glycogen can also be transported and stored in the muscle, with the kidneys and intestines adding yet other minor storage sites. With up to 10% of its weight as glycogen, the liver has the highest glycogen content of any body tissue. These stores of glycogen can be quickly converted to glucose for use in most body tissues. Muscle glycogen is only used by working muscles because of a lack of specific enzymes needed to convert the glycogen for use in other tissues.

According to nutritional researchers, although one might assume that simple carbohydrates are absorbed most quickly, digestion and absorption do not happen at the same rate for all carbohydrates in a particular grouping. Nutritionists working with persons who have diabetes have used the glycemic index to evaluate the rise in blood glucose following ingestion of food (see table 9.4). This same concept of the glycemic index has been applied to people who do not have diabetes in an effort to understand the types of carbohydrates that are more readily usable during exercise. Research in this area will continue to shed light on the relationships between types of carbohydrates and physical performance (Rankin 1997). Current concepts of the use of the glycemic index in exercise suggest that carbohydrates that empty quickly into the bloodstream (high glycemic index) should be used immediately after training to help replace the glycogen stores in the body. The remaining meals of the day should be derived from other natural complex sources of carbohydrates such as beans, vegetables, grains, and fruits. These yield a slower, steadier flow of glucose into the bloodstream (low glycemic index), promoting glycogen replacement hours after exercise.

Fats in the Diet

The average American's diet may be surprisingly high in fat even with the number of "light," "low-fat," and "fat-free" products available (see figure 9.2). It would not be unusual to find

Table 9.4
Glycemic Index of Common Foods

High-glycemic foods	Moderate-glycemic foods	Low-glycemic foods
Carrots	Corn	Apples
Honey	All-Bran	Fish sticks
Corn flakes	Potato chips	Butter beans
Whole meal bread	Peas	Navy beans
White rice	White pasta	Kidney beans
Shredded wheat	Oatmeal	+Lentils
Brown rice	Sweet potatoes	Sausage

From McArdle, Katch, and Katch 1999.

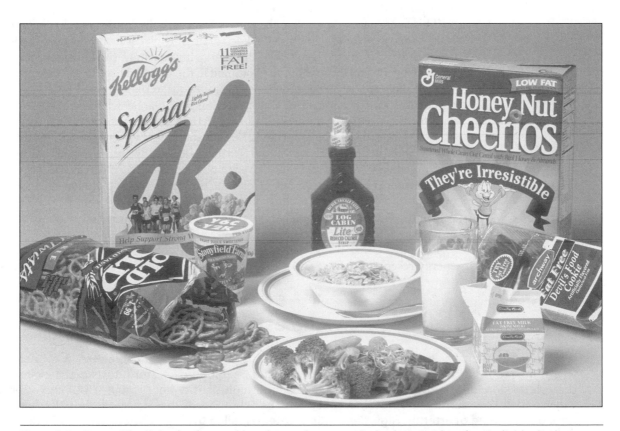

Figure 9.2 Even with all the fat-free and low-fat products, a typical caloric intake of an individual's diet could be made up of 40% to 45% dietary fat. Even though it is recommended that 30% or less of the daily caloric intake come from fat, it is very important that we realize how essential fats are in providing energy for exercise. Light to moderate exercise and exercise of longer duration depend on energy from fat stores. Remember, carbohydrates are the main source of energy for short bursts or intense bouts of exercise; the less intense or longer-lasting exercise utilizes fatty acid fuels.

40% to 45% of the daily caloric intake represented by dietary fat. Most nutritionists agree that 30% or less of the daily caloric intake should be from fat. In addition to the overall percentage of calories, it is important to understand the types of fats available. Similar to the carbohydrate categories, fats are grouped into three different categories: saturated, mono-unsaturated, and polyunsaturated. It is well known that the type of fat is just as important as the total amount of fat you eat.

Dietary fats, or lipids (see table 9.5), are found in our bodies predominantly in the form of triglycerides: Each triglyceride is a molecule of glycerol bonded to three molecules of fatty acid. The breakdown of the triglyceride occurs mainly in the small intestine. The stomach and pancreatic enzymes (working in the small intestine) remove two of the three fatty acids from the glycerol molecule, thus forming a monoglyceride. Some short-chain fatty acids (those with fewer than 12 carbon atoms) will be absorbed by the process of diffusion into the bloodstream. However, most of the fatty acids are long-chain fatty acids, which, along with the monoglyceride, require bile for their absorption. These dietary triglycerides reach the bloodstream by dissolving into a tiny sphere called a micelle, which is a carrier of bile salts. The micelles provide a transport service for the fatty acids and monoglycerides, virtually transporting them through the intestine without any change to the micelle. Further in the process, the monoglycerides (glycerol) and the fatty acids recombine as triglycerides. These triglycerides are transported in the bloodstream as one of three lipoprotein particles: very low-density lipoproteins (VLDLs), low-density lipoproteins (LDLs), and high-density lipoproteins (HDLs). When the individual lacks bile salts because of an obstruction or the loss of the gallbladder, lipid absorption is diminished and the lipids are lost into the feces. If the lipids fail to be absorbed, the excellent source of energy from fats is diminished, as is the absorption of fat-soluble vitamins A, D, E, and K.

This energy from lipids, like the energy from carbohydrates, is in the form of ATP (ATP is the "energy currency" of the cell). Each gram of triglyceride produces about 9 kilocalories of energy. If the body doesn't need the energy immediately, the lipids are stored in adipose tissue (fat deposits) throughout the body and in the liver. Adipose tissue (the body's fat layers) is the storage area of triglycerides until the individual requires the ATP for work, but adipose tissue also provides insulation and protection in the areas where it is present. The major sites for the storage of the unneeded triglycerides are the subcutaneous tissue (about 50% of that being stored), the kidneys (12%), the abdominal viscera (10-15%), the genital areas (20%), and the spaces between muscles (5-8%). The triglycerides stored in adipose tissue are exchanged very rapidly, and thus there is a new storage of triglycerides in our adipose tissue every two or three weeks. At any given time the triglycerides stored in the tissues the previous month will have been used or moved out and replaced by other triglyceride molecules. All triglycerides are continually released from storage, transported in the bloodstream, and redeposited in another storage site.

Remember that triglycerides are an excellent energy value and that about 98% of all energy reserves are from the triglycerides stored in adipose tissue. Glucose is not stored as

Cholesterol

Almost every adult has heard something about cholesterol levels. Blood cholesterol has been studied to attempt to understand its relationship to heart disease. Blood cholesterol tests often evaluate total cholesterol, low-density lipoprotein (LDL) cholesterol, high-density lipoprotein (HDL) cholesterol, and triglycerides. Low-density lipoprotein is called the "bad cholesterol" because it deposits fats and cholesterol on the lining of arteries. High-density lipoprotein is called the "good cholesterol" because it carries the fat and cholesterol away.

Knowing this, most of us would want to decrease our LDL and increase our HDL, but how can that be done? The answer is diet and exercise. So, what foods contain this bad cholesterol? Saturated fats contribute to LDL levels and should be reduced in our diets. Generally, meats and dairy products contain mostly saturated fats. Foods that are less apt to increase LDL levels and may in fact lower the blood cholesterol include unsaturated fats: either monounsaturated (canola, olive, and peanut oils) or polyunsaturated (corn, soybean, and sunflower oils). Additionally, some whole foods that contain unsaturated fats are avocados, olives, and peanuts. Reducing total fat and replacing some saturated fat with unsaturated fat should be a goal of every healthy person. In fact, nutritionists are finding that if we replace some saturated fat with monounsaturated fat, LDL cholesterol and total cholesterol are lowered without decreasing HDL cholesterol levels or raising triglyceride levels.

Table 9.5
Lipid Content of Some Common Foods

Food	Percent fat
Meats	
Veal	10
Chicken	10-17
Beef	16-42 (depends on cut)
Lamb	19-29
Ham, sliced	23
Pork	81
Plant sources of fat	
Potato chips	35
Cashew nuts	48
Peanut butter	50
Margarine	81
Oils	100
Other fats	
Baked beans	31
2% milk	35
Cream cheese	89.5
Hard-boiled egg	61
Cheesecake	63

easily as triglycerides, making fats an excellent resource for energy stores. Although many of the body's cells prefer to use glucose, the heart muscle is one of the organs that uses fatty acids as its energy source.

Dietary Protein

As mentioned previously, the physically active individual needs only slightly more protein than the average person. Proteins provide our bodies with essential amino acids (see table 9.6). "Essential" actually means that the amino acid cannot be manufactured in the body but must be ingested from foods. There are 22 different amino acids in proteins, and various foods supply those amino acids in various amounts. One of the best sources of dietary protein is in dairy products such as milk. Meat is a good source of protein, and vegetables such as legumes and grains offer a partially complete protein in that they lack one or more essential amino acids or contain less than the required amount of the amino acid.

Physically active people who choose not to consume animal products should understand the essential amino acids that are lacking in their diets and attempt to find sources of those missing components. A vegetarian often experiences more difficulty in consuming the appropriate number of calories in the diet than in finding the proper nutrients. This is related to the fact that animal proteins are usually of a higher caloric value than non-meats. This may be more obvious to you if you consider the amount of fat contained in most meat products. The total caloric value of the meat is obtained from the number of protein calories as well as the number of fat calories.

Proteins ingested from the diet are broken down into amino acids, which are absorbed into the bloodstream and transported to the liver. Unlike fats and carbohydrates, proteins are not stored to be used later. Amino acids are used by the body to produce ATP or as the building blocks of new proteins used for growth and repair processes. Excess amounts of dietary amino acids are converted into glucose or triglycerides and stored in the adipose tissues of the body.

Excess Dietary Protein

Some dietary fads encourage high protein intake with very low carbohydrate consumption. This type of diet can actually cause a condition called "ketoacidosis" or "ketosis," which is a by-product of metabolism when ketones are excreted from the burning of fats in an attempt to maintain the body's acid–base balance. Actually ketosis designates a pathological condition that is potentially dangerous to one's health. The advocates of the high-protein diets insist that the burning of ketones is a good thing in that the process of breaking down the fat into ketones requires energy, which translates into calories burned. Most dietary specialists agree

Table 9.6
Recommended Dietary Allowances (RDAs) of Dietary Protein

Recommended amount	Adolescent males	Adult males	Adolescent females	Adult females
Grams of protein per kg body weight	0.9	0.8	0.9	0.8
Grams per day based on average weight	59 g (145 lb = average weight)	56 g (154 lb = average weight)	50 g (123 lb = average weight)	44 g (125 lb = average weight)

that short-term ketosis is usually not a problem; long-term ketosis (several weeks) can create an accumulation of uric acid, which can cause gout or kidney stones in people predisposed to those conditions. Severely restricting carbohydrate consumption is apt to lead the patient into danger much more quickly than diets allowing greater consumption of carbohydrates.

PLANNING THE ATHLETE'S DIET

The nutrition needed for optimal performance does not depend on the meal preceding the event but depends on the nutritional habits of the individual in the days and weeks prior to the competition. In choosing food products to be consumed to maximize the energy for training and competition, it is important to understand the energy requirements of the activity. The role of carbohydrates and fats as fuel sources during exercise depends mostly on the intensity and duration of the activity. Generally, carbohydrates are utilized more as the intensity of the exercise increases, and less as the duration of the activity increases. Long-duration, low-intensity exercise would be expected to rely on fat as the energy source, but actually there is interplay between fat and the carbohydrate utilization during all exercise. Good daily nutritional habits in the weeks preceding the competition provide the best opportunity to build the carbohydrate stores to the maximum while also providing fatty acids that act to increase the utilization of fat as an energy source.

Pre-Event Meals

When the physically active individual prepares for a competitive event, the nutritional habits of the days prior to the event are more important than the meal consumed immediately before the contest. Endurance athletes often begin changing their dietary habits several days before an endurance event. In the common practice of carbohydrate loading, the athlete increases the carbohydrate intake from the usual 60% to 70% to 80% of the total caloric intake. The athlete usually begins this practice three days prior to the event and continues the training schedule as customary. This practice is designed to maximize the carbohydrate stores to allow the athlete a greater reserve of energy.

The last meal before the contest cannot significantly alter the energy stores built up in the preceding days, although it should provide two functions: (1) The foods should be easily digested to allow gastric emptying prior to the start of participation, and (2) the food should satisfy the athlete's feelings of hunger. Thus, the high-carbohydrate pre-event meal is beneficial for two reasons: Carbohydrates are easily and quickly digested and may provide a source of energy for the upcoming physical performance. Proteins and fats, on the other hand, are more difficult to digest and often require a longer period of time to convert to usable energy. Generally, if fats and proteins are included in the pre-event meal, 3 to 4 hr must be allowed between the time of the meal and the start of the event to ensure sufficient digestive time. Most people become focused, or even anxious, as the start time nears, making it even more important to plan the meal to allow sufficient time for the digestive processes. Participants who experience gastric upset after ingesting a meal before exercise or competition may find it beneficial to use a liquid carbohydrate drink to build the energy stores with less need for digestive activity. In any case, the pre-event meal should be supplemented with fluids to aid the participant in the attempt to maximize physical performance.

When a back-to-back competition schedule limits the amount of recovery time between exercise bouts, it is more imperative for the participant to replenish body fluids than to build energy stores. If the ingested fluids contain carbohydrates as well as water, however, both functions will be served. The amount of fluid consumed should exceed the amount of body weight that has been lost during the exercise period preceding the rest break.

The psychological issues surrounding performance come into play with regard to menu selection in the pre-event meal. Some athletes disobey all rules concerning when and what to eat before the contest, yet insist that their performance is best when they consume the unconventional diet. This points to the fact that the pre-event meal is not as important as the meals on the days preceding the contest (see figure 9.3). In the pre-event meal it is important to avoid foods that irritate the bowel, pull fluids from the intestine, or cause bloating or other signs of indigestion. You can usually count on the athlete to avoid foods that cause distress, because the participant will not enjoy the consequences of bowel distress. The foods that cause distress are not the same for all people.

Managing Weight: Gaining and Losing

Athletes place considerable pressures on themselves to perform well. These pressures don't end when the individual leaves the playing area but continue in everyday life. One such nonsport pressure comes from body weight. It would not be surprising to you if you overheard a female gymnast talking about needing to lose weight. Equally common might be the football interior lineman who is challenged with ways to keep his weight on during the intense practice sessions.

Changes in body weight can be very difficult for the athlete to accomplish during a competitive season. Athletes must realize that changes in body weight during the season may occur very slowly. Good nutritional habits are important to establish and maintain throughout the season. A diet low in fat and high in carbohydrate should be employed, with the total calories consumed either higher (to gain) or lower (to lose) than with the current practices.

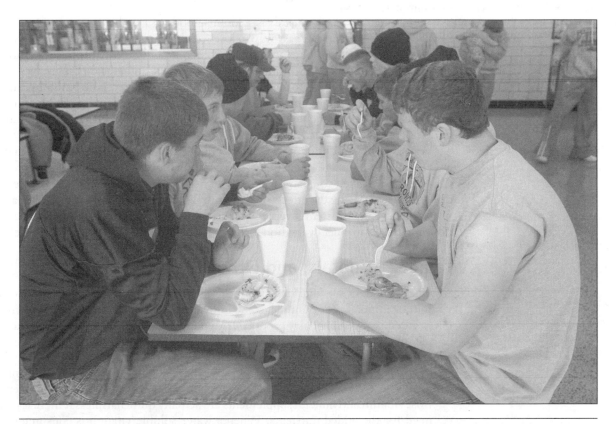

Figure 9.3 For optimal performance and protection from injury, physically active persons should practice good daily nutritional habits, not just rely on pre-event meals.

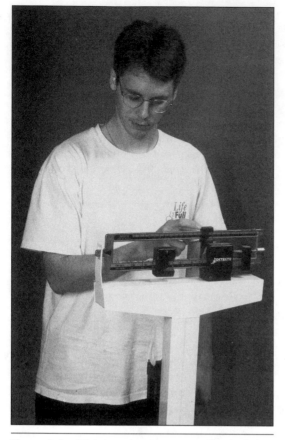

Figure 9.4 Athletes who are attempting to lose weight during the competitive season should anticipate no more than a 2 lb per week loss.

Weight Loss and Fluid Levels

Sports that set limits to the participant's weight through the weigh-in process certainly encourage fasting and other undesirable dietary practices. Rapid weight losses are usually the result of fluid loss in the body. This fluid loss can lead very quickly to dehydration and very serious outcomes. Wrestling has been such a sport, requiring weight limits for competitors of various weight classes. This practice in wrestlers has been so unsafe that late in 1997, three wrestlers' deaths were related to intentional weight loss and dehydration (CDC 1998).

Athletes who are attempting to lose weight during the competitive season should anticipate no more than a 2 lb (0.9 kg) per week loss (see figure 9.4). The diet should be high in carbohydrates, and plenty of fluids must be consumed. Rapid weight loss is a sure sign of a loss of body fluids and could spell disaster if the fluids are not replenished before exercise begins.

Weight gain is sometimes a difficult issue for the athlete because of the access to food at various times throughout the day. The key factor in gaining weight while burning significant amounts of energy is to consume more calories than one is using. The athlete who is able to supplement the normal meals should do so with high-carbohydrate food choices to provide a source of energy for the workout. Snacking throughout the day allows athletes to consume more calories than if they attempt to increase calories only at mealtimes.

Special Diets, Fads, and Supplements and the Athlete

A fast fix is seldom a good fix. Food fads and supplements that offer an easy way to lose weight, gain weight, or gain performance advantages are seldom able to hold up to the promises without a person's significant dedication to a workout regimen. People who dedicate themselves to an exercise program for improved performance, weight control, or even bodybuilding can rest assured that the changes brought about by hard work and dedication are much healthier than those brought about through chemical means. Nothing will replace the effect of hard work and good nutrition.

As an example, one might look at the product ephedrine. Ephedrine is used in many dietary aids as well as in supplements intended to give you more energy (table 9.7). Ephedrine (ephedra) has been linked to death in otherwise healthy professional athletes. One of the many difficulties in studying the effects of ephedrine-containing products is the fact that many of the products have inconsistent levels of ephedrine in each batch or lot. Inconsistencies in content not only make product evaluation difficult but also put the consumer at greater risk.

Vitamins, Minerals, and Other Dietary Supplements

Anyone who lacks specific items from the diet can potentially develop a deficiency of that vitamin or mineral. For example, some individuals are lactose intolerant, meaning that they have difficulty digesting dairy products. As you realize, dairy products are an excellent source of calcium, and unless a person makes an effort to consume other sources of calcium, he or she could run the risk of a calcium deficiency. In this situation, supplementing the normal well-rounded diet may be indicated. On the other hand, if the individual is consuming a well-rounded diet with adequate calories, there should be no real need to supplement the diet.

Most vitamin and mineral supplements are actually quite harmless if there is no physiological need for the added nutrients. When a water-soluble vitamin is consumed in quantities

Table 9.7

Products Containing Ephedra

Product name	Supplier
Carb Cutter	HNS Labs
Diet Fuel	Twin Laboratories
Diet Pep	Natural Balance, Inc.
Diurlean	ISS Research
Dyma-Burn Xtreme	Dymatize Nutrition
Extreme Ripped Force	American Bodybuilding
ETA Stack	Nutra Sport
Fat Cutter Plus	HNS Labs
Herba Fuel	TwinLab Laboratories
Ma Huang	Gaia Herbs, Inc.
MetaCuts	Metaform
Metabolife 356	Metabolife International
MetaboLift	TwinLab Laboratories
NVE Stacker	NVE Pharmaceuticals
Ripped Fuel	TwinLab Laboratories
Thermogenic Power	Nature's Herbs
UltraCuts	BioPlex

greater than the body's need, the excess is excreted into the urine. On the other hand, if the vitamin is fat soluble, the extra vitamin consumed is stored in the body's fat layers where it can build up to a point of being harmful to the person's health. If the vitamin is water soluble and is not needed, the body excretes it into the urine. If a vitamin is not water-soluble, it will be stored in the body's adipose tissues and is termed a fat-soluble vitamin. The fat-soluble vitamins are A, D, E, and K. These vitamins are stored, rather than excreted, and can build up in the body to dangerous levels. People must take care to ensure that they need a supplement and that excess amounts will not be harmful to their general health.

When an individual is diagnosed with a nutritional or metabolic disorder, a health care provider may prescribe nutritional supplements. These prescribed supplements should always be taken under the supervision of the physician or other knowledgeable nutritional or health care professional. Unfortunately, there may be supplements that appear to be safe and according to advertisements are not banned substances but that in actuality have been outlawed by the individual's athletic conference or league. In addition to the possibility that a particular substance is banned, some chemicals interact with others to produce a banned substance. Extreme care must always be taken to understand any and all chemicals to be ingested. The best method to ensure a drug-free body is to stay away from fast fixes and instead depend on hard work and good nutritional habits.

The American Dietetic Association (ADA) has very up-to-date information at www.eatright.org. In addition, you may call the ADA at 800-366-1655, and a recorded voice will provide a referral to a registered dietitian in your area.

NUTRITIONAL CONCERNS IN INJURY OR ILLNESS

Nutrition is often used to help people recover from injury or illness, as rightfully it should be. You probably recall hearing that milk builds strong bones. This is certainly true in that calcium is essential for healthy bones. Milk, an excellent source of calcium, is generally advocated when people experience a fracture. Drinking milk and consuming other products high in calcium help to increase the level of calcium in your body, but drinking milk only after the fracture is not a sound dietary practice. Good nutrition, just like proper calcium intake, should be for every day and not only after an injury or illness.

Nutritional Aspects of Fractures

Stress fractures are one type of fracture that may be due in part to low calcium levels. Low calcium levels are associated with low bone density (osteoporosis) and thus a higher potential for fracture (see figure 9.5). Additionally, Highet (1989) found a decreased level of circulating estrogen a common factor in women suffering stress fractures. Not only is calcium available in the foods we eat; some common foods contain estrogen-like compounds that may supplement low levels of circulating estrogens. These foods include carrots, yams, cheese, milk, yogurt, cottage cheese, and eggs.

Deficiency Diseases

Specific vitamin, mineral, or amino acid deficiencies are well established and often show a direct relationship to nutrition. Some of the well-known deficiencies include anemia (iron deficiency), scurvy (vitamin C deficiency), and rickets (vitamin D deficiency). A person may develop a deficiency disease due to diet or because of an inability to absorb the missing nutrient during digestion, yet recovery is usually very quick once the deficiency is understood and the diet is supplemented. The key to avoiding problems associated with these deficiencies is prevention through good nutrition and early medical evaluation once symptoms are observed.

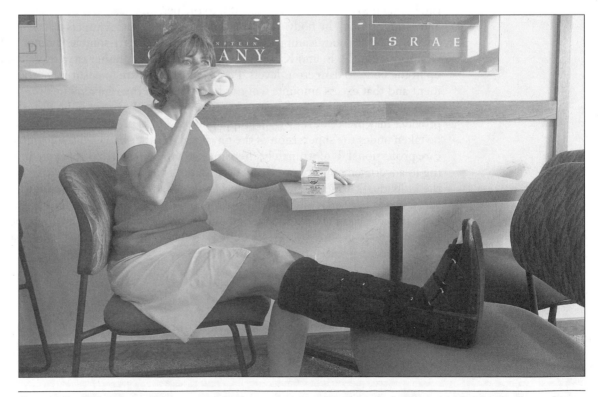

Figure 9.5   Milk, an excellent source of calcium, is generally advocated when an individual suffers a fracture.

Nutrition and the Diabetic Participant

When we think of a physically active individual who must observe nutrition closely due to an illness or injury, we naturally think of the patient with diabetes. Although it may be true that participants with diabetes need not alter their diet from what is customary for other competitors, people who have diabetes must pay much closer attention to their nutritional habits. People with some types of diabetes use insulin along with their dietary habits to control blood glucose levels. These individuals require very consistent mealtimes, as they must monitor their blood glucose level throughout the day to ensure that it remains normal. An insulin dose that is not followed by food intake could cause a serious hypoglycemic reaction. Athletes with diabetes must ensure that their insulin dose matches their food intake to prevent extreme highs or lows in the blood glucose level. Keeping the blood glucose levels from dropping too low during exercise often requires considerable planning and discipline on the part of the athlete. Anyone working with a diabetic athlete must be aware of the possible dangers associated with changes in blood glucose levels. It could be quite dangerous for a diabetic athlete to go home after a workout and take an insulin dose, but then fall asleep before consuming a meal. The high insulin level pushes the glucose to a dangerously low level. Recognizing the potential problems and being prepared to prevent them is the best method of care possible.

Nutritional Aspects of Growth and Repair Processes

A well-balanced diet is essential for normal growth and following injury when tissue repair is required. Individuals who experience frequent injuries or who seem to heal slowly should seek nutritional evaluation. Only after evaluation and detection of areas of deficiency can the proper diet and supplements be understood. With the physician's knowledge of the healing difficulties, referral to a nutritionist is often recommended when other medical issues are ruled out. Nutritional evaluation and consultation, however, can be very helpful regardless of any relation to an injury.

Fracture Healing

As discussed earlier in this chapter, calcium plays a large part in the growth and repair of bones. Additionally, calcium can assist in blood-clotting mechanisms following injury as well as being a potential factor in the regulation of blood pressure. Calcium is obtained from most dairy products (including cheeses and yogurt), calcium-enriched tofu, tortillas made from lime-processed corn, dark green leafy vegetables (spinach, broccoli, turnip greens, and kale), and canned fish containing soft bones that are normally eaten. There are quite a number of dietary sources of calcium, in addition to those mentioned here, that are certainly important for some individuals. One thing we must realize, however, is that some foods act to reduce the absorption of calcium while other minerals and nutrients can affect how well your body is able to absorb and utilize the calcium you consume. Adequate vitamin D enhances calcium absorption while excessive meat, salt, caffeine, and alcohol consumption reduce the absorption of calcium from foods. Anyone who incurs frequent or unusual fractures would be wise to consult a nutritionist to evaluate the diet thoroughly.

SUMMARY

1. *Discuss the recommended dietary intake of carbohydrates, fats, and proteins, and explain how one would calculate the caloric content of a meal or diet.*

   We can calculate calories from food if we know how many grams of each energy source are in a food serving. Each gram of fat is equal to 9 calories, while carbohydrates and protein are 4 calories per gram. Of the total number of calories consumed in one day, no more than 30% should be from fats, 10% to 15% from protein, and about 60% from carbohydrates.

2. *Explain the role of carbohydrates as an energy source and list the types of carbohydrates found in foods.*

Carbohydrates are the energy source used during short-duration exercise as well as for intense exercise. Because carbohydrates play a critical role in providing fuel for exercise, it is important that athletes consume adequate amounts of carbohydrates for their exercise program. Carbohydrates exist as monosaccharides (fructose, galactose, or glucose), disaccharides (in which two or more of the monosaccharides are chemically linked), or polysaccharides (hundreds or thousands of linked monosaccharides). All carbohydrates are broken down into monosaccharides during digestion, a process that typically requires energy. The monosaccharides are converted to glucose in the liver. The rate of carbohydrate digestion and absorption varies for different foods and is the subject of continued research.

3. *Discuss the recommended amount of water that should be consumed daily and explain suitable alternatives to plain drinking water for the replenishing of body fluids.*

As a general rule, the average person should consume eight 8-oz glasses (64-oz total) of water each day. Active individuals require even more water to make up for the water lost in perspiration. Some drinks, such as caffeine products, can increase a person's need for water because the caffeine acts as a diuretic and depletes the body of fluids. Since people tend to drink more of a beverage that tastes good, sport drinks can serve as a viable alternative to water. A flavored sport drink with 6% carbohydrate (60 g of carbohydrate per liter of drink) will be well tolerated and will aid in replenishing body fluids, as well as providing an additional source of energy from the carbohydrates.

4. *Explain the difference between "good" and "bad" cholesterol and suggest the method one might use to minimize the negative effects of cholesterol.*

Cholesterol includes low-density lipoprotein (LDL) cholesterol, high-density lipoprotein (HDL) cholesterol, and triglycerides. The LDL is called the bad cholesterol because it deposits fats and cholesterol on the lining of arteries; HDL is called the good cholesterol because it carries the fat and cholesterol away. Reducing total fat and replacing some saturated fats with unsaturated fats should be a goal of every healthy individual.

5. *Discuss the concepts of a "pre-event meal" versus "pre-event nutrition" and explain why some people may feel they are able to eat anything they want prior to competition.*

Nutrition in the days preceding the event is more critical to athletic performance than the last meal before the contest. Adhering to a well-balanced meal plan will always prove to be the best option. Pre-event meals should be high in carbohydrates due to the need for that type of fuel and ease of digestion. That meal should be consumed between 3 and 4 hr before the event. Psychology plays a large part of all performance, and as such has an influence on the ability to perform regardless of the type of food consumed. As long as the food ingested does not cause gastric distress, some athletes are able to consume very controversial meals without an observable reduction in performance.

CRITICAL THINKING QUESTIONS

1. Compare and contrast two current diet fads. Identify the pros and cons of each of the diets.

2. One of your gymnasts is concerned with her body image and feels that she looks terrible in her competition leotard. She wants you to help her in designing a diet to lose weight. She is 19 years old and currently taking in 2,800 calories per day on average; she is 5 ft 2 in. and weighs 124 lb (56 kg). Make recommendations for the total caloric intake needed during this off-season and design her meals for one day.

3. One of your track distance runners returned from summer vacation and confided in you that her mother was on a protein-only diet, and that she herself had followed the same diet program for the past several weeks. Now that the athlete is back on campus and responsible for her own meals, she wants to know what you think about the Atkins-type diet in which one tries to eliminate carbohydrates. Explain your view of high-protein, low-carbohydrate diets.

4. Design the meals for a basketball team for a seven-day trip in which they will be traveling on day 1 and day 7 with games on days 2, 4, and 6.

5. The female distance runner of question 3 is quite thin, and you suspect that her diet may be partly responsible for the stress fractures in her left foot (last year) and her right foot (this season). Explain the dietary elements you would suggest that she include in her diet to help strengthen her bones.

CITED SOURCES

CDC. 1998. Hyperthermia and dehydration-related deaths associated with intentional rapid weight loss in three collegiate wrestlers—North Carolina, Wisconsin, and Michigan November-December, 1997. *Morbidity and Mortality Weekly Report* 47(06):105-108.

Highet, R. 1989. Athletic amenorrhea: An update on aetiology, complications, and management. *Spts Med* 7: 82-108.

McArdle, W.D., F.I. Katch, and V.L. Katch. 1999. *Sports and exercise nutrition.* Philadelphia: Williams & Wilkins.

Rankin, J.W. 1997. Glycemic index and exercise metabolism. *Gatorade Spts Sci Exch* 10: 64, No. 1.

ADDITIONAL READINGS

Clark, N. 1997. *Nancy Clark's sports nutrition guidebook: Eating to fuel your active lifestyle.* Champaign, IL: Human Kinetics.

Coleman, E., and S. Nelson-Steen. 1996. *The ultimate sports nutrition handbook.* Palo Alto, CA: Bull.

Grandjean, A.C. 1997. Diets of elite athletes: Has the discipline of sports nutrition made an impact? *J Nutr* 127(4): 874-877.

Shi, X., R.W. Summers, H.P. Schedl, S.W. Flanagan, R.T. Chang, and C.V. Gisolfi. 1995. Effects of carbohydrate type and concentration and solution osmolality on water absorption. *Med Sci Spts Exerc* 27: 1607-1615.

Appendix A

National Athletic Trainers' Association Code of Ethics

Preamble

The Code of Ethics of the National Athletic Trainers' Association has been written to make the membership aware of the principles of ethical behavior that should be followed in the practice of athletic training. The primary goal of the Code is the assurance of high quality health care. The Code presents aspirational standards of behavior that all members should strive to achieve.

The principles cannot be expected to cover all specific situations that may be encountered by the practicing athletic trainer, but should be considered representative of the spirit with which athletic trainers should make decisions. The principles are written generally and the circumstances of a situation will determine the interpretation and application of a given principle and of the Code as a whole. Whenever there is a conflict between the Code and legality, the laws prevail. The guidelines set forth in this Code are subject to continual review and revision as the athletic training profession develops and changes.

Principle 1

Members shall respect the rights, welfare, and dignity of all individuals.

1.1 Members shall not discriminate against any legally protected class.

1.2 Members shall be committed to providing competent care consistent with both the requirements and the limitations of their profession.

1.3 Members shall preserve the confidentiality of privileged information and shall not release such information to a third party not involved in the patient's care unless the person consents to such release or release is permitted or required by law.

Principle 2

Members shall comply with the laws and regulations governing the practice of athletic training.

2.1 Members shall comply with applicable local, state, and federal laws and institutional guidelines.

2.2 Members shall be familiar with and adhere to all National Athletic Trainers' Association guidelines and ethical standards.

2.3 Members are encouraged to report illegal or unethical practice pertaining to athletic training to the appropriate person or authority.

2.4 Members shall avoid substance abuse and, when necessary, seek rehabilitation for chemical dependency.

Principle 3

Members shall accept responsibility for the exercise of sound judgment.

3.1 Members shall not misrepresent in any manner, either directly or indirectly, their skills, training, professional credentials, identity, or services.

3.2 Members shall provide only those services for which they are qualified via education and/or experience and by pertinent legal regulatory process.

3.3 Members shall provide services, make referrals, and seek compensation only for those services that are necessary.

Principle 4

Members shall maintain and promote high standards in the provision of services.

4.1 Members shall recognize the need for continuing education and participate in various types of educational activities that enhance their skills and knowledge.

4.2 Members who have the responsibility for employing and evaluating the performance of other staff members shall fulfill such responsibility in a fair, considerate, and equitable manner, on the basis of clearly enunciated criteria.

4.3 Members who have the responsibility for evaluating the performance of employees, supervisees, or students are encouraged to share evaluations with them and allow them the opportunity to respond to those evaluations.

4.4 Members shall educate those whom they supervise in the practice of athletic training with regard to the Code of Ethics and encourage their adherence to it.

4.5 Whenever possible, members are encouraged to participate and support others in the conduct and communication of research and educational activities that may contribute knowledge for improved patient care, patient or student education, and the growth of athletic training as a profession.

4.6 When members are researchers or educators, they are responsible for maintaining and promoting ethical conduct in research and educational activities.

Principle 5

Members shall not engage in any form of conduct that constitutes a conflict of interest or that adversely reflects on the profession.

5.1 The private conduct of the member is a personal matter to the same degree as is any other person's except when such conduct compromises the fulfillment of professional responsibilities.

5.2 Members of the National Athletic Trainers' Association and others serving on the Association's committees or acting as consultants shall not use, directly or by implication, the Association's name or logo or their affiliation with the Association in the endorsement of products or services.

5.3 Members shall not place financial gain above the welfare of the patient being treated and shall not participate in any arrangement that exploits the patient.

5.4 Members may seek remuneration for their services that is commensurate with their services and in compliance with applicable law.

Reprinted from National Athletic Trainers' Association 2002. http://nata.org/publications/brochures/ethics.htm

Appendix B

Historical Perspective on the National Athletic Trainers' Association

1939

First attempt to form a national association by athletic trainers attending Drake Relays, Des Moines, Iowa (association disbanded in 1944).

1940s

Athletic training associations formed within athletic conferences throughout the United States. Regional associations provided impetus for formation of the National Athletic Trainers' Association (NATA).

1950s

NATA sponsored and financed by Cramer Chemical Company (until 1955).

1950

NATA held first national meeting, Kansas City, Missouri.

Charles Cramer, Cramer Chemical Company, appointed as first National Secretary (1950-1954).

1951

NATA Constitution and By-laws adopted.

1952

Official NATA logo adopted.

1953

First honorary member selected.

1954

John Cramer, Cramer Chemical Company, appointed as second National Secretary (1954-1955).

1955

Committee on Gaining Recognition formed to study means of promoting athletic training (*William E. "Pinky" Newell*, Chair). Provided impetus for current NATA Professional Education Committee and Certification Committee.

William "Pinky" Newell, Purdue University, appointed as third National Secretary. First active athletic trainer to hold position (1955-1968).

1956

First publication of *Journal of the National Athletic Trainers' Association*. Forerunner of current publication, *Athletic Training: The Journal of the National Athletic Trainers' Association*.

1957

NATA Code of Ethics adopted.

1959

Board of Directors approval of first program of undergraduate education for athletic trainers submitted by Committee on Gaining Recognition (revised in 1969, 1972, 1977, 1980, and 1983).

1962

First group of athletic trainers inducted into Helms Foundation Hall of Fame.

1969

Jack Rockwell, St. Louis Cardinals football, appointed as fourth Executive Secretary (1968-1971).

Professional Advancement Committee (formerly Committee on Gaining Recognition) divided into two separate committees: Professional Education Committee (*Sayers "Bud" Miller*, Chair) and Certification Committee (*Lindsey McLean*, Chair).

American Medical Association (AMA) resolution recognizing importance of the role of the athletic trainer and commending NATA for efforts to upgrade professional standards.
Plan for structural reorganization of NATA submitted to the Board of Directors. Ad hoc committee appointed to review.

1970

NATA Board of Certification created and authorized to administer certification examination in conjunction with Professional Examination Service.

First NATA certification examination given, Waco, Texas (July 1970).

First undergraduate athletic training curricula approved by NATA Professional Education Committee

Structural reorganization plan approved by membership. Established four Divisions (Professional Services, Professional Advancement, Information Services, National Program and Business Affairs) and office of the President (divisional organization subsequently discontinued).

Bobby Gunn, Houston Oilers football, elected to newly created office of the President (1970-1974).

1971

Otho Davis, Philadelphia Eagles football, appointed as fifth Executive Director (formerly Executive Secretary) (1971-1990).

1972

First graduate athletic training curricula approved by Professional Education Committee
Sherry Kosek Babagian, first female athletic trainer to become certified by NATA.

1974

Frank George, Brown University, elected as second President (1974-1978).

1975

NATA 25th Annual Meeting, Kansas City, Missouri.

1978

Bill Chambers, Fullerton Junior College, elected as third President (1978-1982).

NATA and American Physical Therapy Association (APTA) representatives held joint meetings to discuss licensure for athletic trainers. NATA Model Legislation developed (1978-1979).

1981

Paul Grace, Massachusetts Institute of Technology, appointed Chairman, NATA Board of Certification (1981-present).

1982

Bobby Barton, Eastern Kentucky University, elected as fourth President (1982-1986). NATA Board of Certification granted membership in National Commission for Health Certifying Agencies.

First Role Delineation Study completed by Board of Certification.

1983

Guidelines for Development and Implementation of NATA Approved Undergraduate Athletic Training Education Programs revised by Professional Education Committee and approved by Board of Directors (established the athletic training major, or equivalent, as requirement for curriculum approval). June 1990 established as deadline date for implementation of athletic training major programs.

Competencies in Athletic Training developed by Professional Education Committee and approved by Board of Directors.

NATA became incorporated.

1985

NATA employed public relations firm to conduct nationwide public relations campaign.

1986

Jerry Rhea, Atlanta Falcons football, elected as fifth President (1986-1988).
NATA Standards of Practice adopted.

1987

Columbia Assessment Services, Inc., hired to manage NATA certification examination.

1988

Mark Smaha, Washington State University, elected as sixth President (1988-1990).

NATA Code of Professional Practice developed (revision of Code of Ethics).

Building purchased for relocation of NATA office to Dallas, Texas.

High-risk sport experience required (25% of required supervised hours) for certification. High-risk sports included football, soccer, hockey, wrestling, basketball, volleyball, rugby, lacrosse, and gymnastics.

Publication of *NATA News* (newsletter) initiated.

1989

Management consultant firm (Lawrence-Leiter and Company, Kansas City, Missouri) employed to provide NATA management consulting. Joint meeting with Board of Directors and other NATA representatives in Dallas, Texas (July 1989).

NATA Board of Certification incorporated.

1990

Otho Davis resigned as NATA Executive Director (18 years); *Alan Smith* hired as first NATA full-time Chief Executive Officer.

NATA national office relocated from Greenville, North Carolina, to Dallas, Texas.

Management consultant firm (Lawrence-Leiter and Company) employed to develop visionary strategic plan.

NATA Education and Research Foundation development plans announced.

Athletic training officially recognized by AMA as an allied health profession (June 22, 1990).

Joint Review Committee (NATA, American Academy of Pediatrics, American Orthopaedic Society for Sports Medicine, American Academy of Family Physicians) established to conduct athletic training education program accreditation under auspices of AMA Committee on Allied Health Education and Accreditation. Joint meeting held to develop *Essentials and Guidelines* governing accredited athletic training education programs (October 20, 1990).

Special task force (delegate from APTA and NATA Board of Directors) formed to study and develop professional relationships between athletic training and physical therapy.

Second Role Delineation Study completed by Board of Certifications.

Conversion of undergraduate athletic training education programs to majors, or equivalent, completed.

1991

Denny Miller, Purdue University, elected as seventh President (1991-1994).

NATA launched national public relations campaign (June 1991).

NATA Membership Classifications restructured (October 1991) (classes: Associate, Student, Certified, Supplier).

Essentials and Guidelines for an Accredited Educational Program for the Athletic Trainer adopted by the Council on Medical Education of the AMA (December 7, 1991).

NCAA Drug Distribution Study conducted (results presented December 1991) by Laster-Bradley et al.

NATA Research and Education Foundation officially incorporated.

1992

NATA membership increased from 14,935 in February 1991 to 16,700 in February 1992.

Revised NATA Code of Ethics adopted (February 1992).

Litigation filed against the American Athletic Trainers' Association (AATA) for unauthorized use of the NATA's logo and credentials.

Alan Smith resigned as NATA Executive Director (October 29, 1992) because of "profound and irreconcilable differences."

1993

Eve Becker-Doyle hired as NATA Executive Director (January 27, 1993).

Settlement between AATA and NATA halted use of "ATC" designation.

Strategic Planning Task Force directed the Professional Education Committee and Joint Review Committee on Educational Programs in Athletic Training (JRC/AT) to guide the development of NATA curriculum programs to meet the diverse needs of athletic training work settings.

AATA found in violation of previous settlement agreement with NATA; further litigation pursued.

NATA initiated lobbying campaign to pursue and advocate NATA's interests in federal health care reform.

NATA Code of Ethics and NATA Membership Standards, Eligibility Requirements and Membership Sanctions and Procedures revised and approved by the Board of Directors (November 1993).

NATA By-laws revised and approved by the Board of Directors.
Second Role Delineation Survey Conducted by BOC.

1994

NATA awarded $30,000 in contempt of court ruling against the AATA.

NATA awarded Advance America Award of Excellence for the NATA Code of Ethics.

AMA disbanded Committee on Allied Health Education and Accreditation (June 1994). New system Commission on Accreditation of Allied Health Educational Programs formed (July 1994).

NATA Board of Directors established Educational Task Force to study perspectives of athletic training education (August 1994).

Role Delineation Matrix published; data collected by Board of Certification from 1993 survey of membership.

1995

The NATA, APTA's Sports P.T. Section, and the United States Olympic Committee host joint educational seminar (February 4-5, 1995).

American Orthopaedic Society for Sports Medicine added as committee member of JRC-AT. Committee role is in accreditation process for entry-level athletic training education.

NATA Reimbursement Advisory Group established.

NATA established Women in Athletic Training Task Force to study issues facing female athletic trainers.

Grants and Scholarship Foundation merged into NATA Research and Education Foundation (May 1995).

NATA Board allocated $15,000 per district to promote state involvement in regulatory practice initiatives/amendments and third-party reimbursement activities (May 1995).

1996

Kent Falb, ATC, PT, elected eighth NATA President (1996-1998).

Educational Task Force made 18 proposals to affect athletic training education (published February 1996).

NATA released results of High School Injury Study (February 1996).

NATA College and University Athletic Trainers' Committee: job survey results published (September 1996).

Dave Perrin, PhD, ATC, appointed Editor-in-Chief of *Journal of Athletic Training* (December 1996).

NATA adopted all 18 recommendations of Educational Task Force regarding athletic training education reform (December 1996).

1997

NATA Foundation: First Annual Professional Educators Conference, Dallas, Texas (February 1997).

2000

March designated as National Athletic Training Month

2004

Internship route toward NATA certification eliminated January 1.

Glossary

acclimatization—A physiological adaptation to environmental conditions such as temperature and humidity.

acquired—A condition that develops over a period of time; not present from birth.

aerobic—In the presence of oxygen; in terms of exercise, characterizing the types of activities that rely on the metabolic process requiring oxygen.

agonist—A drug that can interact with specific sites in cells and initiate a therapeutic response. The same term applies to muscles that work with other muscles to produce a desired action.

alimentary—Relating to food or nutrition.

allopath—The medical system based on the treatment of symptoms. The allopath (MD) is often a member of the sports medicine team.

AMA (American Medical Association)—The governing body for physicians.

anaerobic—In the absence of oxygen; in terms of exercise, characterizing the types of activities that use metabolic processes producing energy without oxygen.

analgesic—Relieving pain. Usually referring to a medication that relieves pain but does not affect consciousness.

antagonist—A drug that, by producing no biological effects of its own, inhibits the action of another drug working on the same receptor sites. The same term applies to muscles that work to inhibit the action of another muscle.

anterior cruciate ligament (ACL)—A ligament on the inside of the knee joint that serves to restrict the lower leg (tibia) from moving too far forward (anteriorly) on the thigh bone (femur). See *Assessment of Athletic Injuries* text for more information.

anthropometry—The study and comparison of measurements of the human body. This term is usually used in anthropology.

anticonvulsant—Medicinal drug designed to reduce or prevent convulsions.

anti-inflammatory—A drug working to inhibit or reduce inflammation (swelling).

antipyresis—Reduction of fever.

antitussive—Providing relief of cough.

aortic valve—The last heart valve prior to the body's arterial network. The aortic valve is between the left ventricle and the aorta.

ATC (Certified Athletic Trainer)—Credentials indicating membership in the National Athletic Trainers' Association and level of expertise of a sports medicine professional in the United States.

atherosclerosis—The most common form of heart disease, also known as coronary heart disease or hardening of the arteries (i.e., arteriosclerosis). It involves deposits in the inner lining of an artery. The buildup that results, called plaque, may partially or totally block the blood's flow through the artery, causing a heart attack or stroke (brain attack).

ballistic—Pertaining to sudden, jerking movements during muscle stretching. Thought to contribute to muscle soreness or even muscle tears. Some believe that controlled ballistic stretching can be beneficial but must be closely monitored.

beta-blocker—Drug used to slow the heart rate and to generally reduce the function of the heart (e.g., reduce output of blood to attempt to control blood pressure) and other organs.

bioavailability—The degree to which the active ingredient of a drug is absorbed by the body in an active form. Indicates both the relative amount of the drug that reaches the circulation and the rate at which this absorption occurs.

bioelectrical impedance—Technique that determines the resistance to electrical current of body tissues. From these data, relative body composition (amount of muscle vs. amount of fat) can be estimated.

biomechanical—Referring to the mechanics of the human body, specifically how the musculoskeletal system works.

bronchodilator—A substance that increases the diameter (the lumen) of the bronchial passages.

bronchospasm—Spasm of the bronchial tubes. Also called bronchoconstriction.

cardiomyopathy—Disease of the heart muscle; a primary disease of heart muscle in the absence of a known underlying cause.

cardiorespiratory—Pertaining to the heart and lungs.

cardiovascular—Pertaining to the heart and blood vessels.

CBC (complete blood count)—Test of the blood to determine the numbers of red blood cells (erythrocytes), white blood cells (leukocytes), and other cells composing the blood.

CDC (Centers for Disease Control and Prevention)—An agency of the Department of Health and Human Services; located in Atlanta, Georgia (Web address: www.cdc.gov).

certification—The attainment of board certification in a specialty area. In this book, certification refers to the credentialing process for athletic trainers.

circumduction—A combination of movements that describe an arc or circle, as seen in the hip and shoulder joints. Can take place only in a ball-and-socket joint structure.

concentric—Referring to a shortening contraction of a muscle.

conformability—The ability of a material to conform or mold to a body part or object.

congenital—Referring to a condition that is present at birth.

contractures—Limitations in the range of motion of a joint due to soft-tissue restrictions.

cutaneous—Pertaining to the skin.

defendant—In law, the person or persons against whom an action (suit) is brought.

dermatitis—An acute inflammatory type of skin reaction caused by one of a number of factors, including chemicals or other substances that cause allergic responses, extreme cold or heat, bacteria or virus, and many others.

DO (doctor of osteopathy)—Designation indicating that the individual has accomplished the required training (usually undergraduate plus four or more years in medical school) in the study of osteopathic medicine.

eccentric—A lengthening contraction of a muscle.

elastin—Within soft tissue, a component that has elastic qualities.

electrodes—Pads used to transmit electrical impulses to or from the human body.

emesis—Vomiting.

ENT (ear, nose, and throat)—A medical specialty area concerned with conditions of and injury to the ear, nose, and throat.

enteral—Within the intestine.

epiphysis—The area that is open during growth to allow bone growth. Upon skeletal maturation, the epiphysis closes and the bone will no longer grow. Bones undergo epiphyseal closure at different times throughout the late teens and into the early '20s in some cases. Boys usually reach epiphyseal closure at a later age than girls do.

erythema—Redness of the skin.

ethics—The branch of philosophy that deals with the distinction between right and wrong, or the moral consequences of human actions.

exacerbate—To make a condition or injury worse.

exercise-induced asthma (EIA)—Bronchial spasm, swelling, and mucus secretion brought on by exercise, particularly in cool, dry conditions. Recovery usually occurs spontaneously within 90 min. The condition is confirmed by medical testing.

exertional—Brought on by physical exertion.

extension—The movement, generally, of increasing the angle between two bones. In some joints flexion appears opposite (i.e., shoulder).C2, P35

flexion—The movement, generally, of decreasing the angle between two bones. In the shoulder, however, raising the arm forward makes the angle larger and this is termed flexion.

generic—Referring to the nonproprietary name of a drug; for example, acetaminophen is the generic equivalent of Tylenol.

ginglymus—A hinge joint such as the elbow joint.

gluteals—Muscles of the buttock region, including the gluteus maximus, gluteus medius, and gluteus minimus.

Golgi tendon organ (GTO)—A sensory network within the muscle and extending into the muscle's tendon. When the muscle size changes suddenly, the GTO senses the change and alerts the body, possibly preventing muscle injury while providing information regarding the status of muscle activity.

helmetry—The athletic term (slang) used to describe the science behind the study of protective helmets.

hematocrit (Hct)—The percentage of the volume of a blood sample that is occupied by cells. Usually evaluated along with the level of hemoglobin in the complete blood count.

hemoglobin (Hb)—The red, oxygen-carrying protein of the red blood cell (erythrocyte). Usually measured along with the hematocrit in the complete blood count.

hepatitis B—A serious disease transmitted through blood and bodily fluids. There is no cure for hepatitis B, but there is a vaccine to prevent one from contracting it.

hernia—Protrusion of a part or structure through the tissues normally containing it (synonym—rupture).

humeral epicondyle—The outward flare of the upper arm bone (humerus) as it approaches the elbow joint.

hydrocollator—Heating device used to warm specially designed heat-retaining pads (hydrocolloid filled) used for the application of superficial heat to a patient's skin.

hyperthermia—Too much body heat. May result from a fever or from exercise or other factors.

hyponatremia—An abnormally low concentration of sodium in the blood. Brought about by excessive consumption of water without the presence of electrolytes.

hypotension—Low blood pressure.

hypothalamus—A region within the brain that plays an important role in heat regulation.

hypothermia—Too little body heat; a body temperature significantly below 98.6° F (37° C).

iatrogenic—Pertaining to a condition caused by the treatment given.

idiopathic—No known cause. Most often relating to diseases or conditions such as "idiopathic scoliosis."

intragastric—Within the intestine.

intravenously—Within a vein, as in intravenous injection (an injection of a chemical into a vein).

iontophoresis—A method of using an electric current to drive ions of a chemical into tissues.

isokinetic—Involving a maximal contraction at a constant speed over the entire range of motion. Isokinetic devices are used in testing and rehabilitation.

isometric contraction—A contraction in which the muscle stays at the same length ("iso," same; "metric," measure) while tension in the muscle develops.

isotonic—Producing a muscular contraction that causes a shortening of a muscle against a constant load.

Legg-Calvé-Perthes disease—In young children, a condition in which the head of the femur fails to fully form.

liability—Indication of responsibility.

licensure—A state credential allowing a group or profession to perform indicated functions legally.

Marfan syndrome—A genetic disorder that characteristically affects the major artery exiting the heart, the aorta. Weakness of the walls of the aorta predispose the artery to rupture. Other genetic characteristics are also associated with this syndrome.

MD (medical doctor)—Designation indicating that the individual has accomplished the required training (usually undergraduate degree and four or more years of medical school) in the study of allopathic medicine.

mitral valve—The heart valve located between the left atrium (containing blood returning from the lungs) and left ventricle (containing blood ready to be ejected into the body's arterial network).

mucosa—The tissue that lines body cavities (e.g., the lining of the mouth, nose, and throat).

musculoskeletal—Pertaining to the bones and muscles of the body.

myocarditis—Inflammation ("-itis") of the muscle ("myo-") of the heart ("cardi-").

NAIRS (National Athletic Injury Recording System)—One of the original data collection agencies studying the epidemiology of sport injuries.

NATA (National Athletic Trainers' Association)—The governing body for athletic trainers in the United States (Web address: www.nata.org; phone: 800-TRY-NATA).

NATABOC (National Athletic Trainers' Association Board of Certification)—A group that represents the NATA and is responsible for credentialing standards for its members.

NCAA (National Collegiate Athletic Association)—The governing body of college athletic programs.

nebulizer—An apparatus that disperses a liquid or chemical mixture in the form of a fine spray.

necrosis—Death of tissue in an area.

negligence—In law, failure to exercise the degree of care considered reasonable under the circumstances, resulting in an unintended injury to another party.

nociceptive—Relating to the ability to perceive painful stimuli.

nonprescription—Referring to a drug that is available without permission from a physician or other licensed health care provider.

nonproprietary—Referring to the name assigned by the U.S. Adopted Name Council for a drug found to have a therapeutic value. The name indicates the chemical composition of the drug and is not protected by a trademark (e.g., acetaminophen is the nonproprietary name for Tylenol).

nonsteroidal—Referring to an anti-inflammatory drug that is not within the steroid classification (e.g., ibuprofen).

oropharyngeal—Referring to the passageway from the mouth ("oro-") to the throat (pharynx).

orthopedics (also, "orthopaedics," British)—The medical specialty area dealing with the health and function of the musculoskeletal system, extremities, spine, and associated structures by medical, surgical, and physical methods.

OSHA (Occupational Safety and Health Association)—A governmental agency focusing on reducing the risks of illness and injury due to occupational hazards.

osteoarthritis—Inflammation of the joint surfaces of bones leading to degeneration of the joint. Can result from joint injury or from repetitive wear and tear of the joint.

osteochondritis dissecans—A fracture of the articular surface (hyaline surface) of the bones. The joint surface (articular surface) is usually a very strong, smooth tissue. Fractures in this surface, due to the weight-bearing status of many joints, result in arthritic changes.

osteoid osteoma—A small, benign (noncancerous) tumor composed of bone tissue. It develops anywhere in the body but most often in the long bones and the spine. Also called osseous tumor. Diagnosis is by X-ray; treatment is often surgical.

osteopathy—The therapeutic system based on the concept that the normal body is capable, when in correct adjustment, of making its own remedies against infection and other conditions. Practitioners use conventional medicine in addition to manipulative measures. D.O. is the designation for Doctor of Osteopathy.

parenteral—Taken into the body via a route other than the digestive tract (e.g., via injection or intravenous method).

pars interarticularis—The section of a vertebra between superior and inferior articular facets.

pectoralis major—A large muscle on the anterior (front) chest wall.

periodization—A weight-training technique that utilizes cycles, or periods, to allow the athlete to maximize opportunities for building and maintaining strength during competitive periods of the season.

petit mal—Epileptic seizure, characterized by brief impairment of consciousness often associated with flickering of the eyelids and mild twitching of the mouth.

pharmacodynamics—The study of the effects of a drug on the body and the mechanism of a drug's action.

pharmacokinetics—The study of the passage of a drug through the body, specifically the extent and rate of absorption, distribution, localization in tissues, biotransformation, and elimination.

pharmacotherapeutics—The use of drugs to prevent and treat conditions, and their use in planned alteration of normal function.

phlebotomist—An individual trained and skilled in drawing blood from a vein.

***Physician's Desk Reference* (PDR)**—Reference book for prescription and nonprescription drugs. Lists drugs by generic and trade names and gives manufacturer information.

plaintiff—The person or persons who institute a suit in a court of law.

plyometrics—A method of training the athlete for power or explosiveness through jumping, bounding, and hopping types of exercises. Plyometrics can also be applied to the upper extremity.

pneumatic antishock garment (PASG)—A garment used to control bleeding and blood pressure to prevent shock in a trauma patient.

PPE—Preparticipation physical examination. A medical examination required of athletes prior to the beginning of sport participation.

preparticipation—Occurring (and usually required) prior to participation in some event or activity.

prodrug—A drug that becomes active only after being metabolized.

prophylaxis—Measures taken to prevent something from occurring.

proprioception—The ability to sense the position of joints and of the body as a result of input from sensory nerve endings in the muscles and joints, called proprioceptors.

proprioceptive neuromuscular facilitation (PNF)—A specialized therapeutic technique that combines sensory stimulation with manual resistance to achieve maximal muscular response.

proximal—Nearest the center, midline, or point of origin.

psychrometer—A device used for the calculation of relative humidity from wet- and dry-bulb temperatures.

rehabilitation—Returning to normal health through guided activities and programs. In sport, after an injury the athlete should undergo rehabilitation prior to returning to the sport.

rehydration—Replenishment of body fluids.

resuscitation—Revival from apparent death; provision of artificial respiration and cardiac care.

rhabdomyolysis—An acute, potentially fatal disease that destroys skeletal muscle. Often due to abnormally shaped red blood cells (sickle cells) within the blood.

rheumatoid arthritis—An inflammatory joint disease that affects synovial joints.

rhinitis—Inflammation of the mucus membrane of the nose accompanied by excessive nasal discharge.

role delineation study—A study conducted by the National Athletic Trainers' Association to determine the areas and scope of practice of members of the association. Information from this study guides schools in establishing and modifying educational objectives to ensure that all aspects of the duties of the athletic trainer are being covered in course work.

scoliosis—A sideways curvature of the spine. Affects girls more than boys and worsens with bony growth. Curve can be mild to severe.

seropositive—Containing a particular antibody in the serum, or fluid portion, of the blood, usually indicating the presence of a particular infection.

spinal cord lesion—Injury to the spine, perhaps affecting the spinal cord (nervous system). The injury, or lesion, may range from a partial cut through the cord to a complete cut. Depending on the level (cervical vs. thoracic or lumbar), the patient has paralysis in either the lower extremities only (paraplegia) or in both the lower and the upper extremities (quadriplegia).

spine board—A specially designed board used to immobilize the spine of a patient.

splanchnic—Pertaining to the abdominal and pelvic organs. Usually referring to the autonomic nerves to the organs.

splint—An appliance used for prevention of movement of a joint or for the fixation of displaced or movable parts. Also used to disperse forces to adjacent areas.

spondylolisthesis—A fracture of the vertebra in a part of the vertebra that connects the upper portion of the bone to the lower portion of the bone. This fracture actually occurs on both sides of the bone. Fracture of both sides allows a forward slippage of one vertebra over another, and correction may require surgery. Usually no treatment is required for this type of fracture if it is on one side only (spondylolysis).

stenosis—A constriction of any opening or canal; especially, a narrowing of one of the cardiac valves.

stressors—Factors that contribute to a person's level of stress. These factors are not actually the cause of the stress; rather the individual allows the situation to cause anger, excitement, or stress in some way. An external force acting on the body in an irritating or injurious manner may also be a stressor.

subdural hematoma—A localized area of bleeding that is relatively or completely confined within a space between the skull and the outer surface of the brain. The pool of blood may enlarge and cause damage to adjacent brain tissue.

sublingual—Beneath the tongue.

supplements—As used in nutrition, additions to the normal diet in an attempt to improve aspects of health or performance. Supplements are often poorly researched prior to their introduction to the public.

surveillance—Within the context of this book, the collection, collation, analysis, and dissemination of data; a type of observational study that involves continuous monitoring of disease or injury occurrence within a population (e.g., sport team).

synovial fluid—A lubricating and nutritional fluid that bathes the surfaces of most of the body's joints. Found contained within a synovial membrane iside most joints.

thermoregulatory—The process by which temperature is controlled.

tinnitus—Ringing in the ears.

topical—Referring to a local application, most often indicating application of a drug to the skin (superficial application).

tort—Damage, injury, or a wrongful act done willfully, negligently, or in circumstances involving strict liability but not involving breach of contract, for which a civil suit can be brought.

toxicology—The study of the harmful, or toxic, effects of chemicals on the body. Includes the symptoms and treatment of poisoning as well as identification of the poisonous chemical.

transdermal—Crossing the skin to penetrate into the tissues.

undescended testicle—Incomplete or improper prenatal descent of a testicle. Not uncommon.

uniaxial—Having one axis of rotation. In the body, a uniaxial joint is able to produce movement in only one plane.

urinalysis—Evaluation of the urine to determine some aspects of a person's health.

urticaria—The eruption of itchy areas, often due to hypersensitivity to foods or chemicals or to emotional factors (also called hives).

ventilation—Replacement of the air or other gas in a space by fresh air or gas, as in artificial respiration given to a nonbreathing patient.

windchill—A still-air temperature that would be equivalent to a given combination of temperature and wind speed.

Index

Note: The italicized *f* and *t* following page numbers refers to figures and tables, respectively.

About the Author

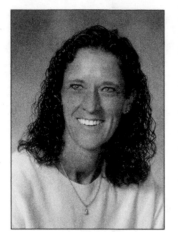

Susan Kay Hillman, ATC, PT, is associate professor and director of Human Anatomy at the Arizona School of Health Sciences, a division of the A.T. Still University. She has more than 13 years of experience as head athletic trainer for the University of Arizona and has served as a consultant, assistant athletic trainer, and physical therapist for the Pittsburgh Steelers as well as the Philadelphia Eagles football clubs.

Hillman has served on the editorial board of the journal *Athletic Therapy Today* and the review board of the *Journal of Sport Rehabilitation*. She is a member of the Rocky Mountain Athletic Trainers Association (RMATA) Program Committee. In 2004, she received the Distinguished Educator Award from the RMATA, and the year before she was named Most Distinguished Athletic Trainer by the National Athletic Trainers' Association (NATA).

Hillman earned a master's degree in physical therapy from Stanford University and a master's degree in physical education and athletic training from the University of Arizona, as well as a bachelor's degree in the same field from Purdue University.

Check out the updated texts in the Athletic Training Education Series

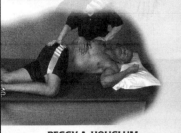

THERAPEUTIC EXERCISE FOR MUSCULOSKELETAL INJURIES

SECOND EDITION

PEGGY A. HOUGLUM

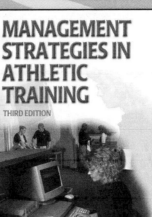

MANAGEMENT STRATEGIES IN ATHLETIC TRAINING

THIRD EDITION

RICHARD RAY

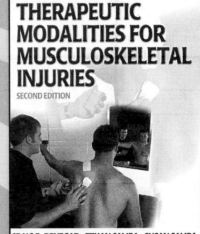

THERAPEUTIC MODALITIES FOR MUSCULOSKELETAL INJURIES

SECOND EDITION

CRAIG R. DENEGAR • ETHAN SALIBA • SUSAN SALIBA

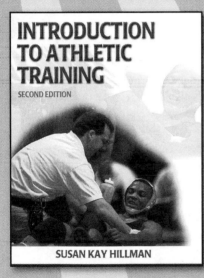

INTRODUCTION TO ATHLETIC TRAINING

SECOND EDITION

SUSAN KAY HILLMAN

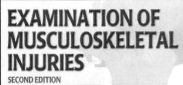

EXAMINATION OF MUSCULOSKELETAL INJURIES

SECOND EDITION

SANDRA J. SHULTZ • PEGGY A. HOUGLUM • DAVID H. PERRIN

Human Kinetics' ground-breaking Athletic Training Education Series includes five outstanding textbooks, each with its own superb supporting instructional resources. Featuring the work of respected athletic training authorities, the series parallels and expounds on the content areas established by the National Athletic Trainers' Association (NATA) Educational Council.

Students preparing for careers as athletic trainers will use these valuable texts not only in the classroom but ultimately as references in the field. Athletic trainers preparing for certification examinations will also appreciate the wealth of information presented.

To learn more about the books in this series, visit the Athletic Training Education Series Web site at **www.HumanKinetics.com/AthleticTrainingEducationSeries**.

For a complete description or to order
Call 1-800-747-4457
In Canada, call 1-800-465-7301
In Europe, call 44 (0) 113-255-5665
In Australia, call 08-8277-1555
In New Zealand, call 09-448-1207
For all other countries, call 217-351-5076
or visit **www.HumanKinetics.com**!

HUMAN KINETICS
The Information Leader in Physical Activity
P.O. Box 5076 • Champaign, IL 61825-5076 USA

Essentials of
Interactive Functional Anatomy

Minimum System Requirements

PC

Windows® 98/2000/ME/XP

Pentium® processor or higher

At least 32 MB RAM

Monitor set to 800 x 600 or greater

High-color display

Mac

Power Mac®

System 8.6 /9/OSX

At least 64 MB RAM

Monitor set to 800 × 600 or greater

Monitor set to thousands of colors

How to Use This Program

PC

The program should launch automatically when the CD is inserted in the CD-ROM drive of your computer. Choose the Install button for IFA Essentials. If you don't already have QuickTime 6 installed on your computer, you should also install that. If the CD does not auto-launch, go to My Computer and double-click the HK_IFA_Ess icon. Install as stated above.

Mac

Insert the CD into the CD-ROM drive of your computer, then double-click the CD-ROM icon. Double-click the IFA Essentials for Power Mac folder, then the IFA Essentials icon. This will launch the program. If you don't already have QuickTime 6 installed on your computer, you should also install that using the QT installer in the IFA Essentials for Power Mac folder.

Quick Start Instructions

Use the Anatomy tab to view the 3D model and click on any anatomical structure to display the relevant text. Click on the red text for hot links to additional and relevant information about the chosen anatomical component. The History function provides access to previous text articles. Use the blue arrow buttons located in the upper right-hand corner of the text interface to move sequentially through the text.

To maximize the model interface, place the cursor over the model/text interface until the double-arrow sign appears, left-click, and drag to the right. To maximize the text interface, drag to the left (PC version only). Rotate the 3D model by using the blue arrow buttons centered under it. The inner buttons rotate the 3D model step by step and the outer buttons rotate it continuously. Strip away anatomical layers, from deep to superficial, using the layer slider centered under the rotation arrows. Change the view of the 3D model by choosing additional views from the drop-down menu located on the lower right-hand side of the model interface.

To help you get started, Help balloons are available. Move the mouse over any button and its function will be revealed. (For a Mac, enable this by selecting Help balloons from the Help menu.) In-depth help is available from the Help menu.